THE
OUTBREAK
ATLAS

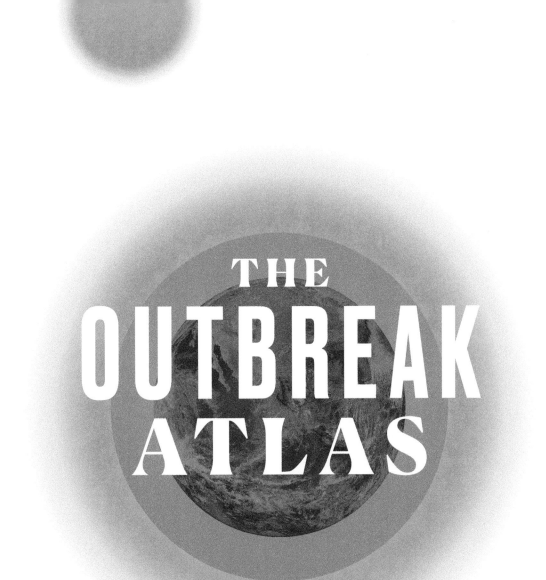

THE
OUTBREAK
ATLAS

REBECCA KATZ

AND

MACKENZIE S. MOORE

VANDERBILT UNIVERSITY PRESS | NASHVILLE, TENNESSEE

Library of Congress Cataloging-in-Publication Data

Names: Katz, Rebecca, 1973- author. | Moore, Mackenzie S., 1996- author.
Title: The outbreak atlas / Rebecca Katz and Mackenzie S. Moore.
Description: Nashville, Tennessee : Vanderbilt University Press, 2024. |
    Includes bibliographical references and index.
Identifiers: LCCN 2023054130 | ISBN 9780826506627 (hardcover) | ISBN
    9780826506610 (paperback) | ISBN 9780826506634 (epub) | ISBN
    9780826506641 (pdf)
Subjects: LCSH: Epidemics--Popular works. | Epidemiology--Popular works. |
    Public health--Popular works. | Epidemics--Prevention--
Popular works.
Classification: LCC RA653 .K38 2024 | DDC 614.4--dc23/eng/20240124
LC record available at https://lccn.loc.gov/2023054130

Cover images: mosquito, Photoongraphy/Shutterstock; bat, dwi putra
stock/Shutterstock

EPIDEMIOLOGY
Who, What, When, Where, Why, and How?

Epidemiology and public health surveillance are the core of infectious disease research, detection, investigation, and response. Epidemiology is the study of how and why diseases occur within a population. Within this field, scientists use defined methodology to explore a myriad of questions: who is getting sick, what type of pathogen is causing a disease, where did the causative agent come from, how does it spread? They identify patterns, examine the frequency of outbreaks, and investigate the risk factors and causes associated with health events. Public health surveillance is one of several valuable tools that feed epidemiological efforts. Surveillance systems capture disease data from a wide variety of sources, notifying health experts of potential outbreaks and providing them with essential information about ongoing disease burden that they can then analyze and use to inform response efforts and inspire future research. In this chapter we outline how epidemiology works in practice to identify and respond to disease events, including epidemiological investigation, attribution investigation, and public health surveillance.

Epidemiological Investigation

When an infectious disease outbreak is suspected, a team of epidemiologists initiates an investigation. Disease detectives work to figure out the origin and extent of the infectious disease outbreak. The data and evidence they gather confirms the existence of an outbreak and provides critical information for health and government officials to use in implementing mitigation and control measures.

An investigation follows several steps, which may occur concurrently or in different orders depending on the nature of the outbreak and the resources available.[1] This process can also be iterative, with some steps being performed multiple times.

1. Verify the existence of an outbreak
2. Confirm the diagnosis
3. Create a case definition
4. Find and document cases
5. Perform descriptive epidemiology
6. Develop hypotheses
7. Plan and perform additional studies
8. Implement control and prevention measures
9. Initiate and/or maintain surveillance
10. Communicate the results of the epidemiological investigation

STEP 1: Verify the Existence of an Outbreak

Is something happening? The first step in an outbreak investigation is to verify whether there is actually an outbreak. A disease outbreak is defined as an increase in disease occurrence beyond what is normally expected for a particular location, time of year, or population. Signals of an outbreak—case reports from clinics or hospitals, laboratory reports, community rumors, etc.—are captured by a public health surveillance system and assessed by a team of disease professionals. They compare the number of cases that would be expected, drawing from health department surveillance records, hospital records, mortality statistics, or clinical reports, to the reported or perceived number and nature of cases.

Sometimes this is very easy to do. For example, if there was a single case of smallpox then you have an outbreak, since you wouldn't expect to see even a single case because it was eradicated decades ago. Sometimes this is hard. Cases of influenza are very common during the winter months. To assess whether something unusual is going on, you would need to look at influenza rates from past winters and compare.

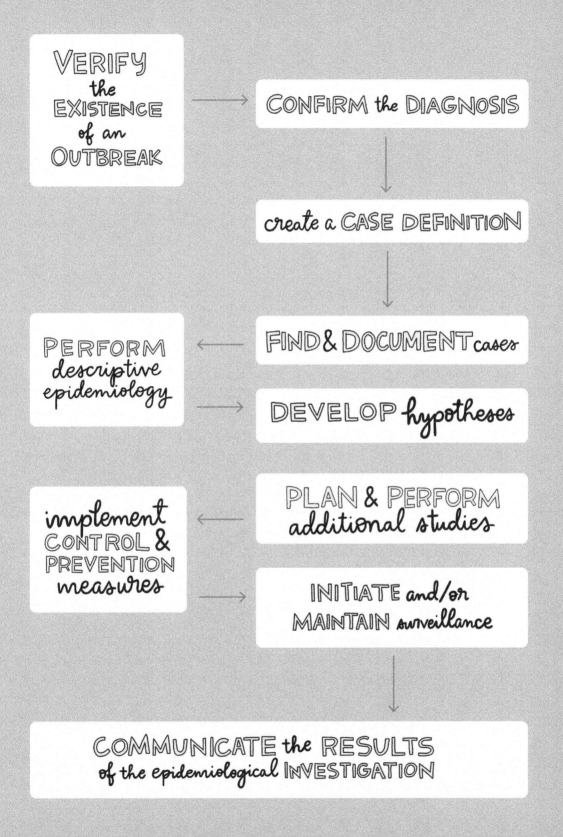

Determining whether the detected rise in cases indicates an outbreak is a complicated process. Epidemiologists must verify the signals and assess their authenticity and reliability by gathering additional information, cross-checking sources, and conducting analyses. There are also many non-disease related factors which can falsely suggest the existence of an outbreak. Changes in local reporting processes, changes in case definitions, increased local or national awareness of a disease, or alterations to diagnostic testing procedures could trigger unexpected numbers of reported cases—all possibilities that need to be assessed by the public health team. Once a health team verifies the signal(s) and concludes that there is a possible infectious disease outbreak, they launch an investigation.

CASE STUDY

Pediatric Hepatitis Cases of Unknown Etiology in the US and UK

One of the earliest steps in outbreak investigation is confirming there is actually an outbreak. However, verifying outbreak signals can be extremely difficult—especially early on. In the autumn of 2021, clinicians in the United States noticed a hospital cluster of pediatric hepatitis of unknown origin, and similar case data was coming from the United Kingdom.[2] In both countries, pathogen testing showed that many of the cases also tested positive for adenovirus, specifically a type of adenovirus that typically causes gastroenteritis (think really bad stomach aches), which had not been associated with hepatitis cases in healthy children.

To establish the existence of an outbreak, public health scientists collected data and analyzed trends on pediatric hepatitis–related hospitalizations, emergency department visits, liver transplants, and the percentage of positive adenovirus samples among children in the US. They compared case numbers to a pre-pandemic baseline to account for the potential changes in healthcare seeking behavior from 2020 to 2022 during the COVID-19 pandemic.

Initial analysis of the data suggested that there was not an increase in pediatric hepatitis cases or adenovirus compared to the pre-pandemic baseline and thus scientists reported in June 2022 that there was no actual outbreak of pediatric hepatitis in the US. Researchers clearly listed the challenges associated with determining the existence of an outbreak of acute pediatric hepatitis, notably the gaps in data coverage, lag between hospitalization outcome and report, and using pediatric hepatitis of unspecified etiology as a proxy.[3] Additionally, they noted this was a rare condition, and analyses of big data sets could miss small but important trend changes. This was especially impacted by the effects the pandemic had on changing healthcare seeking behavior.

But the case was not solved. New case reports and data from eleven countries around Europe suggested this was, in fact, a new problem, and investigations continued.[4] Further investigation in the US and retrospective case identification by December 2023 revealed an additional 290 cases, bringing the total case count in the US to 401, compared to 111 in May 2022.[5]

The US Centers for Disease Control and Prevention (US CDC) issued a nationwide request for clinicians and public health authorities to report any cases of children under the age of ten with particular laboratory results and unknown etiology for clinical hepatitis. Investigators continued to conduct surveillance, monitor case trends, and explore the possible role of concurrent or previous adenovirus and/or SARS-CoV-2 infection on new hepatitis cases.

STEP 2: Confirm the Diagnosis

What is the something that is happening? Initial identification of cases in an outbreak may come from clinician reports of patients' signs and symptoms, or diagnostic laboratories—all providing information that then needs to be further explored through an epidemiologic investigation. Confirming disease diagnosis, which means ruling out any clinical misdiagnosis or laboratory error, enables clinicians to optimize treatment decisions and allows for effective disease-specific control measures.

To confirm diagnosis, health officers review and verify individuals' clinical histories, bolstering data with additional case, family member, and physician interviews to capture additional details on possible etiology and transmission. They also may collect samples from the patients and/or the environment for laboratory processing. This can include samples of sputum (spit), blood, stool, or food or water samples following established sample collection, transport, and diagnostic protocols. There are many laboratory methods for identifying and typing a pathogen, including microscopy, antigen detection, and serology, as well as analysis of DNA or other chemical or biological fingerprinting.[6] Laboratory diagnosis is important to avoid incorrectly attributing the etiology of an outbreak, particularly when so many disease agents cause general or unclear clinical symptoms.

In cases where an outbreak is caused by a known pathogen, health professionals diagnose cases based on already established case definitions and approved laboratory diagnostics. When an outbreak has an unknown etiology or is caused by a novel pathogen, initial diagnoses may be uncertain and laboratory confirmation may not be possible. In these situations, confirming disease diagnosis may just include meeting the clinical case definition and being epidemiologically linked to another confirmed case.[7]

STEP 3: Create a Case Definition

Can we describe the something that is happening? Case definitions standardize criteria used by epidemiologists and health personnel to identify and classify cases. There are three categories of case definitions: *suspected*, *probable*, or *confirmed* cases, based on clinical, laboratory, and situational criteria.[8]

Suspected cases display typical clinical features without laboratory results or epidemiologic information; probable cases show typical clinical features of the illness and have an epidemiologic link to another laboratory-confirmed case, but are not laboratory confirmed; and confirmed cases have laboratory confirmation of the agent through isolation of the causative agent or a positive serological test.

Clinical criteria include a combination of symptoms, physical signs, etiologic agents, and confirmatory diagnostic tests.[9] Laboratory criteria can include presence of pathogen type or subtype, serologic evidence, and detection of specific levels of antibodies or antigens in a sample. Importantly, laboratory criteria might also include the absence of another pathogen that might otherwise explain symptoms, such as testing negative for malaria. A case definition can also include criteria relating to person, place, and time.[10]

Person describes key characteristics the patients share, such as, age, sex, race, and occupation.

Place describes a specific geographic location or facility associated with the outbreak.

Time delineates a period of time associated with illness onset for the cases under investigation. Limiting the period enables exclusion of similar illnesses that are unrelated to the outbreak of interest.

Case definitions may also identify the "at-risk population," meaning the group of individuals who have an increased potential of contracting the disease by either being exposed to the infectious agent or being especially susceptible to the disease. Factors that impact risk of exposure include the geographic location, social groupings, occupation, immunization status, age, or gender.[11] Factors that can increase susceptibility to a disease may include immune status of a population, comorbidities, behaviors like smoking, or other conditions such as pregnancy.[12]

Constructing a case definition requires balancing between including all possible cases (sensitivity) and excluding persons without the disease (specificity). During early stages of an outbreak investigation, when the goal is to identify as many cases as possible, a more sensitive case definition may be used.[13] While a *sensitive* case definition increases the likelihood of detecting cases, it may also count individuals who do not have the disease as cases. A *specific* case definition is often more resource dependent as it can rely on diagnostic or laboratory confirmation, but it minimizes false positives by including only confirmed cases. However, it is possible to miss some cases with a highly specific case definition.

The components of a case definition may vary depending on the nature of each outbreak, and the case definition may be modified as the outbreak evolves. Early on in an outbreak, interim case definitions may be issued and then updated as more information becomes available; for example, a case definition might be changed to include a more specific laboratory component as new diagnostics are developed or an exposure source is identified.

SIMPLIFIED CASE DEFINITION

Sometimes it is helpful to create simplified or community case definitions. These are clear and concise versions that use key signs and easily identified symptoms of the disease or public health event to help the public recognize when a person should seek testing or treatment at a health facility or notify local health personnel of a suspected case.

The advantage of using community case definitions is that they are simpler and broader (lower specificity) than standard case definitions, which means that more suspected or probable cases will be identified, and fewer cases will be missed.

Simplified case definitions are a key part of improving community-based surveillance (CBS) and actively engaging the community in detecting, reporting, monitoring, and responding to health events.[14] The community case definitions, though, are often overly broad and will capture lots of potential cases that can then be ruled in or out based on the more technical definitions.

For more information about the real application of case definitions, see the "Surveillance" section later in this chapter, and the "Community-Based Disease Surveillance" section of the Community Engagement and Humanitarian Response chapter.

STEP 4: Find and Document Cases

Where are the cases and what do we know about them? Field epidemiology comes into practice once the investigation team begins actively searching for cases and gathering information. When cases are identified, they are interviewed and contact tracing begins. If the patient is deceased, relatives may be interviewed or information may be taken from medical records. Information on the suspected, probable, and possible cases and contacts is organized and managed in lists to inform the ongoing investigation, develop hypotheses, and provide data for additional studies.

ACTIVE CASE FINDING

Using the specified case definition, public health investigators actively search for and identify as many cases as possible in order to establish the magnitude and scope of the outbreak.[15] To find cases, outbreak investigative teams review hospital and clinic records, laboratory reports, surveillance reports, and public reporting systems.[16] The first stages of active case finding are often done in partnership with healthcare practitioners and facilities where diagnoses are made. In some communities, informal or unregulated healthcare providers or traditional healers may be the best sources of information for finding cases.

Examples of Standard Case Definition versus Community Case Definition

This table compares some standard case definitions with community case definitions, to illustrate the differences.

DISEASE	STANDARD CASE DEFINITION	COMMUNITY CASE DEFINITION
Yellow Fever	**Suspected case:** Any person with acute onset of fever, with jaundice appearing within fourteen days of onset of the first symptoms. **Probable case:** A suspected case AND one of the following: (a) epidemiological link to a confirmed case or an outbreak, or (b) positive post-mortem liver histopathology	Any person who has fever and two or more other symptoms (headache, vomiting, running stomach, weak in the body, yellow eyes) or who died after serious sickness with fever or bleeding
Typhoid Fever	**Suspected case:** Any person with gradual onset of steadily increasing and then persistently high fever, chills, malaise, headache, sore throat, cough, and, sometimes, abdominal pain and constipation or diarrhea. **Confirmed case:** Suspected case confirmed by isolation of Salmonella typhi from blood, bone marrow, bowel fluid, or stool.	Any person with a prolonged fever during the previous three weeks or more
Measles	**Suspected case:** Any person with fever and maculopapular (non-vesicular) generalized rash and cough, coryza, or conjunctivitis (red eyes) or any person in whom a clinician suspects measles. **Confirmed case:** A suspected case with laboratory confirmation (positive IgM antibody) or epidemiological link to confirmed cases in an outbreak.	Any person with fever and rash

Adapted from the WHO Africa Regional Office's standard case definitions for priority diseases and conditions and community-level case definitions as described in the *Technical Guidelines for Integrated Disease Surveillance and Response in the African Region* (Atlanta: CDC; Brazzaville: WHO Regional Office for Africa, March 2019), https://apps.who.int/iris/bitstream/handle/10665/312317/WHO-AF-WHE-CPI-01-2019-eng.pdf.

Public health workers contact local clinical and laboratory professionals to collect information on any additional cases.[17] They may even go door to door if an entire community might be at risk. When individuals matching the case definition are identified, they are interviewed.

INTERVIEWING INITIAL CASE(S)

Public health officials attempt to interview initial case(s) as soon as possible in order to increase the probability of identifying epidemiologic links between cases and possible exposure.[18]

Epidemiologists often utilize questionnaires or interview guides during case and contact investigation to standardize data collection. Questionnaires may be administered by an interviewer or self-administered by cases and contacts either electronically or on paper. Interviewing initial case(s) is a key step during the early stages of the outbreak investigation to gather information that can be used to generate hypotheses about the origin and type of disease and help investigators understand important factors like how someone became infected.

The following types of information from cases and/or contacts is gathered during interviews:

- demographic and identifying data (age, sex, location, occupation),
- clinical history (date of onset, duration, and severity of symptoms),
- contact history, and
- risk factor information (contact with other ill persons, food consumption history, travel history, possible initial exposure).

CONTACT TRACING

Contact tracing is a core strategy during early outbreak investigation and response to interrupt chains of transmission. It is a public health tool used to identify individuals (contacts) who may have had contact with an infected person (case), notifying them of their exposure, monitoring them for symptoms, and providing additional support so that they may avoid possibly transmitting the disease to others.

Identifying contacts of confirmed cases is the first step in contact tracing. Contacts can be anyone who has been in contact with an infected person: family members, work colleagues, friends, or health care providers. Contact tracing is triggered when a probable or confirmed case or other source of infection (e.g., mass gathering, food source) is identified. Contacts are identified during interviews with confirmed cases or analysis of deceased cases' information and interviews with their family. Trained contact tracing teams then reach out to identified contacts either through in-person home visits or virtually via phone or video calls.

Once they reach an identified contact, a member of the contact tracing team confirms an individual's exposure, assesses whether they have any symptoms, and provides the contact with preventive behavioral guidelines to limit the risk of further exposing people around them.[19] Contacts continue to be monitored for symptom development and are given information about how to report and seek care should they develop symptoms.[20] In some situations, quarantine, either at home or in a hospital or other special facility, is required for contacts who are at particularly high risk of becoming ill.[21] In these situations, contacts should be provided with guidance for how to best self-quarantine and given information about any additional support that may be available (like food delivery).

CONTACT LISTING

Contact tracers keep track of identified contacts using a standardized (usually electronic) contact listing form, where data is entered, managed, and analyzed.

CONTACT FOLLOW-UP

A team of contact tracers and public health staff follow up with all listed contacts either in-person or via phone to monitor for symptoms, test for signs of infection, and provide additional support. If a contact develops symptoms during the established monitoring period based on date of exposure, they are then guided to test, isolate, or seek other treatment depending on the nature of the disease. Once a contact is considered a confirmed case, health personnel initiate contact tracing for that case, and the cycle starts again.

CASE STUDY

Contact Tracing during the West African Ebola Outbreak

During the 2014 through 2016 West African Ebola virus disease (EVD) outbreak, contact tracing was a key strategy used to contain the spread of disease by identifying and isolating potential EVD cases.[22] Contact tracing for EVD began with the identification of each person an Ebola patient came into contact with.

Health workers notified the contacts of their exposure and followed up with them daily for twenty-one days after their last exposure to EVD (the duration of the maximum incubation period of the virus). During follow-up visits, health workers monitored contacts' temperatures and symptoms, and symptomatic contacts were transported to a treatment center or hospital for testing and isolation if needed. By removing suspected cases from environments in which they could easily infect others, the goal was to stop transmission and eventually contain the outbreak.[23]

While contact tracing is a major epidemiological strategy to control the spread of disease and has demonstrated effectiveness in successfully containing EVD outbreaks, a combination of factors complicated contact tracing efforts during the West African EVD outbreak, minimizing its effectiveness in containing the outbreak.[24] The sheer scale of the outbreak and the level of EVD contact tracing was unprecedented.[25] Barriers to effective tracing included the inability to establish a comprehensive list of contacts and inefficient paper-form contact tracing.[26] Incomplete contact tracing allowed for unmonitored transmission, and processing paper-based contact tracing data took days and ran a high-risk of human-error during manual entry, slowing the ability of responders to identify data trends and respond appropriately.[27] Another challenge to effective contact tracing was the dense, urban populations of most of the affected areas, impeding the ability to identify everybody who an EVD patient interacted with.[28] Additionally, insufficient public health infrastructure and workforce and inadequate training of contact tracers made it almost impossible to keep up with the exponential increase in EVD cases.[29]

Further, contact tracers struggled with community distrust, noting that contacts sometimes would resist communication due to mistrust of the government and the fear of being stigmatized within their communities.[30] In the Western Area district of Sierra Leone, communities were quarantined in an attempt to simplify the process of contact tracing and contain the spread of EVD. However, a lack of provisions for basic needs such as food and water fostered resistance that contributed to an incomplete contact tracing database, where as many as 75 percent of confirmed EVD cases had not been listed as contacts prior to the onset of their symptoms. This resistance prompted Sierra Leone's government to pass a law in August 2014 that made it illegal to hide Ebola patients.[31]

During the outbreak, responders tracked the challenges and instituted rapid adjustments, such as piloting a mobile contact tracing program in Guinea to enable immediate data analysis and data-driven response.[32] After the outbreak, researchers examined the strengths and weaknesses of the response, documenting the lessons learned, which included the importance of hiring contact tracers directly from affected communities and compensating them adequately, the need for better training and supervision, and the necessity of adequate delivery of food, water, and other basic needs to individuals and communities in isolation or quarantine.[33]

Digital Patient Notification for Sexually Transmitted Infections

Cases of sexually transmitted infections (STI) of chlamydia, syphilis, and gonorrhea are sharply rising around the world.[34] Partner notification is a form of contact tracing designed to help prevent reinfection of patients and reduce further spread of the infection to other partners. When a patient tests positive for an STI, they can inform their sexual partner(s) directly, or their health providers/health department can notify partners of their anonymous exposure; in either case facilitating testing, and if necessary treatment. Increasingly, STI contact tracing is done through electronic notification, often using a digital tool that sends an email or text to the sexual partner.[35]

Quick Reference: STI versus STD

The terms sexually transmitted infection (STI) and sexually transmitted disease (STD) are often used interchangeably; however, most STIs do not get to the disease stage—either the infection does not develop into a disease, or patients receive medication to treat or cure it.

Taking Infection to the Grave

Some infectious diseases appear in the archeological record. There are numerous cases of archaeologists finding skeletons with unique bone lesions, indicators that they had venereal syphilis.[36] In early 2022, scientists were able to trace the origin of the Black Death pandemic to fourteenth-century Kyrgyzstan by sequencing archaeological remains in a cemetery and isolating DNA from the bacterium behind the plague.[37]

COUNTING CASES AND DEVELOPING LINE LISTS

Following the established case definition, epidemiologists track the number of cases and organize the information for each case in a line list—which is just what it sounds like: a line-by-line listing of each case and their relevant information. The case count is derived from sources such as public health agency surveillance data; medical system records from hospitals, laboratories, or ambulatory care settings; institutional setting records (e.g., school and workplace attendance records); and special surveys.[38] In resource-limited settings, however, the case count may rely more heavily on active case finding (including contact tracing) or community-based surveillance systems. Case information is then captured in a line list, a table used by epidemiologists to record and organize information on each identified case in an outbreak. In a line list, each row represents a separate case with an assigned unique identifier (CaseID), and each column represents a variable of interest. This includes demographic, epidemiological, and clinical information such as the following:

- Case ID number (an assigned number)
- Case-patient initials (or another identifier)
- Age
- Sex/gender
- Location (may be exact home address or aggregated location, like a county, district, etc.)
- Symptoms (column per symptom)
- Date of symptom(s) onset
- Case status (suspect, probable, confirmed, secondary, not a case)
- Epidemiologic links / exposures
- Risk factors / underlying conditions
- Tests conducted
- Type of specimen collected
- Date of specimen collection
- Results of laboratory testing
- Date reported by laboratory[39]

This information is used to conduct descriptive epidemiology, further epidemiological investigation, possibly attribution investigation, and hypothesis generation and testing.

STEP 5: Perform Descriptive Epidemiology

Describe everything we know about the cases. All the information captured over the course of the investigation thus far, interviews, case data, laboratory results, and so on, is used to complete a descriptive analysis of the outbreak. Descriptive epidemiology orients the events of an outbreak in terms of time, place, and person, answering critical questions of who, what, when, where, and how. Analyses involve calculating descriptive statistics, drawing epidemic curves, and creating maps of the outbreak.

Case information recorded in line lists is used to calculate frequency distributions of various variables, compare prevalence and spread among different groups, and identify the potential source of the outbreak, mode of transmission, or risk factors. Epidemiologists can look for patterns or identify "hot spots" to better understand if certain demographic information strongly relates to exposure and risk of contracting the disease.

An epidemic curve, or epi curve, is the standard visual tool used to analyze changes in the number of cases over time. Epidemiologists use epi curves to

More information is available about the management of data collected over the course of an epidemiological investigation, including storage and privacy, in the "Data Management" section of the Outbreak Data chapter.

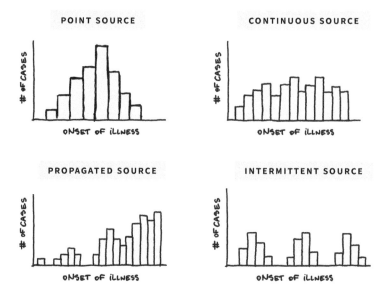

identify modes of transmission by analyzing the shape of the curve and whether it is point source, continuous common source, or propagated (person-to-person spread).[40] In a point source outbreak, people are exposed to the same source over a brief time period. This is observed on the epi curve as the number of cases rising rapidly, peaking, and then gradually decreasing, with most cases occurring within one incubation period of the disease. During continuous common source outbreaks people are exposed to the same source for a prolonged period. The epi curve gradually rises and can plateau. Intermittent source has multiple peaks related to exposures to same source over a period of time. In person-to-person transmission, the epi curve exhibits tall peaks, each representing an incubation period. These curves can provide important clues to investigators regarding the source of an outbreak.[41]

Another important element of descriptive epidemiology is building an outbreak map to show the geographic extent of the public health event by plotting where cases live, work, or were exposed. Epidemiologists can use outbreak maps to compare disease frequency by location, revealing clusters or patterns that lead to a better understanding of the nature and etiology of the event.

Early Outbreak Mapping

Outbreak maps pre-date epidemiology as a recognized science. Physician Valentine Seaman published a map of yellow-fever cases in New York in the *Medical Repository* journal in 1798, demonstrating the possible connection between the outbreak epicenter and waste sites.[42] John Snow is famous for his investigation into the transmission mechanisms of cholera in 1854. Snow postulated that cholera was a water-borne illness, contrary to the common belief at the time that it was caused by miasma (bad air). He used mortality reports, case interviews, and a map of cholera deaths in the Soho district of London and proposed that a single water pump on Broad Street was the source of the cholera outbreak.[43] His solution—remove the pump handle!

Modes of Transmission

Transmission of an infectious agent can occur via a number of ways and can be direct or indirect.

Direct transmission: The infectious agent is transferred from a reservoir to a susceptible host by direct contact or droplet spread. For *direct contact*, the agent is transmitted by physical contact between individuals through skin-to-skin contact, kissing, and sexual intercourse. Some kinds of direct transmission are site specific—for example, you have to touch an infected wound. *Droplet spread* of a pathogen to a new host refers to spray with relatively large, short-range aerosols produced by sneezing, coughing, or talking.[46]

Indirect transmission: A pathogen is transferred by a vector or vehicle. *Vector transmission* occurs when a living organism (vector), like a mosquito, flea, or tick, transmits an infectious pathogen between humans and/or from other animals to humans. *Contaminated vehicles and environments* can transmit pathogens indirectly via food, water, biologic products, and surfaces, also known as fomites. *Airborne transmission* involves particles known as aerosols suspended in air that carry infectious agents.

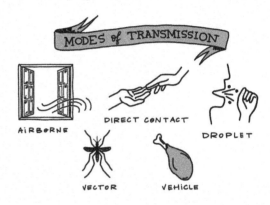

STEP 6: Develop Hypotheses

Given what we know, what do we think is happening and why? Part of the scientific process of epidemiology is developing hypotheses, continuing to reconsider, refine, and re-evaluate them as needed. Information collected during the investigation, the results from descriptive epidemiology, and a review of the literature are used to develop hypotheses about the source or reservoir of the pathogen, the agent's mode of transmission, and risk factors. Hypotheses should be testable, verifiable, supported by literature, and clearly state the relationship between an exposure and disease.[44]

The first step in generating a hypothesis is typically reviewing the preliminary data collected from the investigation. By looking for patterns, differences, and commonalities among responses about cases' personal characteristics, occupation, activities, travel, or location, investigators can build a hypothesis about the cause, source, or mode of transmission.

A literature review of reports and studies can provide valuable insight into potential causative agents, risk factors, or sources of exposures observed during past outbreaks.[45] Literature reviews can help investigators understand the biological drivers behind an outbreak, pathogenic organisms, incubation and infectious period, mode of transmission, and whether reservoirs (animal or environmental) may exist.

R_0: Measuring How Contagious a Pathogen Is

R_0 (pronounced "r naught"), is a numeric value that epidemiologists calculate to characterize the transmissibility (contagiousness) of a pathogen. They consider the infectious period (the length of time an infectious person is contagious), mode of transmission (remember the modes of transmission illustration?), and the contact rate (the number of people an infected person is estimated to come into contact with).

The basic reproductive number, R_0, of a disease thus characterizes the average number of secondary cases an infected person will cause within a susceptible population (e.g., those who lack immunity, are unvaccinated, etc.).[47] It can be used to identify which public health measures to use during an outbreak response and calculate immunization thresholds to control an infectious disease. For example, infectious agents that are airborne spread more easily than ones that require direct contact, so they tend to have higher R_0. Measles is widely considered to have one of the highest R_0, 12 to 18. This means that one person with measles will likely infect 12 to 18 other people who are susceptible. Measles, which is highly contagious, can live in the air for up to two hours after a person carrying it has left the room and infects roughly 90 percent of susceptible people who are exposed to it. This is one of the reasons that vaccination against measles is so essential to preventing the transmission of a pathogen that can spread incredibly easily. Ebola's R_0 is estimated to be between 1.5 and 2.5, however its case fatality ratios have ranged from 25 percent to 90 percent in past outbreaks, with an average case fatality ratio (CFR) of 50 percent.

Many also use R_e (also called R_t), known as the effective reproduction number. This measures the number of people in a population that may be infected by another individual at a specific point in time. The R_e will change over the course of an outbreak, as some people develop immunity or the exposed population size changes.

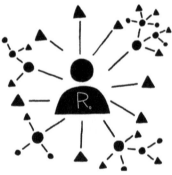

Superspreaders

For pathogens that spread between people, the R_0 can vary. Measles has a particularly high R_0. For COVID-19, the original strain was approximately 1 to 3, meaning each person infected between 1 and 3 additional people. The Omicron strain of COVID-19 was particularly infectious, with an estimated R_0 several times that of the original strain.

Occasionally, though, we will witness transmission outside of the expected R_0, including "superspreader events." These are incidents where one person or multiple people infect many more individuals than would otherwise be expected from the R_0. In 2015, for example, a traveler to South Korea was sick with Middle Eastern Respiratory Syndrome (MERS), and went to multiple clinical centers before being treated. That one person led to 22 cases, which then led to 111 secondary cases.[48] In other examples, funerals of Ebola patients became superspreader events when large communities touched a deceased person (unknown at the time to have died of Ebola).

 Perhaps one of the most famous superspreaders is Mary Mallon, or "Typhoid Mary," suspected of infecting at least 122 people in New York.[49]

STEP 7: Plan and Perform Additional Studies

Try to fill in the gaps of what we don't know yet. Parallel to the outbreak response, scientists carry out studies based on the hypotheses developed during the investigation to effectively explore and refine them or generate new ones. Before initiating a study, researchers conduct literature reviews to identify studies that have already been conducted in a particular area, which methodologies have been used, and relevant background information. There are several kinds of studies scientists conduct based on epidemiological investigation, namely observational studies such as cohort, case-control, cross sectional, or ecological studies.

Cohort study: Individuals are selected and studied based on their exposure status to see whether they develop the disease or health condition of interest over time. Cohort studies are particularly useful for exploring incidence in a specified group of individuals.[50] They can also be performed retrospectively, meaning after both the exposure and outcomes have occurred. Just as with normal cohort studies, during retrospective cohort studies scientists calculate and compare rates of disease among participants based on their exposure histories.

Learn more about public health surveillance in the "Surveillance" section of this chapter.

Case-control study: Used to ascertain whether an exposure is tied with contracting a disease. During a case-control study, investigators simultaneously track a case-patient group (individuals with a disease) and control group (individuals without a disease). Their previous exposures are then compared.

Cross-sectional study: Measures exposures and health outcomes simultaneously. The cross-sectional study tends to assess the presence (prevalence) of the health outcome at that point of time without regard to duration. With this study, however, it can be difficult to distinguish between risk factors for the incidence of the disease and risk factors for survival.

Ecological study: Environmental or microbiological investigations can also be used to further test epidemiological hypotheses to identify other contributing factors of disease. This can include collecting food, water, and/or environmental samples, collaborating with local agencies, and interviewing suspected cases to determine what happened with the suspected source.[51]

Conducting statistical analysis is a core part of testing and evaluating the hypotheses that drive the studies listed above. It allows researchers to quantify the association between various exposures and disease. Depending on the study design, various frequency and effect measures are used, including incidence, prevalence, mortality, relative risk, and odds ratio.[52]

The two primary measures of association are odds ratio (OR) and risk ratio (RR), which demonstrate the strength of association between two variables, such as exposure and disease, for example.[53] The RR and OR are interpreted the same way:

- **RR or OR = 1:** exposure has no association with disease (Start over with a new hypothesis.)
- **RR or OR > 1:** exposure may be positively associated with disease (You are on to something—use this to inform response measures.)
- **RR or OR < 1:** exposure may be negatively associated with disease (Huh. Is the exposure protective? Unsure? Keep investigating.)

The purpose of conducting detailed systematic studies lies in expanding knowledge of the causative agent and improving the sensitivity and specificity of the case definition. It can also refine the defined risk population to allow for more effective and targeted public health efforts.

The 2×2 Table

A 2×2 table is used in epidemiology to evaluate the association between variables, that is, the relationship between a possible risk factor and an outcome—the likelihood that a specific exposure led to a disease. Using a 2×2 table, epidemiologists can calculate:

- OR = (A/B)/(C/D)
- RR = (A/(A+B))/(C/(C+D))

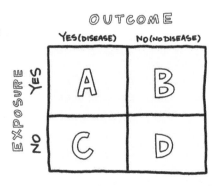

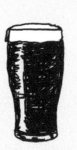
STEP 8: Implement Control and Prevention Measures

Try to stop the outbreak. Based on the findings of the epidemiological investigation, health officials and decision makers implement disease control and prevention measures. This includes nonpharmaceutical interventions (NPI) like hygiene guidance, disinfection practices, or physical distancing, and medical countermeasures (MCM) like drugs and vaccines.

See the Disease Prevention and Mitigation chapter to learn more about specific examples of NPIs and MCMs and their use, procurement, and distribution.

STEP 9: Initiate and/or Maintain Surveillance

Make sure you can monitor how you are doing trying to stop the outbreak. Surveillance and epidemiology go hand in hand. Once an outbreak is detected or an epidemiological investigation ends, public health surveillance does not stop. It is critical to continue collecting information throughout the outbreak because the nature of an outbreak can change, new variants and clades of diseases emerge, and additional risk factors can appear. It also allows health officials to track whether the control and prevention measures implemented were effective.

STEP 10: Communicate the Results of the Epidemiological Investigation

Make sure all relevant stakeholders know what they need to know about the outbreak. It is critical to communicate with both the public and the scientific community at all stages of an epidemiological investigation, disseminating information through a mix of trusted media to keep public health personnel, clinical care workers, the public, and government officials informed. It ensures accountability and provides justification for public health control measures. Communication of epidemiological findings like mode of transmission or new risk factors can be done through press releases and briefings, traditional media, social media, data dashboards, designated disease websites, and publications, papers, and preprints. Results should be presented in a clear, scientifically objective way using language that is accessible to individuals without a scientific background.

A more formal communication step taken at the end of an investigation is the creation of a written after-action report (AAR). Public health officials are responsible for summarizing the findings and providing actionable guidance in a final outbreak investigation report following standard scientific format, including an introduction and sections on background, methods, results, discussion, and recommendations.[56] These reports are important references and documentation of actions for future similar outbreaks and contribute to the public health literature and knowledge base.[57]

From Guatemala to Canada and the US

Tracing a Cyclospora Outbreak in Raspberries

In 1996, large numbers of cases of cyclosporiasis, a gastrointestinal disease caused by the parasite *Cyclospora cayetanensis*, were reported to the US CDC and Health Canada.[58] The outbreaks were unusual given that cyclosporiasis cases were usually only seen in foreign travelers. Prior to 1996, the US had documented only forty-five laboratory-confirmed cases across three small outbreaks. During the spring and summer of 1996, 1,465 cases were reported in the US and Canada.[59]

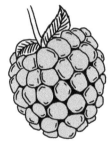

Local health officials initiated an investigation. They solicited healthcare workers and laboratories for cyclosporiasis case reports (1. Verify the existence of an outbreak; 4. Find and document cases) and worked with the US CDC to test case stool specimens for laboratory confirmation (2. Confirm the diagnosis). Investigators noted that clinicians used varying case definitions for probable cases, but that an overwhelming majority of cases demonstrated diarrhea, loss of appetite, fatigue, weight loss, abdominal bloating, gas, cramps or pain, and nausea. Further, health investigators considered a cyclosporiasis outbreak cluster to be two or more cases, at least one of whom had to be laboratory confirmed, who between May 1 to August 31, 1996, ate a food item at an event and experienced gastrointestinal distress twelve hours to fourteen days later (3. Create case definition).

Investigators found that:

A total of 1465 cases of cyclosporiasis—725 cluster-associated cases (49.5 percent) and 740 sporadic cases (50.5 percent)—were reported by 20 states, the District of Columbia, and 2 provinces. All sites were east of the Rocky Mountains except the one in Colorado. A little more than half the cases were in females (772, 52.7 percent), 41 (2.8 percent) were in children under 18 years of age, and 3 (0.2 percent) were in persons known to be infected with the human immunodeficiency virus. Twenty-two hospitalizations (1.5 percent of cases) but no deaths were reported. . . . The median of the event-specific attack rates among persons who ate the berry items that contained or may have contained raspberries, with or without other berries, was 93.3 percent.[60]

(5. Perform descriptive epidemiology)

They also carried out retrospective cohort studies and one case-control study, calculating relative risk and odds ratios to determine the source of the outbreaks (7. Plan and perform additional studies). Health officials hypothesized that imported raspberries were the common source of illness and that the cases of cyclosporiasis were the result of a food-borne outbreak (6. Develop hypotheses). Scientists traced the source of the raspberries through an environmental investigation, analyzing purchase, shipment, and farm records. They hypothesized that the outbreaks could be traced to "as few as five Guatemalan farms," but the way in which the raspberries were contaminated was not determined.

The results of the investigation, "An Outbreak in 1996 of Cyclosporiasis Associated with Imported Raspberries," were published in 1997 in the *New England Journal of Medicine*, by Dr. Barbara L. Herwaldt, Dr. Marta-Louise Ackers, and the Cyclospora Working Group (10. Communicate the results of the epidemiological investigation). The researchers highlighted the importance of identifying and investigating food outbreaks early (9. Initiate and/or maintain surveillance). They also reported that the Guatemalan berry farms implemented several control and prevention measures, including monitoring hazards, using potable water for handwashing and spraying mixtures, and cleaning surfaces that berries touch, as well as overall improved hygiene and sanitation facilities and measures for workers (8. Implement control and prevention measures).

CASE STUDY

Long-Dormant Bacteria Causes a Deadly Anthrax Outbreak

in Reindeer and Humans

During July and August of 2016, in the isolated Yamal Peninsula above the Arctic Circle, more than 2,300 reindeer died as a result of an anthrax outbreak, a deadly infectious disease that had not been seen in this region of Siberia in seventy-five years. This event demonstrated a direct impact of climate change on human health, the spread of disease between animals and humans, and the importance of having strong systems in place for outbreak response.

Disease and Mode of Transmission

The *Bacillus anthracis* bacteria that causes anthrax is found in the soil on nearly every continent. Humans and animals can become infected when anthrax spores are inhaled or ingested. There are several types of anthrax infections based on the manner in which spores enter the body. Cutaneous anthrax occurs when spores enter the body through a cut or scrape; inhalation anthrax is the deadliest form and results from breathing in spores; and gastrointestinal anthrax comes from consuming raw or undercooked meat from an infected animal.

ANTHRAX TYPES

TYPE OF ANTHRAX	MORTALITY WITHOUT TREATMENT	MORTALITY WITH TREATMENT
Inhalation	Almost 100%	45%
Gastrointestinal	>50%	40%
Cutaneous (skin)	20%	Almost 0%

Adapted from the CDC's "Types of Anthrax" web page (last modified November 20, 2020), https://www.cdc.gov/anthrax/basics/types/index.html.

Animals can get infected when they ingest anthrax spores from contaminated soil, plants, or water sources.[61] Anthrax spores can then be transmitted from an infected animal to a human in a number of ways—when people eat infected meat, inhale spores from contaminated hides or carcasses, or handle an infected animal and spores enter the body via a cut.

Outbreak Origin

The Russian Ministry of Agriculture reported that the cause of the animal and human outbreak was the thawed carcass of a reindeer that had died seventy-five years ago from anthrax.[62] Officials speculated that unprecedented high temperatures, reaching 35 degrees Celsius (95 degrees Fahrenheit), thawed the permafrost, revealing long-dormant anthrax in the previously buried carcass. Herds of reindeer were then exposed to the infected carcass, contracting anthrax, and passing it to humans. Several scientific studies from international researchers corroborated this hypothesis.[63] Other hypotheses, though, suggested that the outbreak was caused by infected human remains from a shallow burial ground.

See the Disease Prevention and Mitigation and Animal Health and Safety chapters for strategies used to stop the spread of disease, like quarantine, decontamination, and culling as was seen during this outbreak.

See the Money chapter for information about allocating money during emergency outbreak response.

Emergency Response

Following the deaths of thousands of reindeer, on July 25 Russian health authorities announced a quarantine around the site of the anthrax outbreak.[64] The government allocated money for safe clearing of the area, fencing off the suspected anthrax source, culling infected animals, and burning the carcasses. Health officials collected samples from infected animals and humans and sent them to the central laboratory in Moscow for analysis.[65] The majority of human samples taken from Nenet families near the outbreak zone, the nomadic herding families of the Yamal Peninsula identified as the at-risk population, were negative for anthrax. The governor, though, issued a mass evacuation and quarantine order of local herders. A government airlift evacuated at least sixty-three people from the quarantine area around the site of the outbreak to a secondary quarantine location for preventive inoculation and monitoring.[66] The *Russian Times* reported that ninety people were evacuated and taken to a hospital to be tested and isolated in case of infection.[67] In all, seventy-two nomadic herders, forty-one of whom were children, were hospitalized and held under close observation for development of anthrax symptoms in the town of Salekhard. Health officials reported the first anthrax-confirmed death on July 30: a twelve-year old boy from a reindeer herding family with intestinal anthrax.[68] Thirteen other anthrax cases were confirmed of the seventy-two individuals that were hospitalized.[69]

By July 30 the defense minister had dispatched troops from the Russian army, specialists from the Chemical, Radioactive, and Biological Protection Corps, to control the spread of disease, confirm the focal point of the infection, and dispose of infected carcasses.[70] Additionally, they established a field lab to carry out onsite tests on environmental and biological samples, in addition to the lab work being carried out in Moscow. The military mobilized transportation vehicles including military helicopters, planes, and off-road vehicles to move military and health responders, the at-risk nomads, and supplies for the response.

Local authorities declared a local state of emergency to mobilize resources and funds, but made additional statements insisting that the outbreak would not impact venison exports, the primary trade in the region.

The reindeer death count from anthrax rose to 2,349 by the end of July. Anthrax vaccination in reindeer herds had been halted in 2007, which increased population susceptibility.[71] The Federal Veterinary and Phytosanitary Surveillance Service (Rosselkhoznadzor) released a statement saying that the government's decision to cancel compulsory vaccination was the cause of the outbreak.[72]

See the Laboratories and Lab Analysis chapter to learn about collecting, transporting, and analyzing samples in labs.

See the Emergency Operations and Logistics chapter to learn more about coordinating emergency operations, including mobilizing resources for emergency response and evacuating patients.

See the Security chapter to learn about how health officials work with military, police, and security sectors to stop the spread of disease.

See the Declarations and Notifications chapter to learn how governments announce an outbreak.

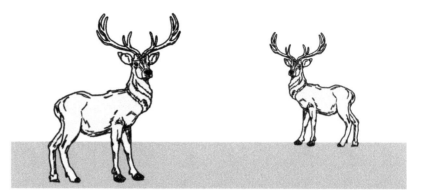

See the Community Engagement and Humanitarian Response chapter for more info about working with and supporting impacted communities during an outbreak.

For more information about sharing public health and risk information during an outbreak, see the Communicating with the Public chapter.

The Emergencies Ministry, Health Ministry, and Military team established an emergency operation site to coordinate the ground response in Yamal. Mitigation and prevention efforts included vaccinating an estimated 4,500 reindeer against anthrax and continuing to incinerate carcasses. Photos from the response show Russian army biological troops in full protective gear while handling the infected animals and carcasses.

By August 2 the confirmed number of human anthrax cases had risen to twenty, and ninety suspected cases were hospitalized.[73] Two-thirds of the anthrax cases had skin anthrax; the rest had the more serious intestinal form. Health authorities expanded the defined at-risk population beyond the original Nenet herding group to include other Nenet nomadic camps in the Yamal district and sent planes to evacuate them. However, some herders refused to move. The Emergencies Ministry announced the establishment of "life sustenance camps," with beds for herders and their families displaced by the evacuation to encourage cooperation. The press service of the governor's office ramped up its public health and risk communication campaign, using social media, radio, and print to explain the symptoms of anthrax infection and modes of transmission. The regional government banned the export of meat, antlers, and skins from the Yamal district amid concerns over black market poaching as a potential risk for further spread of infected biological materials.[74]

As the response unfolded and investigation into the origin of the outbreak continued, the deputy head and senior veterinary regulator from Rosselkhoznadzor claimed there had been a five-week delay in issuing warnings of the anthrax outbreak. Senior officials complained that this was in part due to the unreliable communication infrastructure between veterinarians and herders, stating that "one of [the herders] had to walk for four days across the tundra to inform about the accident."[75]

Laboratory analysis continued to confirm the presence of *Bacillus anthracis* in reindeer carcasses, and the emergency response team continued to incinerate carcasses to stop the spread. The human case confirmation rose again by August 3 to twenty-three cases, six of them with intestinal anthrax. Before the end of the month, two more anthrax outbreaks were reported, another on the Yamal peninsula and the third 155 miles east of the epicenter of the initial outbreak.[76]

Health officials hypothesized that gadflies and mosquitoes were responsible for spreading the disease from infected animals to other herds, or that separate soil contamination spots were exposed during the permafrost thaw. Fortunately, the human death toll remained at one, although three dogs died of anthrax infection, and while the hospitalization total increased to 115, there were no additional confirmed cases. A compulsory vaccination program was instituted for the at-risk group—now considered to be anyone working with reindeer.

In September 2016, Russian officials proposed culling a quarter of a million reindeer by December to reduce the possibility of further anthrax outbreaks by decreasing population density to minimize disease spread.[77] While culling is an annual occurrence in the region for population sustainability, this number would be a massive increase from normal culling. The Yamalo government countered with one hundred thousand. Following extensive debate between Rosselkhoznadzor, the Yamalo government, and other stakeholders on what the culling number should be, it ended up being roughly sixty thousand.

There was also debate on the best way to compensate the nomadic herders for participating in culling. Different proposals included providing herders with mortgages to buy apartments in return for turning their reindeer in for culling, limiting reindeer herds to fenced pastures, or moving herds south.[78] The proposals drew substantial criticism, notably from the anthropological community, who perceived this as the destruction of nomadic lifestyle and cultural traditions.[79] Reindeer are central to the nomadic Nenet people's means of existence; they eat their meat and blood and use reindeer hides and sinews for clothing and tents.[80] Taking away the reindeer would fundamentally change their livelihoods and culture. Watchdog groups also warned that eliminating herding in the north coincided with gas licensing in the region.[81]

Case Management and Treatment

Over the course of the outbreak, 115 suspected cases were hospitalized and observed for anthrax infection symptoms. Between July 25 and August 31, twenty-three confirmed anthrax cases were treated at the hospital in Salekhard where all evacuated cases were brought.

Recovery

In December 2016, as part of a $600,000 anthrax infection recovery program, the government reimbursed forty-five nomadic herding families whose reindeer had died during the anthrax outbreak.[82] A further 90 million rubles (US$1.47 million) in government funds were allocated to support the hundreds of nomadic herders who had been evacuated during the response to assist in building a new settlement of chums (tents).[83] The "Cooperation of Yamal" foundation raised 65 million rubles (US$1.06 million) to help herders replace the possessions they lost when they were evacuated, such as clothing, shoes, personal hygiene items, medicines, and snow mobiles.[84]

See the Community Engagement and Humanitarian Response chapter to read about the role of anthropologists in outbreak response.

For more information about medical services during an outbreak, see the Treating Patients chapter.

See the Money chapter to learn about compensating populations impacted by an outbreak.

Human and Animal Impact

- 2,349 reindeer died
- 115 people hospitalized

- 1 person died (twelve-year-old boy)
- 3 dogs died

Attribution Investigation

Whenever an outbreak happens, everyone wants to know what caused it. In a naturally occurring disease event, this is answered through the epidemiologic investigation to figure out what the pathogen is and how did it lead to an outbreak.

If the outbreak is not naturally occurring, then an attribution investigation can be conducted to determine if an event was accidental or deliberate, and if deliberate, who the responsible party might be. These investigations are conducted by a multidisciplinary team that includes public health and medical professionals as well as security and law enforcement partners.

Attribution investigators draw from a variety of sources to try to identify the agent, characterize the incident, attribute the incident to a specific perpetrator, and, when relevant, explore possible violations of law. They analyze intelligence data, biological and environmental samples, toxicology analyses, clinical reports, medical records, laboratory reports, epidemiologic findings, eyewitness accounts, and expert judgement as part of their investigation to ascertain causal attribution. The findings and any decisions resulting from the investigation may need to stand up to political, scientific, and legal scrutiny.[85]

CASE STUDY

Yellow Rain and the Origins of UNSGM

Starting in the late 1970s and into the early 1980s, there were allegations that Soviet-backed groups were using a toxin called trichothecene mycotoxin against the Mujahidin in Afghanistan, the Hmong in Laos, and Khmer resistance groups in Cambodia. Several countries investigated the allegations into what became known as Yellow Rain—named because Hmong and others described small airplanes that released yellow clouds that look, felt, and sounded like rain.

The United Nations put together an ad hoc investigation, which several years later they codified into a process called the United Nations Secretary General's Mechanism for Investigating Allegations of Chemical or Biological Weapons Use (it's a mouthful. Normally it is referred to as UNSGM or just SGM). The UNSGM has been used about a dozen times since the 1980s to conduct "fact finding" missions into alleged biological or chemical weapons use events, including during the Iran/Iraq war, and to investigate allegations of chemical weapons use in Syria.

Surveillance

Public health surveillance is the continuous, systematic collection and analysis of disease data. The information collected during surveillance enables public health professionals and decision-makers to implement prevention programs before an outbreak occurs, and also to determine the best course of action to contain and mitigate the impact once one does happen.

Disease surveillance is what—most of the time—tells us we have an outbreak and allows us to differentiate between an event we need to go into "outbreak mode" for versus normal or expected cases of a disease. Ongoing surveillance throughout an outbreak provides critical information to inform response and recovery decisions. There are multiple types of disease surveillance employed by public health systems, including actively searching for disease events and more passive data collection. Below we discuss the types of surveillance critical to outbreak detection and response.

Conduct Event-Based Surveillance

Event-based surveillance (EBS) is a type of active surveillance conducted by public health departments in order to have early warning of disease events.[86] EBS involves collecting, monitoring, and assessing usually ad hoc information about unusual events that might signal the beginning of an outbreak.[87] Sources of information might come from social media, rumor logs, public hotlines, or other informal communication networks. EBS captures informal signals that may provide early warning of an evolving threat to public or veterinary health—sometimes providing warning of a disease event even before people start seeking medical care.[88]

EBS systems look for alerts that can signify a range of potential risks. Some examples include:

- unexplained clustered cases of a disease, unusual disease patterns, or unexpected deaths in either humans or animals;
- events related to potential exposure for humans, such as diseases and deaths in animals, contaminated food products or water, and environmental hazards;
- and alerts of potential exposure to chemical hazards, or occurrence of natural or man-made disasters.[89]

Since EBS data can come from lots of places, the first phase of EBS is to identify information from an array of sources, including media, information networks, and communities.[90] Notifications from these sources must then be verified in order to ensure information is credible and to then assess risk.[91] This is often accomplished by an event assessment team that evaluates reported

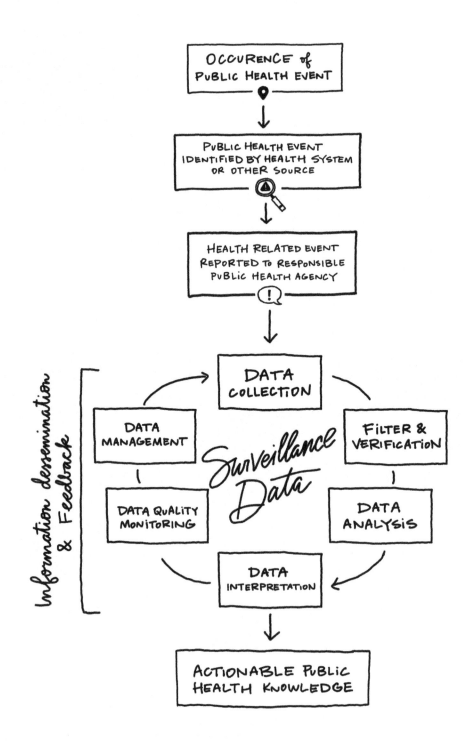

events and triggers rapid response activities.[92] Once the reliability of the information is established, the EBS information needs to be communicated to stakeholders across and outside the healthcare sector.[93]

Mountain-Biking Web Forum Aids Detection
of Campylobacteriosis Outbreak in British Columbia, Canada

On June 16, 2007, 787 individuals participated in a mountain bike race in British Columbia, Canada. Two days after the race, participants began posting on a mountain-biking web forum noting diarrheal illness, sharing symptoms, and asking if anyone else had a similar experience. Increasing numbers of comments and posts about illness among race participants prompted race organizers to reach out to the local health unit on June 20, notifying them of a possible outbreak five days before *Campylobacter jejuni* was confirmed through positive laboratory results.[94] The web forum also served as a valuable resource for investigators, who reviewed detailed posts to identify possible exposures to the bacteria, such as water delivery systems, shared face-wiping cloths, and inadvertent mud ingestion. They also used the forum to establish a case definition based on the symptoms identified by forum participants, generate hypotheses, and develop a questionnaire as part of a retrospective cohort study. Of the 537 racers included in the study, the outbreak investigators identified 225 ill individuals, representing one of the largest campylobacteriosis outbreaks in Canada.[95] Investigators concluded that the outbreak was a result of ingesting mud during the race.

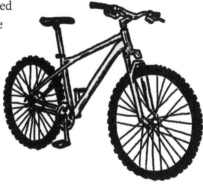

Ingesting mud isn't the only outbreak-related hazard in sporting events. Since 1998, there have been several documented outbreaks of leptospirosis—a bacterial disease spread through the urine of infected animals—linked to the swimming portion of triathlons. This includes ninety-eight athletes who became ill at an Illinois triathlon; five cases in a 2006 triathlon in Germany; and an outbreak at a Reunion Island triathlon in 2013.[96] Inadvertently swallowing water, heavy rainfall, and open wounds have all been associated with contracting leptospirosis.

Conduct Indicator-Based Surveillance

Where event-based surveillance is often unstructured, indicator-based surveillance (IBS) is a structured, standardized way of collecting data.

Indicator-based public health surveillance is a more traditional way of reporting diseases to public health officials. Indicator-based surveillance involves reports of specific diseases from health care providers to public health officials using standardized forms. An example of information obtained through indicator-based surveillance might be reports received on a regular basis and entered routinely into a disease-reporting database on the number of laboratory-confirmed cases of influenza identified at a hospital laboratory.

IBS data provides information about the frequency, origin, and distribution of reportable diseases.[97] This form of surveillance often alerts public health officials to spikes in known diseases (as opposed to EBS, which can help with both knowns and unknowns), and focuses on a list of notifiable diseases that clinicians and laboratories are required—either legally or through regulations—to report on through a structured database.[98]

The primary types of surveillance data that generally feed into IBS systems include the following:[99]

Conventional disease-specific (**biologic**): based on highly specific case definitions that usually include biological and clinical components

Syndromic: based on case definitions made up of associations of symptoms; permits wide surveillance coverage for emerging infectious diseases

Comprehensive (**facility-based**): requires all identified sources to report; usually used in disease eradication programs or for diseases requiring immediate public health attention

Sentinel: requires only a fraction of health care structures to report; usually used for endemic diseases, epidemic-prone diseases, diseases not requiring immediate public health action, and frequent diseases for which a change in pattern might be noteworthy

Laboratory-based: conducted at laboratories to detect events or trends

Case-based: ongoing and rapid identification of identifiable cases for the purpose of case follow-up

Community-based: systematic detection and reporting of events of public health significance within the community, by community members

Structured health data can come through standardized channels such as regular disease incidence reports and mortality data from hospitals or local public health jurisdictions up to higher levels. Sources include health care facilities, laboratories, death registers, and non-health sources like school absenteeism rates or medicine sales.[100] The data generate indicators that correspond to notifiable diseases or conditions; indicators typically include number of cases, survival status of cases, number of laboratory diagnoses, and classification of cases (suspected, probable, and confirmed).[101]

IBS data are useful not only for early warning but also for other objectives, like measuring the impact of health programs or identifying priority health problems.[102]

IBS and EBS Working Together to Slow Nipah Outbreaks

in Bangladesh

Routine IBS at ten designated government hospitals in Bangladesh works jointly with EBS to identify, notify, and investigate cluster cases of encephalitis in order to capture potential Nipah virus outbreaks early on.[103] Nipah virus is a deadly zoonotic pathogen, with fatality rates ranging from 40 to 75 percent. It can be transmitted through contact with infected animals and their by-products, consumption of contaminated food products, and person-to-person close contact. There is no treatment or vaccine currently available for animals or humans.

Health officers from the government of Bangladesh's Institute of Epidemiology, Disease Control and Research and the International Centre for Diarrhoeal Disease Research run simultaneous case-based surveillance in hospitals by collecting and analyzing blood samples from encephalitis cases during the January-through-March Nipah season and cluster-based surveillance in communities linked temporally and geographically to cases in an effort to identify person-to-person transmission.[104] The integration of IBS and EBS systems allows for rapid and targeted surveillance and epidemiological investigation to detect pandemic threats in resource-limited settings.

Fruit bats, particularly bats from the *Pteropus* genus like flying foxes, are the animal reservoir for Nipah virus. In Bangladesh, bats have been observed drinking from spigots and peeing into collection pots used to collect sap from the trees. Bat-to-human transmission of the virus occurs primarily when people drink raw date palm sap or fruit contaminated with urine or saliva from an infected bat. The first documented case of Nipah virus was in 1999 in Malaysia. The outbreak originated from fruit bats whose contaminated saliva got into fruit that fell to the ground and was eaten by pigs. The pigs then transmitted the virus to humans.

Conduct Syndromic Surveillance

One of the goals of surveillance for outbreak response is to identify an event happening as soon as possible. In order to do that, public health officials need to collect information available at the earliest possible stages of an event. Syndromic surveillance is when public health officials track real time information on disease trends or health-seeking behaviors, often even before they know the diagnosis or specific pathogen causing the symptoms. For example, they may collect clinical data on high fevers or flu-like symptoms. They may collect information on emergency room visits. They may track over-the-counter sales of drugs like aspirin or antidiarrheal medication, or school absenteeism. This data can help identify early clusters of outbreaks even before confirmed diagnosis; it can also help monitor severity or clinical changes in an ongoing outbreak.

Using School Absenteeism to Track Influenza

Lessons from the H1N1 Pandemic

The 2009 H1N1 pandemic increased awareness of the value of school absenteeism data as a syndromic surveillance tool. Research across several countries, including the US, UK, and Japan, showed that disease-specific absenteeism data could be used to improve surveillance of illnesses like influenza and support health providers in planning response activities and deliver services.[105] Schools are breeding grounds for the spread of germs and disease, and studies have shown that they are "primary venues of influenza amplification with secondary spread to communities."[106] As a result, school absenteeism data can be used for early detection of influenza before significant community spread occurs.

Conduct Surveillance at Points of Entry into a Country

Conducting disease surveillance at points of entry (PoE) into a country can help control the international spread of diseases and other health hazards. PoE are defined in the International Health Regulations (IHR) as "a passage for international entry or exit of travelers, baggage, cargo, containers, conveyances, goods and postal parcels, as well as agencies and areas providing services to them on entry or exit." PoE surveillance plays a key role in managing and preventing the importation and exportation of health hazards.[107] But PoE surveillance is also really hard. Countries often identify certain airports or land crossings to conduct surveillance activities. Some countries may only have a few places where people and goods enter the country. In other countries, there may be hundreds of official and unofficial land or sea crossings.

Communicating standardized data generated at PoE to the national health systems and other PoEs allows for coordinated efforts to control the spread of health hazards between nations. Surveillance at PoE involves the additional challenge of sharing information across borders and sectors. A goal of PoE surveillance is to not only identify events to prevent further spread of disease by goods or travelers, but to do so in a manner that respects human rights and limits interference with travel and trade as much as possible.[108]

PoE-specific surveillance activities include screening luggage, cargo, and postal goods to confirm that they are free of sources of infections, as well as performing vector control, disinfection, and decontamination. Additional surveillance of passengers can include gathering information upon arrival from health forms, temperature checks, symptom screening, and rapid diagnostic tests, and carrying out medical examinations of airline passengers.

Under the IHR, countries only are responsible for disease surveillance and control at designated PoEs. A country may have hundreds of points of entry but may only decide to designate international airports or major land crossings for the IHR.

CASE STUDY

Screening for Ebola Virus Disease at Uganda Points of Entry

The Ministry of Health of Uganda, along with the International Organization for Migration (IOM) and the Uganda Red Cross Society, manages a coordinated effort to track point of entry (PoE) screening preparedness for Ebola virus disease (EVD) in different districts as part of routine surveillance.[109] They map each formal and informal PoE and its resources (smartphones, laptops, infrared thermometers), noting if active screening for EVD is carried out. The PoE surveillance system captures key data, including the total number of screenings conducted (disaggregated by gender and age), number of persons isolated, and number of persons referred. It also considers the land configuration (mountainous, forest, etc.), the type of access road (main or rural), and the reasons behind PoE crossings, including agricultural and trade activities, migration, and so on.

Triage of Surveillance Information and Verification of Signals

Triage is a process for screening surveillance data and information based on their relevance for the early detection of acute public health events. The triage process is crucial for differentiating between data that relate to non-acute events, like changes in endemic disease patterns, and data that correspond to an acute event of public health importance. Triage helps prevent the epidemic intelligence system from getting overwhelmed by filtering information that is not relevant for early warning.[110] Triage steps include checking data quality (like deleting duplicates), performing descriptive and analytical epidemiology, and sorting information by priority disease.[111] When a surveillance system captures data suggesting an acute problem, it is considered a signal, alerting health professionals of a potential public health event. The signals must be verified. Verification confirms the authenticity of a signal by cross-checking the validity of the information using reliable sources, contacting the original source, and collecting additional information required to validate the signal.

Assessment of Surveillance Systems

Surveillance systems need to be constantly assessed to evaluate the overall effectiveness and accuracy of the system in early detection of acute public health events, as well as to understand the timeliness and effectiveness of a response. This is an ongoing process, as public health officials must constantly refine, adapt, and improve surveillance systems. Frameworks and guidelines for conducting assessments of surveillance systems are available from organizations including the US CDC and World Health Organization (WHO).[112]

A comprehensive assessment of surveillance systems should look at

- Acceptability
- Completeness
- Flexibility of the existing system
- Representativeness
- Simplicity

- Timeliness
- Usefulness
- Sensitivity
- Specificity
- Positive predictive value[113]

While most of the above indicators are usually expressed as ratios, percentages, or other quantitative descriptors, it is also important to consider collection of qualitative data on the performance of the system, for example through stakeholder consultations and key informant interviews. Routine assessments of the surveillance system can also enable more effective resource allocation, inform understanding of achievements as well as surveillance failures, and help guide any modifications to the system.[114] In this way, ongoing assessment, as well as evaluation, of a surveillance system is a critical tool for ensuring its relevance to national health priorities within the context of continuous improvement.

As a second step, the data from the surveillance assessment should be used to perform a gap analysis. The gap analysis uses a SWOT (strengths, weaknesses, opportunities, and threats) approach to analyzing the existing surveillance system, taking into consideration the context of the country's specific needs and priorities. The gap analysis allows for the identification of key actions and resources needed to address identified gaps and strengthen early detection and response to acute public health events.

Example of a Surveillance System Assessment

Assessing Cholera Surveillance in the Greater Accra Region of Ghana

In January 2014, in the Osu Klottey District in Accra, health officers from the Ghana Field Epidemiology and Laboratory Training Programme and Ghana Health Services conducted an assessment to evaluate the attributes and performance of the cholera surveillance system. Using US CDC guidelines, the investigators examined district level surveillance data records, interviewed stakeholders and key informants using structured questionnaires, and reviewed data registries at health facilities at the district, regional, and national levels. They analyzed surveillance data against the calculated frequencies of cholera cases. Findings indicated that the surveillance system was achieving set objectives for cholera detection and that the system was sensitive, simple, stable, flexible, and timely, and that it operated in a way that encouraged participation and reporting within the surveillance system.[115] The evaluators also highlighted the contributions of clear field guidelines and well-trained health staff to the success and good predictive ability of the surveillance system. Moreover, the surveillance data was useful and of relatively good quality. The assessment concluded that better education on the transmission and prevention of cholera was needed within communities, and it identified the need to strengthen disease control officer training on data management.

Notification of Cholera

Cholera is an acute diarrheal illness caused by the toxigenic bacterium *Vibrio cholerae*. The International Health Regulations (IHR) decision instrument for the assessment and notification of events lists it as a disease with "demonstrated ability to cause serious public health impact and spread rapidly internationally." Thus, when a cholera outbreak is detected by a national surveillance system, it always triggers utilization of the IHR algorithm to determine notification to the WHO.

To learn more about notification of IHR events, go to the Declarations and Notifications chapter.

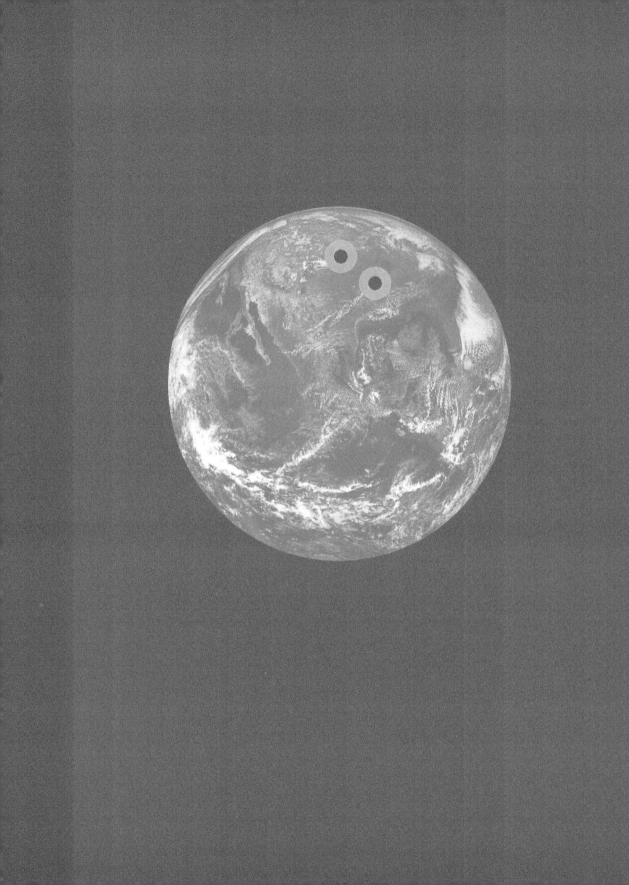

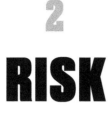

2

RISK

Should We Be Worried? And Who and What Should We Be Worried About?

Disease events happen all the time. Organizations like the WHO and regional Centers for Disease Control, and civil society efforts are constantly tracking signals for outbreaks.[1] In 2022, the WHO was screening approximately 43,000 signals of public health events around the world every month. They followed up on about 4,500 events each month and verified 30—meaning a public health event of some significance occurred every single day.[2]

Risk assessments are the processes required to take those disease event signals, determine which are significant events, and define core questions like, Which event poses what type of risks to populations? Who needs to be worried about the event? What should be done about it? Are the risks different to different populations? Is it possible that the disease will spread beyond a community? Beyond a country? Beyond a continent?

In this chapter we describe the multiple stages of risk assessment carried out to try to answer these questions.

Collect Data to Assess the Magnitude and Nature of the (Disease) Event

You need information to assess risk. The initial signals of a potential outbreak often will not have all the data necessary to figure out what is going on and answer those questions about who is at what level of risk. The original signal might also come from a nonofficial source that will need to be verified. The type of data collected at this stage will vary depending on the event, but in general the desired information includes:[3]

- What is the nature of the event/agent/disease? (If known. And if known, how?)
- Who reported the incident?
- How was the incident detected?
- Where is the location of the event / where have cases occurred?
- What is the potential origin (infectious, chemical, radiological, nuclear)?
- Is the disease typical/expected in this region or within this population?
- Over what time period have cases been detected?
- How many cases/deaths have there been, and what is the severity of the cases?
- What are the symptoms?
- Have samples been taken? If so, what lab is examining them? When will results be available?
- How many people have potentially been exposed to the hazard?
- What groups are affected (e.g., age, occupation, gender)?
- What are the common clinical/laboratory characteristics among the affected?
- Where are cases being managed? What is being done to prevent new cases?
- What is the likelihood of group intoxication/contamination?
- Who (agencies/organizations) is involved right now?

Read the Literature

Once scientists collect basic information about an emerging event, they must get smart. At this stage, they need to conduct a literature review and collect information on what is known about a disease, including where it has happened in the past, the reservoir (is it in animals?), whether specific groups are more susceptible than others, how it spreads, and known clinical presentations. The literature will also have information about existing laboratory tests, treatments, and control measures.

Any gaps in the literature should be filled by reaching out to known experts—particularly those who have documented experience with a given disease.

CASE STUDY

Early Warnings of Mpox 2022 (Previously Named Monkeypox)

In September 2017, a clinician in Nigeria saw a patient with a rash and sores that he eventually determined was mpox.[5] Over several weeks, Dr. Ogoina and his colleagues continued to see more cases across the region. They familiarized themselves with what had been documented in the past, including the epidemiologic and clinical characteristics of past outbreaks. The literature guided initial treatments and containment efforts, but after combing through the resources, they realized the outbreak they were seeing was abnormal and not following predictable patterns of transmission. Nigeria CDC and collaborating partners started warning the world of an outbreak of mpox that was behaving differently than outbreaks in the past and called for epidemiologic research and wide dissemination of findings.[6] Unfortunately, many in the global health community ignored the warnings from Nigeria and by summer 2022, the virus had spread to more than eighty nonendemic countries.

Learn more about disease naming in the Governance chapter.

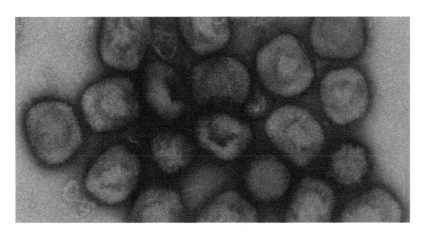

Mpox Virus.
Credit: NIAID

Assess the Evidence and Determine Risk

Once officials have collected all of the pertinent information available about a potential outbreak and done their homework on the disease, they have to assess the evidence and characterize the level of risk based on the nature, probability, and scale of the threat.[7] This is an iterative process that should continue as the outbreak evolves and more information is confirmed, as changing assessment of risk should guide outbreak response over time.[8]

All of the known evidence about the emerging event should be assessed to determine the level of confidence in the information, focusing on the disease event itself—or the hazard—what is known about exposure, and the context of the situation including the physical and ecological environment, as well as socio-economic and cultural norms of the affected population. Then risk is assessed based on a combination of *probability* and *impact* of the health threat. This can be tricky when a situation is evolving, and some information may be unknown or unverified.

Probability should capture routes and likelihood of exposures, susceptibility of the population to infection, and transmissibility of a pathogen. *Impact* may capture whether a significant number of people might be affected, if the disease will be severe, and if there are effective control measures, including drugs or vaccines, available.[9]

Based on the findings of the assessment, the risk level is then characterized, typically on a scale from Very Low to Very High. This may be visualized using a risk matrix that compares estimates of the probability of the event or outcome versus impact or consequences of the event to produce the level of risk. The qualitative definitions of probability and impact used in a risk assessment take into consideration the event's national and sub-national context.

Precautionary Principle

The 1992 Conference on Environment and Development introduced the precautionary principle, which means using risk mitigation for policy making, noting that when faced with serious threats, decision makers should not wait for full scientific certainty before taking measures to mitigate the threat.[10] Applied to public health emergencies or outbreaks, this means that if there is a public health threat, even if uncertain, preventative action should be taken.

Assign Actions to Risk Levels

Risk assessment is tied to specific actions. A risk assessment could conclude that the event—as understood at a point in time—is not a threat to human health and can be disregarded. It may be decided that a specific response isn't necessary yet, but that the event should be closely monitored. Another option would be to send a field investigative team to further asses a situation or even start control measures.

If a risk assessment finds that the public health community should respond, the assessment will often delineate the importance of rapid action and include options for next steps, including plans for escalating decision making, transmission and infection prevention and control measures, and treatment strategies.[11]

The risk assessment should be assessed, revised, and refined based on the characteristics of the public health event whenever additional data becomes available. This requires active and ongoing communication with public health professionals. This could be daily or along a regular timetable.

CASPER

Public health needs assessments are conducted in parallel with the risk assessments to assess public health needs during an outbreak. One example of a public health needs assessment is the US CDC Community Assessment for Public Health Emergency Response (CASPER) process, designed to help guide a community needs assessment to prioritize resources in an emergency response. CASPERs are generally used when the response team has limited or no information on aspects of a disaster, such as its overall effect on a population or the current health status and basic needs of that population.

In a CASPER, public health practitioners and emergency management officials rapidly characterize the health status and basic needs of the affected community.

The main objectives of a CASPER are to:
• determine the critical health needs and assess the impact of the disaster,
• characterize the population residing in the affected area,
• produce household-based information and estimates for decision-makers, and
• evaluate the effectiveness of relief efforts through conducting a follow-up CASPER.[12]

Multiple public health departments in the US performed CASPER assessments for Zika virus (ZIKAV) around general mosquito prevention and breeding, knowledge of Zika, and travel histories. This assessment then helped guide both messaging to the population as well as response efforts.[13]

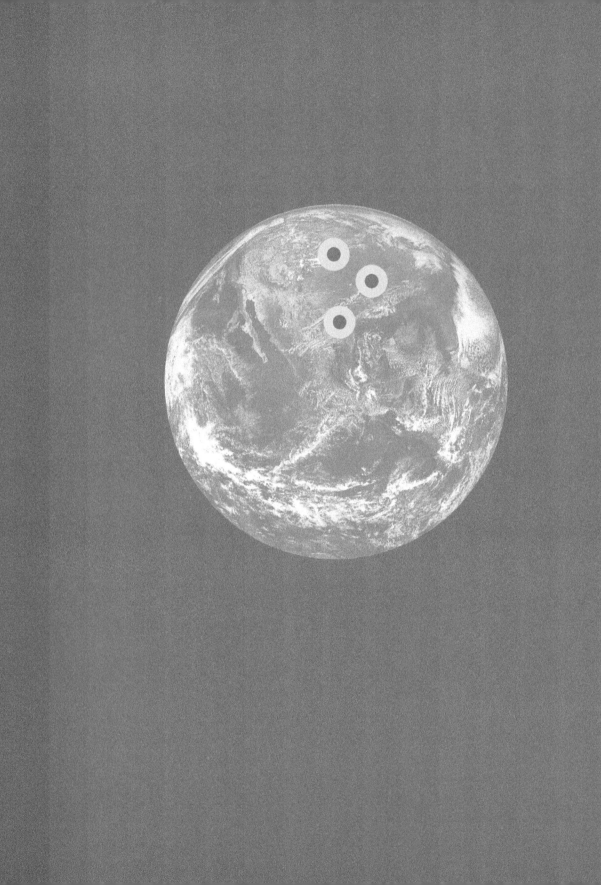

LABORATORIES AND LAB ANALYSIS

Getting to Know the Pathogen

Laboratories play a key role in outbreak surveillance, monitoring disease trends and detecting and investigating outbreaks. One of the first steps of outbreak investigation, verifying the existence of an outbreak, is supported through laboratory confirmation. An increase in laboratory reports may be the first sign that an outbreak is occurring.

Laboratories provide essential testing and analytic services for surveillance and investigation, as well as for disease response and preparedness. Lab confirmation of an outbreak informs public health mitigation efforts and clinical response. Laboratories play a critical role in research and development of diagnostics and medical counter measures like treatments and vaccines. There are many different types of laboratories—diagnostic, hospital, clinical, environmental, national and local, research, and academic, among others. They operate at local, regional, national, and international levels.

This chapter breaks down the collection, transport, testing, and analysis of samples in a public health laboratory system, as well as the biosafety and biosecurity measures central to laboratory activities.

Ensuring Biosafety and Biosecurity

Working with infectious, potentially deadly agents carries a clear risk. The scientists and health personnel that work with such pathogens follow clearly defined biosafety and biosecurity protocols during both routine disease surveillance and disease outbreaks. In laboratory contexts, these guidelines relate to the processes and equipment needed for secure handling of biological agents during collection, storage, transport, and analysis, according to their countries' national regulations and international best practices.

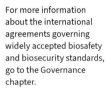

For more information about the international agreements governing widely accepted biosafety and biosecurity standards, go to the Governance chapter.

Human error, flawed technique, and insufficient infrastructure are the primary causes of contamination and exposure in laboratory settings. Laboratories and staff are provided with strict guidelines relating to sample handling and storage to avoid mistakes that jeopardize workplace safety. In addition to the key biosafety procedures, laboratories also conduct risk assessments to identify potential risks and implement steps to mitigate them.

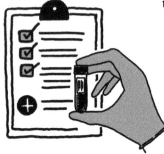

The US CDC classifies laboratories according to four biosafety levels (BSL), increasing from BSL-1 to BSL-4 based on the level of risk of the biological agents stored and analyzed there. Each BSL designation relates to the biosafety practices, containment controls, infrastructure, and safety equipment required to work with biological samples of varying risk. While this classification is still used around the world, the WHO, in the fourth edition of its *Laboratory Biosafety Manual* moved toward a more fluid framework that included balancing the risk associated with working with each pathogen and important safety measures on a case by case basis.[1]

Learn more about animal biosecurity in the Animal Health and Safety chapter.

The term *biosecurity* is used slightly differently across industries. In general, it includes security measures designed to prevent and reduce the risk of intentional transmission of infectious diseases. For laboratory contexts, biosecurity refers to the safe and secure management and storage of biological samples to prevent theft, loss, or unintentional use or release of a pathogen. This includes physical security for laboratory infrastructure and equipment, trained and reliable personnel, and data security to protect sensitive details about the pathogens stored.

Biosafety and biosecurity involve the appropriate use of personal protective equipment (PPE), disinfection procedures, personal hygiene, infrastructure

---

Quick Reference: Biosafety versus Biosecurity
Biosafety is about keeping people safe from bad pathogens
Biosecurity is about keeping pathogens safe from bad people

adaptations that minimize disease spread based on a pathogen's mode of transmission, and monitoring for and reporting possible infections.

Public health officials ensure biosafety and biosecurity through routine trainings and assessments, laboratory design and maintenance, and proper decontamination and waste management practices.

While collecting, transporting, storing, and working with samples, health and laboratory personnel are expected to follow the strict biosafety and biosecurity guidance set by their labs, their governments, and relevant international agencies.

For more information on sharing genetic sequence data, and specimen and data sharing policies in general, go to the Governance chapter.

Biosafety and Lab-Acquired Infections

Working with pathogens is dangerous. Biosafety measures, like training in appropriate handling of biohazardous materials, using proper containment devices and facilities, and wearing personal protective equipment (PPE) can help protect the people who work with infectious agents against lab-acquired infections (LAIs). Fortunately, LAIs are incredibly rare thanks to improved biosafety standards in laboratories around the world.[2] In the twenty-first century, there have been a handful of LAIs, with incidents typically limited to infection of a *single* individual, including West Nile Virus, Severe Acute Respiratory Syndrome (SARS), plague, dengue, vaccine-resistant meningitis, Zika, and variant Creutzfeldt-Jakob disease.[3]

CASE STUDY

Breach in Biosafety Protocol Leads to Mass Infection of *Brucella*

More than ten thousand people contracted brucellosis after a biopharmaceutical plant in Lanzhou, China, broke biosafety protocol.[4] Brucellosis is caused by the *Brucella* bacteria usually seen in animals, but it can be transmitted from animals to humans, causing flu-like symptoms including fever, sweats, aches, and weakness, and in serious cases, permanent damage to the central nervous system or even death.

In November 2019, several laboratory students at the Lanzhou Veterinary Research Institute contracted brucellosis.[5] By the end of the month, at least 181 workers at the academic institute had tested positive for the disease. Investigation into the outbreak revealed that a nearby biopharmaceutical factory, China Animal Husbandry Industry, had been using expired sanitizers and disinfectants for months to treat waste gas from the facility. This allowed contaminated gas carrying aerosolized *Brucella* to spread to the academic institute where the outbreak first was noticed, as well as into the local community, where thousands more people were infected over the course of the next year.[6]

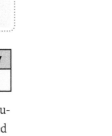

Brucella melitensis

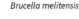

Collect Samples

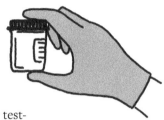

As part of disease surveillance and active outbreak response, health care providers, technicians, and field epidemiologists routinely and safely collect biological and environmental samples for laboratory testing. Biological samples typically include (human or animal) blood, urine, a nasopharyngeal (nose) swab or saliva, vomitus, or feces. Environmental specimens include food, water, soil, and swabs from surfaces (fomites). Depending on the type of outbreak, biological samples may also be collected from animals, particularly in cases where a disease can jump between animals and humans.

The type of sample collected, and well as the method of collection, depends on the suspected pathogen and nature of the outbreak. Trained health personnel collecting samples are equipped with appropriate sample collection equipment, transport media, and PPE relevant to the specific type of collection following standard operating procedure guidance, as provided through academic training or national accrediting bodies. For example, to assess the presence of a bloodborne pathogen, blood samples will be needed, which require materials like alcohol wipes, hollow needles, and collection tubes or vials in addition to the PPE used by the sample collector.

CASE STUDY

Tularemia in Martha's Vineyard

Tularemia is a rare, zoonotic disease caused by the highly infectious bacteria *Francisella tularensis*. It causes a nonspecific febrile illness that can last weeks to months. In 2000, there was an outbreak of tularemia in Martha's Vineyard, an island off the coast of Massachusetts. Fifteen people fell ill, eleven of them developing pneumonic tularemia, the most severe form of the disease.

Tularemia can be acquired a number of ways, through bug bites (mosquitoes, ticks, or flies), direct contact with an infected animal (usually rabbits or rodents), or inhalation of contaminated soil, water, or air particles.[7] While the bacteria does not form spores (unlike anthrax), it can survive for weeks, if not months, even at low temperatures, in soil, water, and decaying animals and plants. Scientists suspect that the bacteria arrived in the 1930s when cottontail rabbits were introduced to Martha's Vineyard by game clubs and tularemia cases began appearing on the island.[8] It is now endemic in the soil of Martha's Vineyard.

The island observed its first major outbreak in 1978, and a second in 2000.[9] As part of the 2000 investigation, scientists collected human and animal samples to test for antibodies and look for evidence of disease. They also collected environmental samples suspected of spreading the bacteria, including air samples, grass clippings from lawn mowing equipment, water, and soil. Investigators found that the cases had mowed lawns or cut brush along the southern coast of the island, the location of the 1978 outbreak.[10] They concluded that landscaping was the primary risk factor for the outbreak, highlighting the importance of taking environmental samples when studying diseases that can survive in the soil and water for decades.

Disease-Specific Guidance for Sample Collection

The WHO publishes disease-specific data sheets that outline technical specifications on the type of samples required for diagnosis, necessary collection vessels (such as swabs, containers, tubes, and boxes), and appropriate transport medium used for priority infectious diseases, including Ebola virus disease (EVD), Marburg virus disease, Lassa fever, Severe Acute Respiratory Syndrome (SARS); COVID-19; Middle Eastern respiratory syndrome (MERS), cholera, influenza (pandemic), meningitis, yellow fever, typhoid, and Shigellosis.[11]

For example, they advise that for surveillance and detection of Lassa fever, a BSL-4 pathogen, blood and nasopharyngeal samples should be collected. These samples can then be used to diagnose cases of Lassa fever using a number of laboratory tests, such as polymerase chain reaction (PCR) or immunoassay. When transporting the samples, they advise using triple packaging boxes. The samples should be collected and stored in vacuum tubes designed for blood collection with EDTA, sterile, capped with vacuum seal, and made of 4 ml and 6 ml plastic. Lastly, a prominently marked, puncture-resistant sharps container is used for collection and disposal of disposable and auto-disable syringes and needles used to collect blood.

Transport Samples

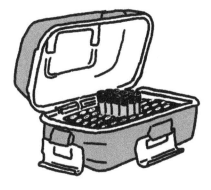

Once samples are collected, they are transported to laboratories that can process, analyze, and store them. Given that they are potentially infectious substances, they must be transported quickly, safely, and securely. Following established biosafety and biosecurity protocols protects the transporters and public, as well as preserves the samples for laboratory analysis. This includes labelling and packaging the samples correctly and using the appropriate bags and containers. Depending on the type of sample collected and its intended use, it may be transported to a close local laboratory, a national

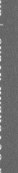

Read more about the legal and governance procedures involved in international sample and specimen transport in the Governance chapter.

laboratory, or an international reference laboratory. When samples require transport across international borders, health personnel follow established international agreements relating to air, rail, road, sea, and post transport of biologically hazardous substances. There are four main steps involved in sample transport.

Determining Sample Category

Countries typically follow the WHO's *Guidance on Regulations for the Transport of Infectious Substances*, which classifies samples as Category A or B based on their potential to cause harm.[12]

A Category A sample is defined as an infectious substance that is "capable of causing permanent disability, life-threatening or fatal disease in otherwise healthy humans or animals." Category B samples are biological agents that, while infectious, do not fall under Category A.

Prepare Shipment for Transport

Based on its classification and method of transportation (air, vehicle, etc.), a sample is packaged, labelled, and shipped along with the proper documentation describing the sample. Samples are triple packaged regardless of category.

Chain of Custody and Cold Chain during Transport

Throughout transportation, samples must be accounted for through a chain of custody.

A chain of custody is a set of procedures and documents that account for the integrity of a sample and allow outbreak investigators and officials to track its handling and storage from the point of collection through transport, laboratory testing, and short- and/or long-term storage, until final disposition. Systematic records of sample chain of custody help health officials identify any problems that may have occurred along the way (e.g., sample misidentification, delivery delays, breach in cold chain) and so prevent them in the future.

Depending on the sample, it may also need to be protected via cold chain, the system of transport and storage mechanisms that maintain optimum temperature to prevent degradation. This may involve using a network of cold boxes, refrigerators, freezers, and cold rooms as a sample is moved from its point of collection to a laboratory and then storage.

Detailed information about cold chains for samples, as well as more information about medical counter-measures and lab reagents, can be found under "Procurement, Supply Chains, and Stockpiling" in the Emergency Operations and Logistics chapter.

Prepare for Spill Clean-Up and Incident Reporting

Should a sample be compromised and impact its storage environment during transportation, the senders, carriers, and receivers involved with sample transport follow established clean-up procedures using appropriate PPE and report the incident, notifying authorities that an event occurred that might have led to human or animal exposure.

Challenges to International Sharing of Zika Samples from Brazil

On February 1, 2016, the WHO declared clusters of microcephaly and associated neurological disorders associated with the Zika virus (ZIKV) in Brazil a Public Health Emergency of International Concern (PHEIC).[13]

Scientists and researchers around the world sought to obtain samples of ZIKV from Brazil to develop diagnostic tests, treatments, and vaccines, and conduct further scientific research on the relationship between microcephaly and ZIKV. However, by February 3, 2016, it was estimated that fewer than twenty ZIKV samples had been shared internationally. Without access to samples from the Brazil outbreak, researchers were forced to rely on strains of ZIKV from previous outbreaks around the world, such as a 2013 outbreak in French Polynesia and a 2007 outbreak on Yap in the Federated States of Micronesia. International health officials conveyed concern that without access to current samples they were less able to predict potential mutations of the Brazilian ZIKV and develop important medical countermeasures.[14]

Challenges in transporting ZIKV samples out of the country was attributed to Brazil's biosecurity and biodiversity legislation. Fears of "bio-piracy" from foreign researchers taking biological samples out of the country without benefit to Brazil drove the adoption of a strict biodiversity law in 2015, aligning with definitions of genetic material ownership and sharing provided in the Convention on Biological Diversity's (CBD) Nagoya Protocol.[15] This legislation made it difficult for scientists to rapidly share ZIKV samples internationally.

Eventually, by February 19, 2016, Brazil sent the US CDC ZIKV samples, including tissue samples from newborns with microcephaly and miscarried fetuses. The women connected to each sample showed symptoms of Zika infection. US CDC scientists used reverse transcriptase-polymerase chain reaction (RT-PCR) to discover that there was evidence of ZIKV RNA and antigens in the brains of the newborns and in the miscarriage placenta—evidence of a link between ZIKV and microcephaly.[16]

Store Samples

Laboratory sample storage is an important step that supports a complete epidemiological investigation as well as attribution investigations and future research and development projects. Responsible and safe sample storage involves proper labeling and appropriate environmental conditions at all stages of sample handling, from collection, arrival at a laboratory, processing, and analyzing, to short- or long-term storage. Trained laboratory staff work to ensure the integrity of samples for immediate and future use through appropriate short- and long-term storage of samples, including protection from

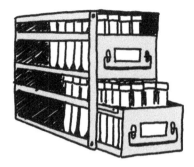

desiccation, temperature fluctuations, ultraviolet light degradation, humidity, contamination, and the potential for loss of identification documentation.[17] They also mitigate identified risks like accidents, theft, or inadvertent loss of specimens. This protects the health of laboratory staff and the public and prevents delays to investigations.

Short- and long-term storage requirements vary by specimen type and the pathogen or other biological target isolated for testing. During short-term storage, samples needed for frequent or periodic access are typically aliquoted (divided into multiple test tubes) to minimize freeze-thaw of the master sample stock and avoid potential problems with repeated retrieval and return.[18] Also, during an outbreak, there may be an increase in demand for short-term storage space while a higher volume of samples wait for processing. Freezer storage at –20°C and –80°C are common for periods that may range from months to five to ten years. Samples for long-term storage may be stored separately from those being used for more frequent access to help preserve their integrity. Ultra-low temperatures (e.g., liquid nitrogen, cryopreservation in freezers at or below –140°C) are optimal for long-term storage, which is critical as investigations may need to return to previously tested samples for additional analysis. Maintaining biological integrity and ensuring samples have appropriate identifiers is thus essential. Well-characterized specimen collections are also critical for future research and development efforts, retrospective studies, and providing reference materials for assay standardization, validation, proficiency testing programs, and potential legal inquiries.[19]

Biobanking

Biobanks are just what they sound like—a collection of biological specimens. Biobanks exist all over the world, bringing together large numbers of high-quality biological specimens with associated data, such as information about the individual the specimens came from, their health records and genetic and family information. These collections, acquired and stored based on the local legal and regulatory environment, are then used to support research efforts.[20]

CASE STUDY

Discovery of Smallpox in a US Lab

Smallpox is a serious infectious disease caused by the variola virus; it is estimated to have caused roughly three hundred million deaths in the twentieth century and has been a documented scourge on humanity for centuries.[21] The WHO led a successful worldwide vaccination campaign, launching an intense effort in 1967, leading to the eventual eradication of the disease by 1980. For strictly research purposes, small quantities of the virus remain stored in two official WHO-designated research laboratories under a 1979 agreement: the US CDC in Atlanta, Georgia, and the VECTOR laboratory in Novosibirsk in Russia.[22] All other facilities around the world were told to destroy their remaining smallpox samples. There have been fears circulating for decades, though, of samples existing outside of these two facilities.

In July 2014, US scientists found vials containing variola along with several other vials with unclear labels in an old cold storage room of a US Food and Drug Administration laboratory on the Bethesda campus of the National Institutes of Health that had inadvertently been left in a freezer and never destroyed. In total, twelve boxes and 327 vials of various pathogens, including dengue, rickettsia, and Q fever, were discovered while scientists conducted a lab clean-up and inventory.[23] Some the vials were dated from the 1950s.

The discovery of untracked smallpox virus raised significant concerns in the public health community, highlighting critical issues regarding appropriate storage of dangerous pathogens and the desire to ensure that smallpox remain eradicated. While all samples remained well-packaged and showed no signs of leakage, testing of the variola-labelled vials by a US CDC team in a BSL-4 lab confirmed that they did indeed contain variola and showed growth tissue cultures, suggesting that the samples were still alive. Upon the discovery that the vials contained viable virus, the variola samples and the vials of unidentified contents were destroyed at a US CDC facility under the supervision of WHO officials.[24] The entire situation was debriefed to the international community, including at the Biological and Toxin Weapons Convention meeting.

Smallpox and the Origins of Vaccination

The origins of vaccines can be traced to an early control effort for smallpox—variolation. Named for the variola virus that caused smallpox, variolation was a process through which individuals who had never had smallpox were exposed to samples taken from smallpox pustules by rubbing it into their arm or inhaling it. Variolation was practiced as far back as the early 1700s in Constantinople and the mid-1500s in China.[25] Individuals would develop similar symptoms to smallpox, and usually be granted immunity from a disease that typically killed 3 out of every 10 people infected.

Milkmaids with cowpox, a virus in the same genus as the variola virus, were protected from smallpox. Based on his knowledge of variolation and observations of milkmaid immunity, in 1796 English doctor Edward Jenner took a sample from a milkmaid's cowpox sore and injected it into the arm of his gardener's son. Later, the boy was exposed to variola several times, but never developed smallpox, supporting Jenner's theory of immunity through deliberate infection—inoculation.

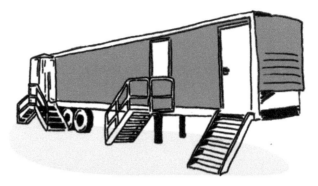

Laboratory Testing and Analysis

Once a sample is collected and transported to a laboratory, lab technicians begin the process of identifying the pathogen or agent responsible for the outbreak. Typically, agent identification and laboratory testing occur at laboratories at the district, regional, or national levels based on the country's infrastructure and organization of its laboratory system. These types of labs have the capacity to perform lengthy and complex testing procedures. Depending

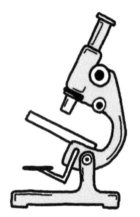

on the resources required for a particular test, field or mobile laboratories may also be used for rapid identification as well as supporting the collection and processing of specimens that go to national laboratories. International reference libraries exist to support the identification of rare or extremely dangerous pathogens using their banks of infrequently used diagnostic reagents and materials that local or regional laboratories may not possess.

Laboratory confirmation is a critical step in outbreak investigation. Once the agent is identified, a cascade of reactions can occur including updating the case definition, verifying case management and treatment protocols, and triggering procurement for additional laboratory reagents and materials required for sampling, diagnostics, and testing. However, laboratory confirmation is not always straightforward and easy. Interpretation of laboratory tests results must be done extremely carefully, taking into account the sensitivity and specificity trade off of the tests performed, and the likelihood of false negatives or false positives. Further, it is possible that multiple causative agents appear present in test results, obscuring the ability to identify which agent is driving the outbreak. This is especially true in unstable, environmentally degraded samples, and resource-limited settings.

Using the sample(s) collected from the infected host or environment, lab technicians isolate the agent. The process of isolation and typing allows scientists to determine how closely related the cases are and whether there is actually an outbreak. (Remember step 1 of epidemiological investigation—verify the existence of an outbreak!) Lab techs determine whether the isolates are unrelated, meaning the observed increase in cases is the result of multiple unrelated disease strains, or if in fact the isolates are epidemiologically related and represent a true outbreak.

After isolation, various phenotypic and genotypic laboratory approaches can be used to identify the agent responsible for an outbreak.[26] Phenotypic methods allow for identification through the analysis of the isolate's expressed characteristics, whereas genotypic methods evaluate DNA and chromosomal characteristics.

Reagent Banks

The International Reagent Resource (IRR) is an entity established by the US CDC as a centralized source of reagents, tools, and information for public health laboratories around the world studying and detecting influenza virus.[27] The IRR can support laboratories that need to build their reagent inventory for influenza specifically. During the COVID-19 pandemic, the organization expanded its scope and made reagents available to the fifty states and US territories.

Quick Reference: Sensitivity versus Specificity

Sensitivity is the ability to yield a positive result for an individual with that disease. However, it can result in false positives, that is, individuals who test positive but do not have the disease.

Specificity is the ability to yield a negative result for an individual who does not have the disease. High specificity can lead to false negatives, that is, individuals who test negative when they in fact do have the disease.

Sensitivity and specificity are inversely related. As one increases, the other decreases. Highly sensitive tests lead to positive findings for patients with a disease, whereas highly specific tests will lead to negative results for people without disease.

Phenotypic Methods

Lab technicians can identify an agent based on its cell structure, cellular metabolism, biochemical, antigenic, or susceptibility properties. Specific methods include culture growth, microscopy, mass spectrometry, spectrometry, chromatography, serological profiles, growth characteristics, susceptibilities to bacteriophage or antimicrobial agents, and other traditional biochemical techniques.[28] While several general phenotypic methods, like gram staining and culture growth, are able to detect a wide variety of pathogens, there are limitations to each test that may result in certain hard-to-detect pathogens being missed. In these cases, scientists conduct tests specific to the suspected pathogen, typically using a particular culture media or stain.[29]

Molecular and Genotypic Methods

Molecular methods analyze the chromosomal or genetic elements of the agent. Polymerase chain reaction (PCR) or RT-PCR (reverse transcription-PCR) are the most commonly used molecular methods for identifying an infectious agent. Other nucleic-acid-based identification tools include whole-genome sequencing (WGS), amplified fragment length polymorphism (AFLP), multi-locus sequence typing (MLST), pulsed-field gel electrophoresis (PFGE), and ribotyping.[300] These methods are highly sensitive and specific, and can produce rapid results. The sequencing methods used vary depending on the type of sample and experimental conditions.

Examples of Recommended Tests for Pathogen Identification

International organizations like the WHO and national-level public health agencies publish guidance for laboratories that break down specifically what types of tests laboratories can use for confirmation of various major infectious diseases.[31] For example, confirmation of Ebola virus infection is recommended through either RT-PCR assay, antibody-capture enzyme-linked immunosorbent assay (ELISA), antigen-capture detection test, serum neutralization test, electron microscopy, or virus isolation by cell culture.

MORE ON GENETICALLY SEQUENCING SAMPLES

What is genetic sequence data?

Genetic sequence data (GSD) is the genetic information that makes up the structure and functions of an organism. Genetic code, the particular sequence of DNA molecules called nucleotides, is what determines a pathogen's transmissibility, pathogenicity, and virulence, as well as its susceptibilities. By reading and analyzing these sequences, scientists gain insight into its origin, relation to other pathogens, and the properties that effect its mode of transmission and virulence.

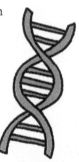

How to sequence data?

GSD is generated through sequencing technology. Nowadays it is mostly obtained through next-generation sequencing, or high-throughput sequencing, which allows for rapid, full sequencing of a pathogen's genome. As with many other laboratory procedures, genome sequencing should be carried out as close as possible to the sample collection time to reduce risk of sample degradation and to produce rapid results for informing outbreak response.

Why is it used?

Genomic sequencing is a powerful tool, increasingly used in public health to detect, investigate, and respond to infectious disease outbreaks. GSD can provide important and useful information on the infectious agent responsible for an outbreak, even if it is a previously unknown pathogen. This includes insight into a pathogen's origins, mode of transmission, and drug resistance. In addition to supporting epidemiological investigation, GSD is an effective tool for attribution and source investigation. Sequencing provides information on chains of transmission and geographic attribution. Understanding the genetic makeup of a pathogen also allows scientists to effectively design diagnostics and develop treatments and vaccines.[32]

Ongoing genome sequencing as part of disease surveillance as well as active sequencing during an outbreak helps to both monitor and predict the spread of disease and the evolution of new strains or antimicrobial resistance. Public health professionals and scientists can adjust response measures accordingly and develop additional diagnostics and treatments as necessary.

Test for Antiviral, Antibiotic, and/or Vaccine Resistance

Antimicrobial resistance (AMR) is a major global health threat—it is estimated that over 1 million people around the world die of AMR every year.[33] AMR refers to the resistance of microbial pathogens—bacterial, viral, fungal, or parasitic—against drugs used to prevent or treat them. Because of the rising threat of AMR, it is critical to conduct laboratory testing to determine if the pathogen responsible for an outbreak is susceptible or resistant to available drugs. This testing should be conducted throughout the outbreak to ensure that resistance doesn't develop over time.

Various laboratory tests are used to detect resistance or reduced suscepti-bility. They include specific functional assays (genotypic or phenotypic) and molecular techniques (sequencing and pyrosequencing).[34] These tests identify genetic changes typically associated with reduced susceptibility. Phenotypic assays are the standard, but are time consuming and depend on an ability to propagate the virus.[35] Genotypic assays, on the other hand, are easier to carry out, but are often unable to detect the mutations that lead to resistance. Genome sequencing, a process by which the DNA sequence of a pathogen is identified in a single process, can also support investigations of resistance.[36]

If AMR is detected, new drugs and vaccines may be required to effectively treat cases.

Laboratory Testing for Antimicrobial Resistance

during the 1999–2000 Shigellosis Outbreak in Sierra Leone

Shigella bacteria are highly infectious and have become increasingly resistant to common antimicrobials. In November 1999, Médecins Sans Frontières (MSF/Doctors Without Borders) personnel in Sierra Leone reported an abnormally high incidence of bloody diarrhea, a symptom of—among other things—shigellosis. An outbreak was confirmed soon after when *Shigella flexneri* were isolated from samples collected in the Western Area district, and *Shigella dysenteriae* serotype 1 (Sd1) were isolated from samples collected in Kenema district, Koinadugu district, and Moyamba district.

Laboratory testing identified the exact drugs the *Shigella flexneri* and Sd1 isolates were resistant to, and in doing so, supported decision-making for treating patients and allowed for the selection of effective medications. This effort also limited further development of AMR in Shigella strains. All isolates were found to be sensitive to ciprofloxacin and nalidixic acid.

The government of Sierra Leone requested assistance from the WHO in January 2000 to help respond to the outbreak. The WHO's Regional Office for Africa sent a two-person team and 103,000 nalidixic acid tablets to Freetown, Sierra Leone. Medical staff at a laboratory in Connaught Hospital received a two-day training in the identification of *Shigella* species and were provided with necessary equipment for testing. Staff began laboratory testing of stool samples collected in the field for drug resistance and found that seventy-two of eighty-two samples were sensitive to ciprofloxacin and nalidixic acid.

Further laboratory testing in February 2000 at the national reference laboratory in Freetown and the field laboratory of Kenema district revealed that the isolates were sensitive and resistant to multiple drugs.

There was debate among outbreak response organizations over which drug should be administered, ciprofloxacin or nalidixic acid, due to both financial and biological reasons. The WHO decided to first administer nalidixic acid, then ciprofloxacin if the nalidixic acid did not take effect. This was done for largely financial reasons; nalidixic acid was available at one-tenth the cost of ciprofloxacin. Médecins Sans Frontières chose to only use ciprofloxacin, which, compared to nalidixic acid in previous Shigellosis outbreaks, had a significantly higher compliance rate (99.7 percent vs. 50 percent) and lower case fatality ratio (CFR) (0.9 percent vs. 13 percent). There was also an argument to be made against the use of ciprofloxacin after nalidixic acid because the mutation in *Shigella* that confers resistance to nalidixic acid also confers resistance to ciprofloxacin. This could result in an expedited acquisition of resistance to ciprofloxacin in *Shigella* strains. MSF urged the WHO to reconsider its recommendation for the use of nalidixic acid in outbreaks of Shigellosis dysenteriae type 1. Because Shigellosis is a self-limiting disease, only severe cases and those who were under the age of five, over the age of fifty, or malnourished were recommended for treatment with antibiotics.

In subsequent years, resistance has developed rapidly. Many strains of *Shigella* are now resistant to the majority of drugs that were used to treat the disease. It is more critical than ever to conduct AMR analysis and continue efforts to find an effective and accessible vaccine.

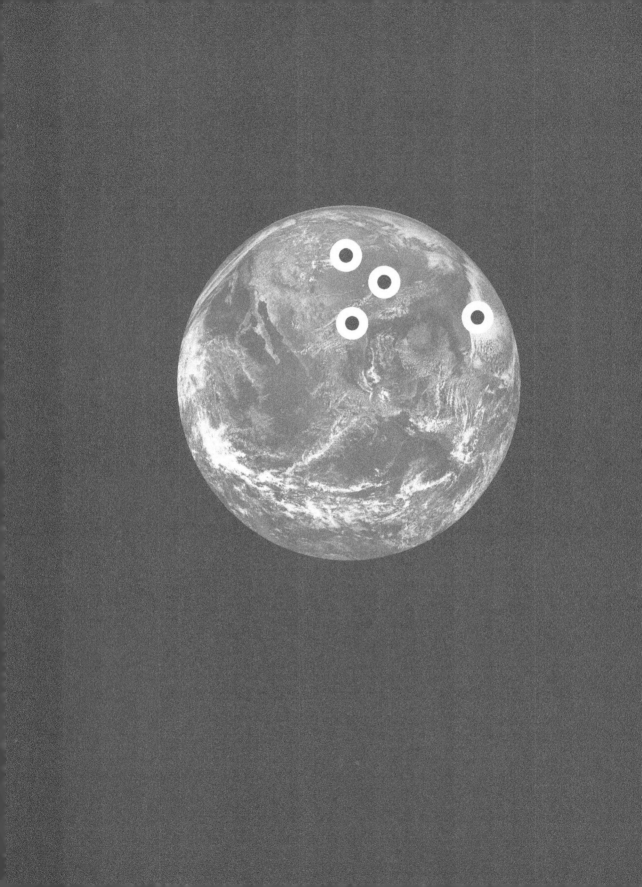

COMMUNITY ENGAGEMENT AND HUMANITARIAN RESPONSE

How Can We Help?

Outbreak response is—at its core—about protecting communities, and the communities themselves must be active participants if an outbreak response is to be successful.

There is a saying in Latin, *Nihil de nobis, sine nobis*. It means, "Nothing about us, without us." We can describe an entire book's worth of activities for successful outbreak response, but unless the community is an active partner, the response is doomed to fail. And this means real partners, real partnerships, heard voices, and real actions.

Community Engagement

Public health professionals work with community members during a variety of outbreak activities, from ongoing disease surveillance through outbreak response and recovery. Community engagement is vital for detecting and responding to outbreaks, as well as for encouraging risk reduction behaviors. By working with communities, public health professionals are able to make better informed decisions and develop response plans that are tailored to each community's unique makeup and situation. Sustained coordination and communication lead to lasting partnerships that empower and educate communities, making them better prepared for the next disease outbreak and more resilient against the effects of a public health event.

CASE STUDY

Community-Based Efforts Help Prevent Rocky Mountain Spotted Fever

The brown dog tick is a known carrier of Rocky Mountain spotted fever (RMSF), a serious and potentially deadly bacterial infection.[1] RMSF was first identified on Arizona tribal land in the early 2000s and disproportionately impacted tribal populations as compared to other demographic groups.[2] RMSF epidemics on two reservations between 2002 and 2011 resulted in an estimated $13.2 million in losses, capturing "medical cost, time off work, and loss of lifetime productivity due to premature death."[3] Between 2002 and 2014, more than three hundred cases and twenty deaths occurred. To combat the spread of RMSF, state, federal, and tribal health and animal authorities implemented local tick control plans. These community-based efforts included regularly treating areas around homes with pesticide and offering community education programs. Public health officials also found that free-roaming dogs were carrying infected ticks, so they fitted the dogs with long-lasting tick collars and "after only 4 months, 99% of dogs were tick-free in the community."[4]

The Tick Bite That Can Make You Allergic to Red Meat

Ticks can carry all sorts of diseases. One can even cause you to become allergic to red meat. The Lone Star tick, primarily found in the southeastern part of the USA, can transfer alpha-gal, a sugar molecule, into a person's blood stream triggering alpha-gal syndrome, a red meat food allergy.[5]

Community-Based Disease Surveillance

Community-based surveillance (CBS) is a key component of disease surveillance, and it hinges on community engagement. CBS is the systematic detection, monitoring, and reporting of events of public health significance within the community, by community members. Through increased public awareness of case definitions (signs and symptoms of a disease), community members can report potential cases to health workers or at a health facility. Information gathered through CBS can provide early warning of an epidemic, support active case finding and mortality counting during an outbreak, and monitor

To learn more about general disease surveillance, go to the "Surveillance" section of the Epidemiology chapter; see the Staffing and Training chapter to learn about how community members are trained.

disease control efforts post-event.[6] It can also play a pivotal role in reporting rumors and misinformation. Public health organizations work with community members to provide training in disease surveillance and reporting.

To learn more about misinformation, see the Communicating with the Public chapter.

CASE STUDY

CBS around the World

CBS programs have been piloted and implemented all over the world, especially to help identify outbreak-prone diseases early and respond quickly.

CBS can fill gaps in national surveillance systems and support both humanitarian and health-event responses, as evidenced by CBS programs in South Sudan, where community-led surveillance is a vital tool in the guinea worm eradication efforts.[7] In 2019, a CBS program in Ekondo-Titi, Cameroon, generated "9 alerts of suspected outbreak prone diseases as compared to 0 by the [traditional surveillance system in the district], with 8 investigated, 5 responses and 3 confirmed outbreaks" of measles, mpox, and tropical ulcer.[8]

International organizations have also operationalized CBS to detect priority diseases and strengthen humanitarian and health efforts. In 2014 and 2015 the Haitian Red Cross implemented CBS through volunteer SMS reporting of potential cholera cases.[9] Médecins Sans Frontières has used CBS to monitor refugee health and for early detection of outbreaks in thirteen Rohingya sub-camps of Cox's Bazar since August 2017.[10] Their indicator-based CBS program operates alongside ongoing health facility surveillance to identify potential cases of diseases like cholera, dengue, diphtheria, measles, and meningitis before they have a chance to spread through the camps. The surveillance program used formal case definitions at two health facilities and simplified case definitions for the community surveillance workers (CSW). MSF recruited and trained CSWs from the camp population and refreshed their training every six months. Trainings covered case definitions, data collection, and referral pathways. Researchers evaluating MSF's CBS program noted that 100 percent of the camp households consented to participate in CBS.

Keeping the Community Informed

Part of making a community an active partner in disease detection and response is consistent and clear communication. An informed community makes for a better partner. Communities should be engaged in an ongoing dialogue with public health professionals about risks and potential exposures that can lead to epidemics and about any ongoing public health events. This means using communication media that are widely accepted and spokespeople that are trusted. Equipped with up-to-date risk reduction measures, communities can be empowered to make decisions to protect themselves during an outbreak.[11]

Go to the Communicating with the Public chapter for more information about how public health communications are developed and distributed.

Identifying and Engaging Local Spokespersons

A valuable tool in community engagement and communication is identifying and working with local champions to raise awareness and improve public knowledge of key health messages and encourage risk prevention behaviors. Key actors and mobilizers in communities impacted by a disease are familiar with the unique situation within their community.[12] They will not be the same in every community, but could include religious leaders, local health personnel, community leaders, educators, entertainers, social media influencers, or local administrators. The position they hold in their community offers a sense of trust that external public health workers have to build over a period of time, time that may not be available during an emergency health event.

Local Advocates Help Discover Lyme Disease in Their Community

In 1975, thirty-nine children and twelve adults in the town of Lyme, Connecticut, and the surrounding areas of Old Lyme and East Haddam, began suffering from puzzling cases of arthritis, severe chronic fatigue, fevers, rashes, and headaches.[13] Two mothers from Old Lyme, unsatisfied with the diagnoses of juvenile rheumatoid arthritis, began their own investigation, taking notes on the locations of the cases (mostly near heavily wooded areas) and common exposures (tick bites), and notified the Connecticut state health department and Yale Rheumatology Clinic about the local epidemic their community was facing.[14] In 1982, after epidemiological, clinical, and laboratory investigation and surveillance, scientists finally identified the mystery bacterium behind the disease, *Borrelia burgdorferi*, and were able to develop serology tests to report cases.[15]

Enhancing Community Resilience Following an Outbreak

During the outbreak recovery process, local and national governments, international nongovernmental organizations (INGOs), nongovernmental organizations (NGOs), and communities ideally work together to apply the lessons learned from an outbreak to build back and strengthen communities. Timely, well-designed, and community-driven solutions can better enable communities to manage future outbreaks more efficiently and proactively by addressing local needs, implementing clear disease reporting mechanisms, and improving access to health services.[16] This requires supporting public health and clinical care systems, managing equitable local financial recovery, and enhancing disease surveillance for early detection of the next potential event.

Public health responders, government officials, and community members use outbreak reports, disease and population impact data, and relevant assessments (risk, health system, anthropological, etc.) to identify a community's strengths and vulnerabilities during an outbreak.[17] By integrating and analyzing information from both the public health response and community experiences, responders can develop a more holistic resiliency plan.[18]

Health and emergency response systems must work within the context of their environment to effectively respond to outbreaks. Understanding how a health system is embedded in the unique social and economic structures of a community is critical to learning from the consequences of an outbreak and building a more resilient and sustainable community.[19] This also benefits the process of constructing and sustaining community-based surveillance systems that are integral to outbreak detection and response.

A health system that is resilient and sustainable is able to absorb the shock of a disease outbreak, respond to the public health threat, and continue to provide quality essential services and routine care.[20] It is thereby able to respond more effectively to future public health crises.

High-impact disease outbreaks, though, often have economic consequences at the community level and may require financial intervention to build back.

For more information on financial recovery from disease outbreaks, go to the Money chapter.

Humanitarian Response

An epidemic can occur anywhere, regardless of a location's security and stability. During severe infectious disease outbreaks, a humanitarian response may be rolled out concurrently with public health efforts. Humanitarian response is the provision of material and logistic assistance to alleviate suffering, protect human dignity, and save lives. Public health workers might also need to coordinate with humanitarian authorities if an outbreak occurs in a humanitarian-disaster response zone.

Infectious diseases are the primary cause of deaths in areas of conflict and among internally displaced and refugee populations.[21] Thus preventing and controlling diseases with outbreak potential is an essential element of humanitarian response. Humanitarian emergencies may involve the displacement of large numbers of people, shortages of food and water, poor sanitation, reduced access to diagnosis and treatment, and security concerns. These environments are ripe for outbreak occurrence and the consequences are compounded when a public health emergency takes place in an already vulnerable area.

This section discusses humanitarian response strictly within the context of infectious disease outbreaks. This includes both outbreaks that occur within a humanitarian crisis area and outbreaks that necessitate a humanitarian response. When operating in conflict settings, or even in locations where tensions are high as a result of restrictive public health measures, it may be necessary to provide protection and security for patients, for healthcare workers, and at health facilities.

Read more about providing security in an outbreak setting in the Security chapter.

Studies and Strategies

Humanitarian response during an outbreak involves a complex map of actors and actions. In order to lead an effective response, multisectoral coordination between the different government agencies, organizations, and affected communities is essential. This requires a clear response plan and coordination strategy to mobilize additional responders, manage supply chains and communications channels, and provide aid such as healthcare, food, water, and housing. Public health and humanitarian authorities determine where to allocate resources and personnel based on a series of assessments and data collection.

For information about the Office for the Coordination of Humanitarian Affairs, see the Governance chapter.

NEEDS AND RISK ASSESSMENTS FOR HUMANITARIAN RESPONSE

A humanitarian assessment is a helpful tool to guide decision making during an emergency and in resource-limited settings. It considers the resources available, response capacity, and the needs and issues of the target audience based on data collected about the event and the geographical, cultural, and political situation. A humanitarian risk assessment considers the likelihood and anticipated scope and severity of an event that adversely impacts the health of a population. These types of assessments help officials decide which response activities should be carried out, where, and when. During outbreaks, these assessments and the integration of their results into response efforts should be ongoing rather than only conducted at the beginning of a response.

ANTHROPOLOGICAL ASSESSMENT

Anthropological engagement in epidemics is crucial to understanding how people experience illness and to help frame disease response strategies. Anthropologists can work alongside epidemiologists and public health and humanitarian responders to understand the ways unique social, cultural, ecological, economic, and political dynamics influence disease transmission, health-seeking behavior, and barriers to care. This is not necessary in a response solely coordinated by people from the community. It becomes critical, though, when external responders arrive, or if a response is centered in a population that is not well understood by others within a geographical region.

Anthropologists typically use mixed methods or qualitative approaches to collect data with and about populations experiencing a disease event. Methods involve in-depth interviews with different community members and leaders as well as with public health officials involved in a response, surveys, observation, and literature review. Through this kind of ethnographic work, anthropologists can identify leadership structures and trusted authorities to engage in community-led responses and public health message dissemination. They also explore communities' understanding of disease and health-seeking processes to help public health and humanitarian workers address areas of community uncertainty or resistance, strategize responses to misinformation, and adjust strategies to avoid clashes between infection prevention control measures and local beliefs.[22]

Anthropological methods should be carried out at the same time as public health studies so as to inform and evaluate appropriate and effective health interventions and humanitarian response efforts. The distinctive insight and methodology anthropologists bring to public health events may help responders consider epidemic control measures, like quarantine and contact tracing, and promote risk reduction behavior, from a socio-cultural and socio-political vantage point. By identifying and addressing socially and culturally driven risk factors for disease, like stigmatization, gender roles, religious customs and rites, colonial legacies, and social and economic inequalities, public health responders can design and implement more effective health programs because they will have considered cultural context and included community members in their creation.[23]

Quick Reference: Medical Anthropology

There is a subfield of anthropology that examines the complexity of health and illness and how they are experienced, shaped, and understood across different social, cultural, economic, and political environments. Medical anthropologists explore the various factors that influence the distribution of disease; the provision, exclusion, and use of health care and medical services; and the experienced and accepted sick role. They also provide critical assessments of the implementation and evaluation of health interventions.

CASE STUDY

Anthropologists in Outbreaks

Studying Kuru and Cannibalism

Kuru is a rare neurodegenerative disease belonging to a family of infectious diseases known as transmissible spongiform encephalopathies (TSEs), or prion diseases. They occur when pathogenic proteins, either inherited or obtained through ingestion or environmental exposure, trigger otherwise normal proteins to fold abnormally, leading to brain and central nervous system damage. TSEs including kuru (humans), Creutzfeldt-Jakob disease (CJD; humans), variant CJD (vCJD; humans), bovine spongiform encephalopathy (BSE, or mad cow disease; cows), chronic wasting disease (CWD; deer, elk, and moose), and scrapie (sheep and goats), can occur in humans and animals.[24] There are no known treatments or cures for TSEs.

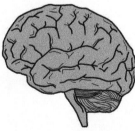

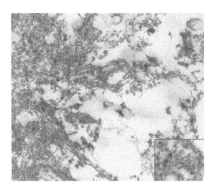

Kuru plaque

In Papua New Guinea between 1957 and 1961, roughly one thousand people died from a mysterious disease, what would later be identified as *kuru*, the Fore word for *shiver*.[25] Historian June Goodfield recounts the anthropological documentation of the "terrible affliction that was decimating the Fore. Sorcerers, they said, had cursed them with a wasting, shaking, demonic disease, which was relentlessly picking off its victims one by one. Soon the entire Fore people would be extinct."[26]

Between 1957 and 1959, 60 percent of Kuru cases were adult females, while only 2 percent were adult males, and the rest both male and female children and adolescents.[27] Anthropologists Shirley Lindenbaum and Robert Glasse and epidemiologist R. W. Hornbrook worked together to consider transumption (ritual eating of dead kin) as the route of transmission, based on the question "What is it that the adult women and the children of both sexes in the Fore tribe are doing that the men are not?"[28] The answer was found in burial preparation rites, which were led by women. The two primary hypotheses as to the route of transmission of kuru were that women would occasionally eat flesh and steamed brain tissue from the bodies, and pathogenic particles from the deceased could be transmitted via open cuts or sores.[29]

See the Epidemiology chapter for more information on epidemiological investigation.

Given the mode of transmission, prevention methods focused on changing behavioral practices among the Fore and explaining the medical etiology of the disease to local leaders. Authorities banned endocannibalism and its practice largely disappeared by the early 1960s. The incubation period of the disease can be as long as fifty years, and the last person with kuru died in 2005.[30]

> **Eating brain matter from the same species may not be the best idea.** Go to the case study on Bovine Spongiform Encephalitis, or Mad Cow Disease, to learn more.

Learn more about how humanitarian and public health data are integrated to inform holistic response and recovery programs in the Outbreak Data chapter.

Humanitarian Data Management

The data collected from humanitarian assessments and surveys capture how disease impacts and spreads through different populations. Responders then use that data to design needs- and evidence-based interventions and appropriately apportion resources. Well-structured data collection efforts can also help communities build resilience against future shocks and keep responders accountable to the populations they aim to serve.[31] As with all public health efforts, responders are expected to practice cultural competency and uphold ethical standards throughout a response, including during data collection and its use.

Humanitarian Workforce and Logistics

The variety of activities and workforces involved in a humanitarian relief response during a public health event mandates coordinated logistics to ensure target groups receive care and resources in an appropriate timeframe, to protect against redundancy, facilitate communication between responders, transport people and resources, and safeguard the health of both impacted populations and the responders serving them. In emergency public health responses it is sometimes necessary for workers from different sectors to be granted relevant credentials or to have expanded scope of practice approved in order to participate in an outbreak response and ensure an adequate public health workforce.

To learn more about the logistics behind providing health and humanitarian resources go to the Emergency Operations and Logistics chapter.

See the Staffing and Training chapter for more about the different personnel involved in response and recovery, as well as strategies for both emergency and long-term staffing plans.

Providing Humanitarian Aid

Governments, INGOs, and NGOs organize and provide various forms of aid over the course of an outbreak and during the recovery phase. Based on the needs assessment(s) conducted, they distribute food, water, and resource support, and offer health services to impacted populations. To ensure that resources are used effectively and appropriately, and are reaching those in need, health and humanitarian officials conduct ongoing monitoring and evaluation efforts. That way, they can measure the impact of the services provided and update the humanitarian response accordingly.

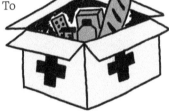

HEALTH CARE

Outbreaks increase demand for health services. Those services need to be maintained and shored up to respond to the increased disease burden while continuing to offer emergency and routine health services. This involves ensuring sufficient staffing of health practitioners, availability of resources (health facilities and other infrastructure, reliable power sources, telecommunications, water, medical equipment and supplies, and medicines), and financing for the health response (compensating staff, purchasing equipment and medical countermeasures, etc.).

To learn more about clinical care and health services operations during an outbreak, go to the Treating Patients chapter.

Particular attention should be paid to ensure access to healthcare and resources for populations that are particularly vulnerable to infectious diseases, including individuals with compromised immune systems or existing health or demographic conditions that make them more susceptible to the outbreak disease, such as pregnant women, children, the elderly, and institutionalized and displaced populations.

FOOD AID AND AGRICULTURAL SUPPORT

Outbreaks, both human and animal, can disrupt agricultural practices and food supply chains. Worker shortages resulting from infection or movement

Learn more about how government and international agencies like the World Food Programme (WFP) operate emergency food distribution and agricultural support during an outbreak in the Emergency Operations and Logistics chapter.

restrictions can lead to food being unharvested, unprocessed, and unable to be distributed; shipping restrictions and border closures limit the transport and import of food products; culling of diseased plants and animals limits the availability of certain food sources and reduces economic earnings. Malnutrition substantially lowers a person's immune system, and without access to food and a nutritional diet, people can be more susceptible to disease. Food shortages and reduced agricultural production can also drive up costs, impacting national and individual economic stability and food access by leaving lower-income countries and individuals at a disadvantage in maintaining food security.[32] To offset rising food costs, organizations may distribute food vouchers or manage points of dispensing for food kits.

> More than 113 million people around the world faced food shortages and famine, exacerbated by the COVID-19 pandemic as a result of loss of income, economic inflation, disruptions to the food supply chain, lockdowns, and travel bans.[33]

CLEAN WATER

Access to a safe and sufficient supply of water is essential not just for community consumption and use, it is critical for health and humanitarian response during an outbreak and basic public health infrastructure.[34] Clean water is necessary for hygiene, sanitation, and hydration, all critical elements of general health as well as disease management. Insufficient or contaminated water thus undermines a population's ability to resist and recover from infectious disease outbreaks and health facilities' ability to provide safe conditions to patients and staff. There are also many kinds of waterborne illnesses which can exacerbate an ongoing outbreak.

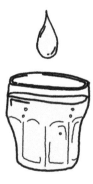

CASE STUDY

WASH Rapid Response Teams Fight Cholera in Yemen

One of the largest cholera epidemics in modern history began in October 2016 in Yemen. During the peak of the outbreak in 2017 it was estimated that cholera was "killing one person nearly every hour."[35] By the end of the outbreak in 2021, there had been more than 2.5 million cholera cases.[36]

Cholera is caused by consuming water or food contaminated with the *Vibrio cholerae* bacterium from an infected person's cholera-infested feces.[37] Without adequate water and sewage treatment systems, cholera can spread rapidly in communities. Yemen faced what was dubbed at the time the "world's worst humanitarian crisis" after two years of civil war.[38] The ongoing conflict compounded issues of food insecurity, chronic malnutrition, and extreme poverty.[39] Broader impacts of the armed conflict included severe disruption of water, health, and sanitation infrastructure and widespread displacement, with more than two million internally displaced people (IDPs) living in temporary camps.[40] Water sanitation infrastructure was destroyed by airstrikes, leaving upward of nineteen million people—two thirds of the country's population—without potable water and access to sanitation facilities.[41] Fighting in Sanaa, the capitol, and government failure to pay municipal workers resulted in the sewer system failing, contaminated waste entering the water supply, and ultimately an outbreak of cholera. Additionally, half of Yemen's health facilities

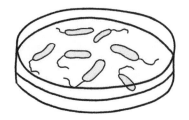

VIBRIO CHOLERAE BACTERIUM

were closed, either having been destroyed or damaged by airstrikes or shut down due to lack of personnel and funding.[42] An estimated thirty thousand critical health workers had not been paid salaries in nearly a year.[43] These factors, directly caused or exacerbated by armed conflict, led to the rapid spread of disease through the population.[44]

In 2016, the Yemeni government stopped funding the public health department. As a result, the response to the cholera outbreak was primarily led by international organizations like the WHO, United Nations Children's Fund (UNICEF), International Committee of the Red Cross (ICRC), International Rescue Committee (IRC), and other NGOs, which brought in medical and water purification supplies and worked with Yemeni health staff to manage

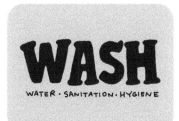

cholera treatment facilities; improve water, sanitation, and hygiene (WASH) conditions; and carry out cholera awareness campaigns for the public.

Cholera can be easily treated with basic oral rehydration. However, if left untreated it can be fatal in just a few hours. One of the most effective nonpharmaceutical interventions to prevent and control cholera outbreaks is immediate improvement of hygiene and sanitation conditions. These efforts can be led by WASH rapid response teams (RRTs), trained professionals who quickly and efficiently respond to global health emergencies by implementing disease control measures in communities.[45] After the cholera case surge in 2017 in Yemen, international organizations like UNICEF trained and dispatched local personnel, usually two-person teams (one man and one woman), as WASH RRTs under the General Authority of Rural Waters Supply Project.[46]

WASH RRTs distributed WASH kits containing soap and chlorine tablets to households and taught residents how to use the chlorine to disinfect water and instructed them in proper handwashing techniques with soap.[47] They also worked with communities to improve common-source water sanitation, through actions such as fixing broken WASH infrastructure, and at the household level, via techniques such as water storage and treatment.[48]

Within five days of a cholera case alert, but often as early as the following day after a case was identified, a WASH RRT would make a house visit to the infected or suspected individual to promote proper WASH techniques to prevent the spread of the disease to other residents in the house, neighbors, and community members.[49]

By the end of 2018, UNICEF had deployed over one thousand RRTs in Yemen spanning across twenty-one of the twenty-two cholera-affected governates.[50] The deployment of RRTs was considered to be UNICEF's most crucial control measure.[51]

HOUSING

Populations displaced by the political, economic and/or social turmoil resulting from an outbreak, as well as pre-existing displaced populations, require housing, particularly during the period of increased risk from an infectious disease outbreak. Best practice is allocating housing to these displaced populations and/or providing rental subsidies. However, when that is not possible, temporary shelters and camp settings should be designed carefully and constructed rapidly.[52] Housing, be it emergency shelter or short- or long-term housing options, should be designed intelligently, in line with infection prevention and control (IPC) measures based on the mode of transmission of the outbreak disease, and consider basic hygiene and sanitation needs. Infectious disease outbreaks are common among inhabitants of temporary shelters, particularly in camp settings.[53] Thus, appropriate management of infectious disease risk through IPC and infrastructure design that limits overcrowding and allows for isolation and/or quarantine when needed is important to mitigate further spread of the ongoing outbreak disease and prevent emergence of a new disease.

For more details about financing humanitarian response and supporting communities during an outbreak, including obtaining emergency funding, providing economic support to impacted populations, and compensating response workers, go to the Money chapter.

CASE STUDY

Repurposing Hotels for Isolation

By providing alternative housing options, organizations can provide infected individuals the ability to isolate effectively and not infect household members without fear of financial burden tied to renting a room. During the COVID-19 pandemic, city governments around the world repurposed hotel rooms to house infectious persons in isolation, as well as hospital workers, to

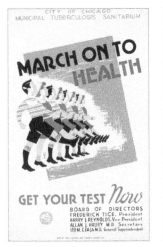

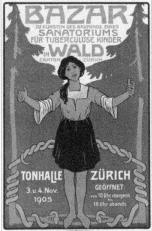

Poster for the City of Chicago Municipal Tuburculosis Sanitarium.

German poster requesting funds for a children's sanitorium.

avoid infecting their families.[54] This was not the first time infectious patients had been isolated outside of a medical center in a hotel facility. Prior to the advent of modern medicines like antibiotics, dedicated infrastructure for the long-term isolation of patients was commonplace. Tuberculosis sanitoriums were designed specifically to house TB patients, often in areas considered to be "healthy climates," like the countryside or the mountains, to prevent the spread of the highly infectious disease.[55]

Mapping Infectious Diseases in Refugee Camps

Researchers from Johns Hopkins University and the United Nations High Commissioner for Refugees (UNHCR) used data from the UNHCR Health Information System to map a total of 364 infectious disease outbreaks in 108 refugee camps between January 2009 and July 2017.[56] According to their report, 75 percent of all outbreaks were caused by just three diseases: measles, cholera, and meningitis. These three diseases are all vaccine preventable and treatable.

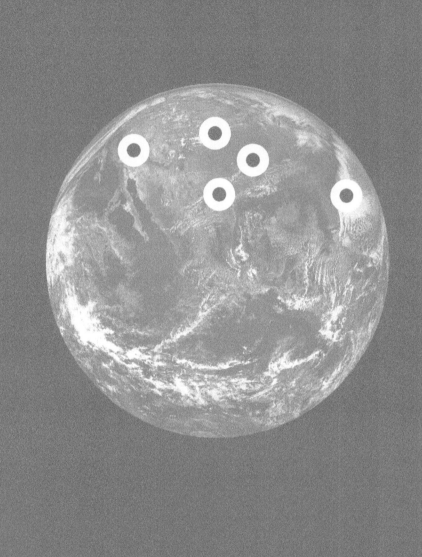

OUTBREAK DATA

Collecting, Managing, and Sharing Disease Data

Leading up to and over the course of an outbreak, an enormous amount of data is collected and analyzed. Public health personnel collect and monitor reported data fed to disease surveillance systems to catch potential outbreaks early on. Civil society actors ingest data, create models, and assess relationships to inform action. Once an outbreak is detected, officials must make prompt, strategic decisions regarding methods of outbreak data collection, management systems, and technologies, as well as determine which data are critical to collect and how best to structure the data. These data are used to track the spread of disease, assess risk, measure impacts to economic and social systems, and inform the design of outbreak preparedness plans and operational response. In this chapter we present the different types of data collected, the data management systems used, operational data sharing among responders, and ways data are shared with the public.

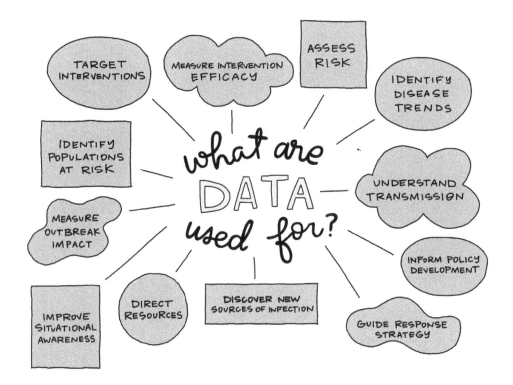

Data Collection

Disease data enable decision-makers to determine courses of action that can best prevent, contain, and mitigate outbreaks. The first step is collecting that data. Epidemiological, surveillance, laboratory, clinical, modeling, anthropological and social science, resource, financial, and security data are collected and reported by different people and sectors before, during, and after an outbreak. Health data can be reported by staff at health clinics, hospitals, laboratories, points of entry, and at the community level. These data can be reported systematically daily, weekly, or monthly into disease data management systems. Data can also be actively collected by disease investigators to answer the who, what, when, where, why, and how of a disease outbreak. The roles

Social Media, Preprints, and Outbreak Data

Increasingly, social media and preprints are being used to post and disseminate public health data used for decision making. Scientists posted long Twitter (X) threads to "publish" early findings during the COVID-19 pandemic. Other scientists utilized pre-prints to "pre-publish" time-sensitive data while still keeping publication rights to the work.

and responsibilities of personnel involved in data collection, the types of data required to be reported and collected, and standards that balance data confidentiality with transparency may be documented in ministry or department of health guidelines.

The processes of active disease data collection and reporting data to public health surveillance systems generates large amounts of information that is essential for evidence-based public health control measures. In order to pursue the best course of action, the data collected must be of sufficient quality, resolution, and timeliness to match the objectives of those who need to make decisions with it, which is why data and information are triaged during the surveillance process.[1] In sum, there can be an overwhelming amount of data. The trick is finding the right data for decision making.

Go to the "Surveillance" section in the Epidemiology chapter to learn how disease data collected during surveillance are triaged.

Electronic Data Collection and Management

To efficiently respond to an outbreak and make data-driven decisions, personnel need to have access to electronic tools for data aggregation and management. Prepackaged technologies exist to collect, store, manage, and analyze outbreak data, including on mobile devices, which can be critical when collecting information in the field.

Types of Data

Epidemiological/Case Data: Case numbers/counts (used to calculate CFR, incidence, prevalence, etc.); mortality/fatality; qualitative data on morbidity and mortality; quantitative data on disease incidence, morbidity and mortality; geographic data; case line data; contact tracing data; syndromic surveillance data (school and workplace closures)

Humanitarian Data: Food security, access to water, security environment, population locations

Laboratory Data: Results of diagnostic tests, environmental assays, presence of antimicrobial susceptibility/resistance, GSD

Observational Studies and Clinical Trials: Results of drug and vaccine trials, vaccine uptake data

Modeling Studies: Results of various outbreak models and predictive analyses

MCM Data: Access to medical countermeasures and outcomes

Non-Case Data: Resource quantities and costs (laboratory materials, PPE, MCMs, etc.), workforce, supply chain, secondary impact data

Data Management

The volume of information collected during disease surveillance and outbreak response can be considerable, making standardized and electronic management essential to ensure all data are properly captured and stored. Once collected, data are cleaned and aggregated in integrated digital data systems that pull from multiple data streams. Disease data collected from all levels and sources have to be integrated and stored properly to be useful and provide disease experts with a holistic picture of an outbreak. Integrated data can then be used to identify patterns and transmission dynamics which allow health professionals to design evidence-based disease prevention and action plans. Flexible, interoperable data platforms and adequate, well-trained staff are critical to effective outbreak management. Integrating a multitude of data streams and types from many reporting channels can be challenging and thus requires coordination and well-structured data architecture and management.

A thoughtfully designed data architecture allows datasets to be efficiently managed and analyzed to then inform an appropriate response. Throughout the data response element to an outbreak, the establishment and maintenance of security, standards, and database backups are essential. This requires protection of technology against data loss and unauthorized access, and determinations of acceptable equipment for use in the public health agency's internal network.

An additional benefit of digital data management is that it also helps facilitate downstream steps including the rapid dissemination of information across the various sectors involved in the prevention, detection, and response to outbreaks.

Sharing Data among Responders

For intelligence to be useful, it must be shared. It is not enough to simply have systems or activities that collect and store data—the individual elements that make up data collection should be capable of coordination and integration. Rapid sharing of data and information can help inform all stakeholders about new outbreak developments and speed the identification and implementation of appropriate mitigation measures.

Ensuring functionality of data sharing platforms between stakeholders involved in outbreak response is essential for proper communication and coordination. Well-integrated public health, laboratory, clinical, humanitarian, and other data helps responders proactively identify outsized impacts on certain populations. Integrated analysis of geospatial data in particular can help both epidemiologists and humanitarian responders recognize patterns and plan logistics.[2] Likewise, humanitarian and population data on needs and impacts should be integrated to increase understanding of the disease at hand and can hint at transmission modalities and the effectiveness of different risk reduction approaches.

Countries develop national protocols for handling and sharing disease data and information prior to an outbreak to provide clarity on the expected methods, frequency, and types of data and how they will be shared across sectors responsible for responding to an outbreak. All data sharing should follow the appropriate policies, laws, regulations and international agreements a country is subject to. Yet, given the various stakeholders, data may be "owned" by entities that might ask for data sharing agreements to ensure the data are only used for managing the outbreak.

Learn more about data and specimen sharing policies in the Governance chapter.

CASE STUDY

GISAID

Sharing GSD during the COVID-19 Pandemic

Scientists around the world can choose to upload genetic/genomic sequence data to one of several platforms in order to share their findings with the rest of the scientific community. Three of the main platforms are hosted by the US government, Japan, and the European Nucleotide Archive. The majority of GSD uploaded throughout the COVID-19 pandemic, however, was to a nongovernmental platform—the Global Initiative on Sharing All Influenza Data (GISAID). GISAID allowed for rapid access to data while also enforcing access agreements that include crediting the scientists and laboratories that submit the data. By the end of 2022, over fourteen million COVID-19 genome sequences had been submitted to GISAID.

Go to the Governance chapter to learn about international treaties around sharing GSD.

Publishing Data

Disease data can be published for direct use by different stakeholders, including health professionals. Outbreak data is also published and shared broadly with the general public, to keep people informed during an ongoing outbreak. This is particularly critical when public health actors require the public to take specific actions to assist in mitigating the outbreak.

PUBLISHING FINDINGS

Data should be analyzed regularly and published, either in regularly timed reports and/or in the scientific literature. Research studies evaluating behavioral, institutional, and socio-political interventions can help inform emergency and long-term policies, legislation, and preventative measures. In a fast-moving outbreak, public websites, media outlets, and even social media can be used to share outbreak data.

Go to the Communicating with the Public chapter to learn more about how public health responders communicate and share key information with a broad audience.

Over time, outbreak data will also be published in peer-reviewed manuscripts to contribute to the broader scientific understanding of the pathogen or disease process. Researchers also study data from past outbreaks to better understand how and why a disease spread within a population the way it did. They can then apply that learning to better respond to future outbreaks. Scientific journals will often try to rush the publication cycle in order to get outbreak-related manuscripts published in a timely fashion.

DATA FOR THE PUBLIC

National response plans and disease data sharing protocols will typically acknowledge how data and information will be summarized and by which channels it will be distributed to the general public. Access to sensitive data will be limited to responders to protect the identities of people involved in clinical studies, infectious persons, and confirmed or suspected cases to avoid stigma and discrimination. However, sharing key data with the public is an important part of keeping them educated, and part of the public health field's larger effort of making the public a partner in outbreak response. Disease data published for the public often focuses on key descriptive data of an outbreak—case numbers, fatality, location of cases, and risk factors for transmission—displayed in table or graph forms.[3]

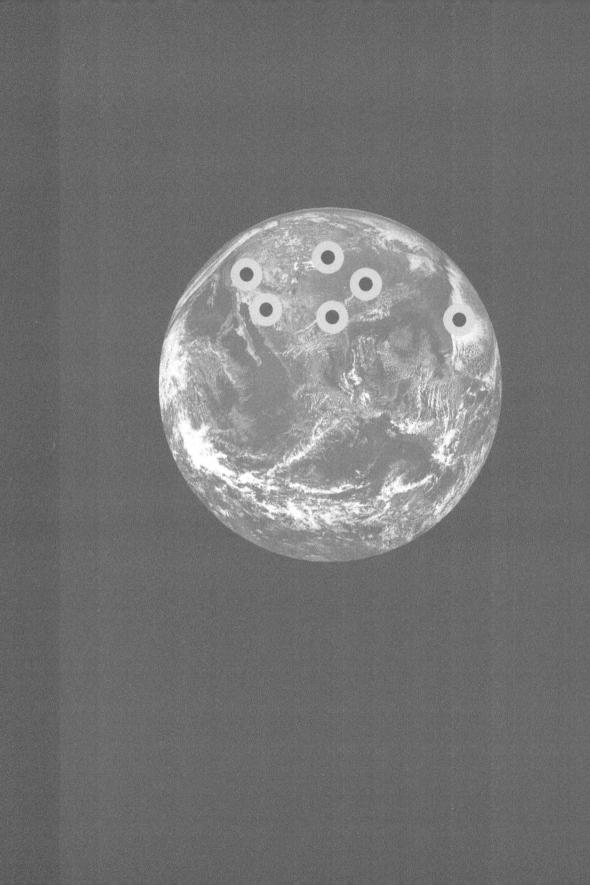

6

DECLARATIONS AND NOTIFICATIONS

Announcing Your Outbreak

If a tree falls in a forest, and no one hears it, does it make a sound?

If a dangerous pathogen spreads through a population and someone does know about it, but doesn't tell anyone, is it an outbreak? (Probably)

Is it a violation of international law? (Possibly)

Are lives at stake? (Most certainly)

Declarations and notifications of outbreaks are critical to outbreak response. Telling the world, neighboring jurisdictions, at-risk individuals, and other impacted populations about an emerging outbreak is critical to mounting an effective response and saving lives.

If you know about it, you can do something about it. If you do something about it (and act fast), you may save lives.

National-Level Notification of a Potential Public Health Emergency

All public health is local. When a clinician sees a patient with strange and severe symptoms, or a laboratory technician finds the same pathogen in a cluster of blood samples, or when suddenly half a school calls in sick, it raises alarms. Local public health officials are responsible for capturing this information and identifying unusual or unexpected disease or deaths, assessing the information, confirming events, initiating control measures, and—importantly— reporting. They have to tell someone.

Suspected outbreaks are reported to an intermediate level—for example, in the United States, this would be the state level—and then to national-level authorities. Events should also be reported back to the impacted community, so the population knows what is happening.[1] Every country has a slightly different method for national-level notification, which will follow local guidelines; national policies, strategies, and regulations; and regional and international agreements. Some situations require using a disease data system with accompanying forms and reports. It may be hard to believe, but postcards and fax machines are still used by some health departments![2] Most jurisdictions, though, have moved to digital reporting systems.

Every jurisdiction has a legal and regulatory regime for who has to report what and when, impacting clinicians, laboratories, and other health officials.[3] Some disease events only need to be reported once a year. Others need to be reported daily.

Read more about keeping the community informed in the Community Engagement and Humanitarian Response chapter, and about distributing public health messages through multiple channels and different media in the Communicating with the Public chapter.

Declare an Outbreak Nationally

Once the national government has been made aware of a possible outbreak through reporting mechanisms, it may decide the event warrants a formal proclamation that an outbreak exists. A national-level declaration is issued when an outbreak is ongoing, illnesses are severe, the number of new illnesses is increasing rapidly, or there is a security threat such as a bioterrorist attack.[4] It may be used to formally notify decision makers at the national, regional, and local level, as well as the general population, about a public health event, and is a key step in governance and operations associated with the response. The declaration often triggers a set of response actions, including establishing emergency services and staffing, ascertaining the availability of funds or economic packages, and accessing stockpiles and other resources.[5]

The tone of these declarations is important, as *how* the outbreak declaration is communicated can set a path for the early response and how information will be shared with the public. Sometimes these declarations are coupled with guidance on what individuals can do to protect their personal health and the health of those around them; any urgent, specific advice to retailers, restaurants, and other businesses; and basic epidemiological information including how many people are sick, the known signs and symptoms of the disease, and other investigation details.

Issue an Emergency Declaration

It may sound strange, but an emergency declaration is not always the same thing as declaring a national outbreak.

While some outbreaks are quickly contained, some become emergencies. Depending on the event, government authorities may issue an emergency declaration. The declaration can be made at a local, regional, or national level. These declarations are often used to mobilize resources and supplement local and regional response efforts.[6] Because these declarations carry legal, financial, political, and sociological implications, it is important to consider the following before issuing an emergency declaration:

- What are the statutory requirements for declaring an emergency at the relevant level (local, regional, national, etc.)?
- Who has the authority to make a declaration?
- What are the legal and programmatic implications of issuing an emergency declaration—what happens next? Does money flow? Do resources flow? Do restrictions get automatically put in place?
- How should the effects of emergency declarations be communicated to the relevant stakeholders and media?[7]

COVID-19 Emergency Declaration in the USA

COVID-19 was declared a Public Health Emergency of International Concern (PHEIC) on January 30, 2020, and a global pandemic on March 11, 2020. It had also been declared a public health emergency in the US on January 31, 2020.[8]

See the Governance chapter to learn more about PHEICs.

By the middle of March, there had already been in excess of 1,600 documented cases in the US, and more than forty confirmed deaths.[9] On March 14, 2020, the president of the US declared COVID-19 a national emergency. Here is the text of the factsheet released by the Federal Emergency Management Agency (FEMA). Note that the emergency declaration under the Stafford Act was tied to specific authorizations, such as sharing and reimbursing response costs.[10]

March 14, 2020. HQ-20-017-FactSheet

On March 13, 2020, the President declared the ongoing Coronavirus Disease 2019 (COVID-19) pandemic of sufficient severity and magnitude to warrant an emergency declaration for all states, tribes, territories, and the District of Columbia pursuant to section 501 (b) of the Robert T. Stafford Disaster Relief and Emergency Assistance Act, 42 U.S.C. 5121–5207 (the "Stafford Act"). State, Territorial, Tribal, local government entities, and certain private non-profit (PNP) organizations are eligible to apply for Public Assistance.

In accordance with section 502 of the Stafford Act, eligible emergency protective measures taken to respond to the COVID-19 emergency at the direction or guidance of public health officials' may be reimbursed under Category B of the agency's Public Assistance program. FEMA will not duplicate assistance provided by the Department of Health and Human Services (HHS), including the Centers for Disease Control and Prevention, or other federal agencies. This includes necessary emergency protective measures for activities taken in response to the COVID-19 incident. FEMA assistance will be provided at the 75 percent Federal cost share.

This declaration increases federal support to HHS in its role as the lead federal agency for the federal government's response to COVID-19. The emergency declaration does not impact measures authorized under other Federal statutes.

FEMA assistance will require execution of a FEMA-State/Tribal/Territory Agreement, as appropriate, and execution of an applicable emergency plan. States, Tribal and Territorial governments do not need to request separate emergency declarations to receive FEMA assistance under this nationwide declaration.

FEMA encourages officials to take appropriate actions that are necessary to protect public health and safety pursuant to public health guidance.

On April 10, 2023, the president of the US signed legislation ending the COVID-19 national emergency.

Notification of Outbreak to International Organizations

Depending on the type of outbreak and membership in international organizations, countries will notify various organizations about different events.

Animal Disease

For animal-disease events of epidemiological significance, countries report to the World Organisation for Animal Health (now going by the acronym WOAH, although it previously went by the acronym OIE, representing the name of the organization in French).[11] WOAH maintains a list of notifiable disease and requires nations to notify the organization after the first occurrence of a listed disease and/or infection, the recurrence of a listed disease after the outbreak has been declared over, the first occurrence of a new strain of pathogen in a WOAH country, or an emerging disease with significant morbidity, mortality, or zoonotic potential. The country's focal point is designated to provide the WOAH with all relevant animal health and epidemiological information.

Human Disease

All nations that are part of the World Health Organization are party to an international agreement known as the International Health Regulations (IHR). The latest revision of the IHR requires nations to report any potential public health emergency of international concern to the WHO within twenty-four hours of a national-level assessment and respond to follow up requests within seventy-two hours.[12] Each country designates a National IHR Focal Point (NFP), which is responsible for conducting the formal notifications and responding to follow up requests.[13]

For events that do not require notification under the IHR, states can still notify the WHO of a public health event through the NFP and consult with WHO on appropriate health measures.

In order to guide countries on what events they should report to WHO, the IHR provides an algorithm in Annex 2. There are some diseases that are always notifiable. For example, if there is a single case of smallpox anywhere in the world, that country must notify the WHO immediately. There are some diseases that are situationally dependent. Countries should always use the algorithm for events like cholera or Ebola to determine if they should make a notification. The algorithm asks questions about the severity of the event, whether it is unusual or unexpected, if there is a risk of international spread, and whether the event may interfere with travel and trade.

WHO Priority Diseases

The WHO has developed a list of priority diseases that pose the greatest public health risk due to their epidemic potential and/or their lack of available vaccines or treatments. As of the time of this writing, the list includes COVID-19, Crimean-Congo hemorrhagic fever, Ebola virus disease, Marburg virus disease, Lassa fever, Middle East respiratory syndrome (MERS) and Severe Acute Respiratory Syndrome (SARS), Henipavirus diseases, Rift Valley fever, Zika virus, and "Disease X." Disease X represents a disease caused by a pathogen currently unknown to cause human disease.

Continual Reassessment of Outbreak Status

Once an outbreak has been declared, it is critical to continuously assess how things are going. The WHO and its Emergency Committee will meet every three months to formally assess whether a public health emergency is still going or not. Other country level declarations have similar processes to assess if the event is ongoing, getting worse, getting better, or headed toward resolution.

Declare When the Outbreak Is Over

Declaring that an outbreak is over is a key step in communicating risk and adjusting operational procedures put in place during a response including demobilizing resources, removing public health restrictions, adjusting staffing levels, or deactivating an emergency operation center (EOC) when relevant.[14] Timing and messaging should be coordinated in all communications regarding the end of the outbreak in order to avoid misinterpretation and confusion among agencies involved in a public health response and the general public.[15] The decision to declare an outbreak over should be made using an evidence-based approach. There are several key criteria used to decide when to declare the end of an outbreak:

- The number of new reported cases drops to the number normally expected, that is, to baseline levels.[16]
- No confirmed or probable cases have been detected for a defined period of time; for example, two incubation periods for the organism have passed since the end of symptoms in the last case or since the last potential exposure to the last case occurred.[17]

Be aware of the possibility of re-emergence and continue to monitor health surveillance networks. If the number of cases increases again, the epidemiological investigation should resume or restart.

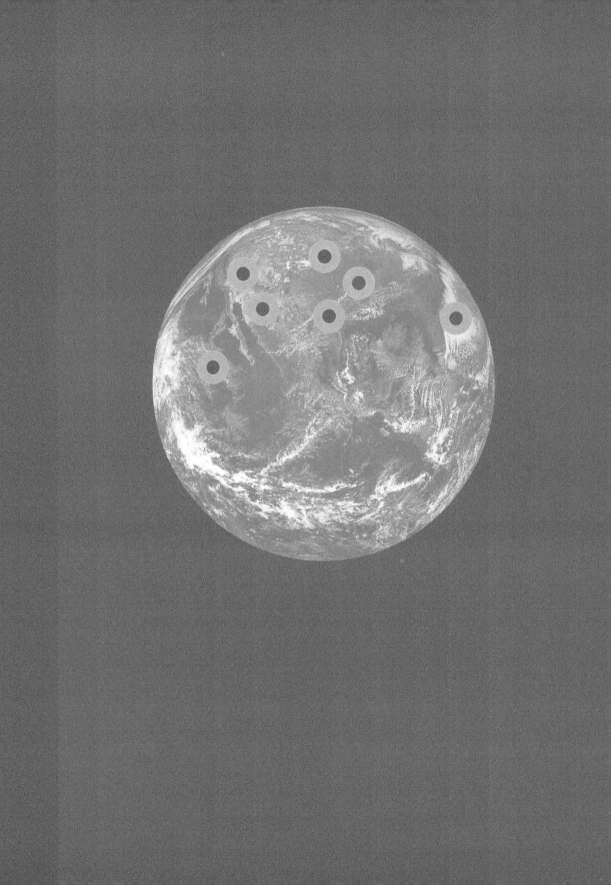

7
COMMUNICATING WITH THE PUBLIC
Spread Knowledge, Not Disease!

Clear, frequent, and honest communication can make or break a successful outbreak response. An informed and educated public is often more engaged. The public can and should be an active partner in an outbreak response, which increases the likelihood that they help detect outbreaks too. This book is part of our effort as public health professionals to reach out and improve public literacy about outbreaks by showing what goes on behind the scenes.

In this chapter we outline what goes into communicating with the public during an outbreak, from developing a communication strategy to engaging the media and community leaders and members to help spread accurate information across multiple channels.

Develop a Communication Strategy

Ideally prior to an outbreak happening, public health offices will develop a communication strategy outlining how they will share information with the media and public in the case of a disease event. With a plan in place, health personnel are able to proactively launch a communications response, sharing information about changes in the spread of disease, recommended infection prevention and control practices, drug and vaccine guidance, and identifying at-risk populations, behaviors, and activities.

A communication strategy clearly defines the roles and responsibilities of health personnel in a communications response and identifies standard operating procedures for coordinating with other important stakeholders.[1] It should also outline procedures for evaluating, revising, and updating the media strategy as an outbreak unfolds. Strategies may change depending on the extent and severity of an outbreak, or to reflect new channels of communication. A key part of a communication strategy is identifying the main information channels a community uses. It is essential that public health messages are delivered using methods and sources that are timely, wide-reaching, and trusted by the community. This can involve a mix of both direct messaging from a public health agency and approved public health messages and information delivered through and by media organizations, community leaders and groups, and individuals. When there are multiple agencies or organizations involved in an event, they must coordinate to avoid releasing contradicting information and guidance.

The dissemination of appropriate and reliable information can help counter confusion, anxiety, misinformation, and exploitation in an emergency situation.[2] By ensuring communities have access to up-to-date guidance and facts about a disease outbreak, community members are more likely to be active participants in a disease response.

Establish Resource Centers

In line with a communication strategy based on transparency, community awareness, and education, health authorities may establish a variety of resource centers where community members can receive and report information about the outbreak. This might include an outbreak-designated website or social media page, or a call center. Core tenants of these resources are that they must be accessible, easy to use, well advertised, and clearly communicate essential information. Resource centers are most effective when there are clearly established goals about their use and their target audience is defined.[3] Potential goals of resource centers include:

- providing accurate public health information and risk communication, including information about infection prevention and control;
- allowing community members to report rumored or suspected cases of a disease; and/or
- identifying trends in public requests or misinformation about an outbreak.

Part of establishing resource centers is staffing them. Public health agencies may choose to build websites designated to a particular outbreak, or instead add a new page to their primary website in the case of smaller outbreaks. Hotlines may be automated, manned, or a combination of the two.[4] Hotline and call center staffing may be employees, volunteers, or a mix. Depending on the resources available and extent of an outbreak, they can be twenty-four-hour operated, or have set hours, in which case hotlines and call centers switch from manned to automated systems outside of staffing hours.

It is important that reporting and feedback mechanisms exist between the information resources and the decision-makers and outbreak responders so that they may coordinate, evaluate, and adapt their response based on the information reported. Similarly, there should be an established routine for updating resource and hotline information when new epidemiological information is obtained, for example, when new epidemiological evidence leads public health officials to update prevention measures.

CASE STUDY

The Call Center Strategy

Identifying Gaps in Vaccination to Eradicate Polio in Chad

Geographic, environmental, and political conditions around Lake Chad posed major obstacles to polio eradication, the biggest problems being the supply and logistic challenges of supplying vaccines to island sub-districts, contacting remote villages, staffing with a limited human workforce, and running a health program where the terrorist group Boko Haram operated.[5] To address gaps in polio vaccination in the Bol district of Chad, a district task force along with the UNICEF district-based team and a WHO support team ran a series of supplemental immunization activities (SIAs) and mop-up campaigns, in line with the Global Polio Eradication Initiative's (GPEI) key strategies.[6] They implemented an experimental strategy during their April 2018 polio SIA centered on the use of call centers to boost immunization coverage in the island settlements.

Researchers studied the use of call centers to identify gaps in immunization and vaccinate missed populations in the twelve sub-districts of Bol where this strategy was used.[7] The study detailed the three phases of the campaign and the multiple rounds of polio vaccination campaigns for children aged zero though ten. The first phase of the project was the development of the "call centers for polio efforts" strategy with the task force and district management teams, and the selection of Banangore sub-district as the April 2018 pilot site for the strategy. During the second phase of the pilot, the team led a community meeting with the various stakeholders in Banangore, including the village chiefs, district and sub-district representatives, and community workers to "raise community awareness of the vaccination campaign, validate the vaccinators' progress plan and develop the telephone directory to include the village chiefs."[8] The third phase of the project was evaluating the results of the Banangore pilot and extending the call center strategy across the Bol district during the May 2018 polio SIA.

To implement the vaccination campaign across the twelve sub-districts, implementers mapped management and vaccinator teams to their responsible sub-district, established a telephone directory of village, ferry, and fishing camp chiefs, and clearly defined and validated progress plans. The health team ensured that before carrying out a vaccination activity, sub-district managers, vaccinators, and social mobilizers validated the vaccination progress plan for each health area and were updated on "the polio situation, route and dosage of the vaccine, the messages to be conveyed to parents and caregivers, [and the] number of teams per area of responsibility."[9] The day before the immunization campaign visit, the main coordinator would call the village, ferry, and camp chiefs to notify them of the visit of the vaccination team. Later, a verification call would then be made to ensure that the vaccination team had visited their designated area. At the end of the day, vaccination visit records from the vaccinators were reviewed against the results of the telephone calls with community leaders at the coordination centers. Data were used to generate lists of fully, partially, and unvaccinated villages to update the vaccination progress plans. Vaccinators would then be asked to return to any community where community leaders did not confirm visits or where children were missed as part of a "mop-up" exercise.

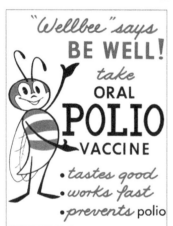

Poster from 1963.
Courtesy of CDC PHIL.

Researchers analyzed the telephone call data and calculated descriptive statistics for the rate at which villages, ferries, and fishing camps were vaccinated. Further, the research team measured the impact of the call center approach by comparing vaccination rates in the Bol district before and after the campaign to demonstrate that the call center had a significantly positive impact on immunization coverage. The number of vaccinated children more than doubled with the call center approach, by 52 percent during the first round and 50 percent during the second round.

Researchers attributed the success of the call center immunization campaign and the doubling of vaccinated children to the active involvement of community chiefs and community empowerment. Bol district has since taken on ownership of the program and extended it to all routine immunization activities.

As of 2023, there were only two countries where uninterrupted transmission of wild poliovirus remained endemic – Afghanistan and Pakistan. The Western Pacific, Eastern Mediterranean, Europe, Southeast Asia, Americas, and Africa are all certified wild polio-free, with Africa receiving the most recent certification on August 25, 2020.[10]

Create Public Health Messages

Communication with the public during an outbreak is typically centered around (1) basic information about the outbreak: type of disease (if known), how it spreads, the symptoms, basic data (cases, hospitalizations, deaths), and who is most at risk and why, and (2) what can be done to prevent exposure and stop the spread of disease.

To learn more about constructing both case definitions and simplified case definitions for community use, go to the "Epidemiological Investigation" section of the Epidemiology chapter.

Details about a pathogen and public health guidance are derived from ongoing or concluded epidemiological investigations, as well as existing knowledge and literature from previous outbreaks. Accompanying guidance encourages change or promotion of certain behaviors to limit disease transmission, raise awareness of risks, and keep populations up to date on current response activities. Public disease communication also includes sharing simplified case definitions to support community identification of cases and encourage individuals to seek testing and/or treatment.

Messages should be clear and concise, in simple language so as to engage effectively with affected populations and should be tailored to the actual level of risk rather than under- or over-reassuring the targeted audience.[11] They are developed directly by or in collaboration with trained public health professionals who represent a range of experience in field investigation, clinical treatment, and infectious disease research. Public health professionals observe the unique characteristics of each outbreak and make real-time decisions about the recommended guidance based on their experience with past outbreaks. As an outbreak unfolds, especially in cases where it is caused by a new or unknown pathogen, new information is discovered and guidance may change, requiring the release of updated messages. This does not mean the previous guidance was made to intentionally mislead the public, it means new information was discovered that changes the way we can prevent transmission and the consequences of disease.

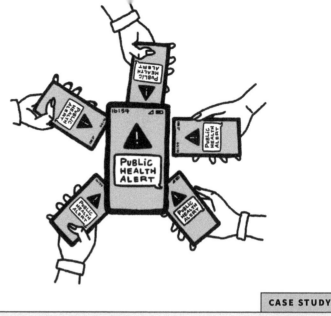

Mass-Texts for Public Information

In 2022, in the Republic of the Marshall Islands (RMI) there was one mobile operator, the National Telecom Authority (NTA). As a result, anyone on the island with a phone had a SIM card from the NTA and could receive mass-text public announcements from the provider in English and Marshallese, including job opportunities, daily weather forecasts, and health notices. The RMI Ministry of Health and Human Services (MHHS) worked with the NTA to send out mass texts as part of the NTA Health Public Announcement system to keep the public informed about ongoing public health concerns and shared prevention measures and simplified case definitions for when someone should seek medical attention. During the summer and autumn of 2022, in response to RSV outbreaks, RMI citizens received daily texts about how to limit the spread of the illness. RSV, respiratory syncytial virus, is a common respiratory virus that causes cold-like symptoms but can lead to serious illness and hospitalization in infants and people with weakened immune systems. The RMI MHHS sent out texts advising "avoiding close contact with sick people, cover your coughs and sneezes, clean and disinfect surfaces, and stay home when sick," because the primary transmission method for RSV is via droplets. The mass texts also provided guidance for monitoring disease in children and advising adults about when to seek medical attention.

2001 Anthrax Attacks

Communication amid Dynamic Uncertainty and Fear

Bacillus anthracis is a spore-forming bacterium that can cause anthrax. In September and October 2001, letters containing anthrax spores were sent to five major news media offices in New York City, New York State, and Boca Raton,

Florida, and to two US senators in Washington DC. At least twenty-two people developed anthrax infections, eleven of whom developed serious inhalational anthrax. Five people died.

The US CDC coordinated the outbreak response, identifying multiple epicenters: Florida, New York, New Jersey, Washington, DC (Capitol Hill and the regional area including Maryland and Virginia), and Connecticut. Investigators recovered four envelopes containing powdered anthrax spores and traced their path through the mail, linking them to nineteen of the cases. The source of infection for three of the victims was never identified. This was the first instance in the US of multiple simultaneous outbreaks caused by intentional release of an infectious agent, and the standard systems for communication between the US CDC and clinicians were poorly suited for adapting and responding to a complex, rapidly changing situation. Anthrax infection is rare in the US, and many clinicians were unfamiliar with diagnosing and treating it. Physicians struggled to reach local and federal public health officials due to phone lines overwhelmed by individuals concerned about their exposure risk (remember this is before social media and mass messaging). All sightings of white powder in mailrooms turned into massive responses from fire, police, and emergency medical services.

Without clear public health communication from the US CDC and due to the evolving nature of the situation, health providers and the public relied heavily on media reports for information, which fostered more confusion.[12] Uncertainty was driven by ambiguous definitions of who was at risk and a lack of details about how anthrax spread. Many Americans were concerned that anthrax was contagious (it is not). Identification of the population at risk was complicated by the number of outbreak epicenters, involvement of stakeholders at different levels, the unclear actor(s) behind the attacks, and the generally unfamiliar nature of the threat. Individuals most likely to have been exposed, including postal workers and Senate staffers, were frustrated about the quality and timeliness of information provided.[13] All of the unknowns about the anthrax outbreaks were compounded by the fear of terrorism in America post 9/11.

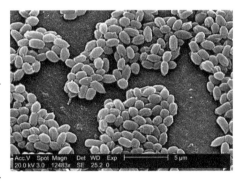

Bacillus anthracis spores. Photo credit: Janice Haney Carr

The complex nature of the crisis and ineffective communication from public health officials resulted in delays in administering the known and effective prevention and treatment for anthrax infection: a prophylactic course of antibiotics. This in itself was complicated by the heightened fear, mistrust, and frustration with the federal government's response by public health professionals, clinical providers, and the public, and concerns with individuals hoarding antibiotics.[14]

Distribute Public Health Messages through Multiple Channels and Different Media

Accurate information must be provided early and often to keep the public informed during a public health emergency. However, simply releasing information does not automatically result in engagement and uptake of public health measures. To this end, public health messages must be distributed regularly, across multiple channels, in accessible formats, with the support and engagement of a diverse network of stakeholders.

Identifying which channels will be effective, appropriate, and trusted requires contextual awareness about the target audience and a holistic understanding of each channel's unique advantages and disadvantages. Depending on the message and type of information conveyed, public health communication may be written, visual, audio, or a mix. Using a variety of media to convey a message can catch different peoples' attention. Around the world there is a wide range of media formats and outlets through which to spread disease knowledge. This includes news releases and briefings, radio or television programs, websites, public address systems and service announcements, designated websites or web pages, printed or digital materials (fact sheets, flyers, brochures, circulars, etc.), telephone hotlines and toll-free numbers, telephone communication campaigns and mobile phone text messaging, and social media.[15] By repeating public health messages across various channels, in the languages spoken by the population, there is a greater likelihood for the information and guidance to be comprehended and heeded.[16] Many people are familiar with hand-washing hygiene posters that appear in the bathrooms of public spaces from hospitals to restaurants. Public-service announcements via television or radio are also common forms of disseminating important public health information.

Coordinating effectively with mass media is an important part of ensuring accurate dissemination of health information as they play a key role in shaping the narrative during a public health crisis. There are different branches of media that public health experts can work with: news, advertising, entertainment, and social media platforms. Public health and medical experts work with journalists to best translate complex epidemiological concepts into accessible, comprehensible, and tangible health news guidance.[17] Social media can be another channel through which to promote disease prevention practices and provide situational updates on an outbreak. Social and traditional media can also bring attention to and pressure leaders, politicians, and government officials to take specific actions on health challenges.[18]

Nurses Challenge Vaccine Misinformation in their Communities

The largest measles outbreak in the US in over a quarter of a century happened in 2019.[19] One of the most severe outbreaks was centered in Orthodox Jewish communities in New York and New Jersey, driven by a rise in vaccine hesitancy.

Misinformation about vaccines causing autism and sudden infant death syndrome (SIDS) and incorrect information about vaccine ingredients were distributed to the Orthodox Jewish community in *The Vaccine Safety Handbook* by the anonymous antivaccination group PEACH (Parents Educating and Advocating for Children's Health) and its community hotline, and further circulated in text chat groups. In response, the community stopped vaccinating their children.

Blima Marcus, a local nurse and member of the Orthodox community in Brooklyn, began spending time researching scientific studies in order to answer questions and refute false claims via text.

Marcus and fellow nurses organized the Vaccine Taskforce of Orthodox Jewish Nurses to challenge the false information targeted at Orthodox Jewish families and address the unique concerns of patients and families in their community. They organized small group sessions for Orthodox women during which they would discredit common anti-vax misconceptions and claims from the PEACH handbook by using scientific literature and research studies "translated" into more approachable terms for their audience. The nurses dissected the false information in the antivaccination handbook to best understand the beliefs circulating, and created their own handbook, dubbed Parents Informed and Educated (PIE), with a rotting peach on the cover in an effort to poke fun at the claims they hoped to refute.[20] Another nursing group organized a confidential hotline where community members could ask questions about measles and the vaccine and request discrete at-home vaccination.[21]

According to Marcus, her communication methods worked because "I wasn't calling them fools. I didn't insinuate that anyone was unintelligent. I didn't accuse anyone of being selfish, and, honestly, I don't think they are. I think they're victims of a lot of scare tactics."[22]

The nurses emphasized the importance of action based on protecting the community by sharing statistics about immune-compromised children unable to be vaccinated, addressing concerns rather than dismissing them, and understanding that parents largely try to do what is best for their children and misinformation plays on their fears. At the same time, the local governments and authorities instituted vaccination audits and mandates, closed child-care centers and schools that were in violation of a city order, and issued $1000 fines. The nurses approach— led by people trusted in the community—helped to spread scientifically correct information. Together, these efforts halted the outbreak.

Monitor and Minimize Rumors and Misinformation

Both the accessibility and the volume of news create challenges in accurately informing the public during health crises. But misinformation has always plagued public health response. It is dangerous and can further the spread of disease, increasing the risk of infection, death, economic loss, and other long-term consequences.

It is thus essential to utilize expert and trusted voices and effective online tools to help curb the spread of misinformation.[23] To counter misinformation, public health professionals may collaborate with celebrities, community leaders, and other nontraditional messengers, as well as target messaging from both official and unofficial sources.

By tracking rumors that are circulating, public health responders can proactively address them. They can identify public posts on social media platforms, reports from clinical care and community health workers and volunteers, and notices from community members when there are misinformation-reporting mechanisms.

CASE STUDY

Zika, 2015 and 2016

Rumors, Conspiracies, and Misinformation

Studies have demonstrated that during threatening situations a common coping response from the public is increased information sharing and seeking.[24] Propagating conspiracy theories about the threat of infectious disease outbreaks arises from a "need for sense making."[25] The 2015 to 2016 Zika epidemic was no different. Public health responders studying the outbreak found that conspiracy theories and pseudoscientific claims were able to spread rapidly over social media platforms.[26] While the majority of Zika cases were so mild that someone may not have known they were infected, the more serious conditions tied to the 2015–2016 outbreak understandably incited fear. The virus led some infected mothers to give birth to babies with a rare birth defect—microcephaly, where babies are born with underdeveloped brains and abnormally small heads. Additionally, there was evidence that infection with Zika triggered cases of Guillain-Barre syndrome in some individuals, which can lead to paralysis.

False and unsupported information shared on social media touted the "true" origin or agent behind the outbreak and cures for disease. The most common theories claimed that it wasn't Zika at all that was causing birth defects, instead claiming it was driven by pesticides or genetically modified mosquitoes. Other conspiracies cited the nefarious goals of international companies and organizations to use Zika as a bioweapon for population reduction.[27] Researchers studying rumor and conspiracy propagation on social media during the Zika outbreak found that rumors were shared three times more often than verified stories.[28] Misinformation posts often contained words like "hoax" and "false flag," invoked "authorities" to back their unsubstantiated claims, or were phrased as clearly leading and/or rhetorical questions.[29] These are recognized characteristics of conspiracy theory patterns, framed as "just asking questions" and using "leading questions to undermine rival explanations without opening oneself up to criticism by providing an alternative."[30]

> ### The Disinformation Dozen
> Researchers studying misinformation on social media about COVID-19 found that 65 percent of the anti-vaccine content could be traced back to twelve people.[35] Their misleading claims and lies promoted anti-vaccine rhetoric and false claims about the efficacy of public health measures like physical distancing.

Researchers found that conspiracy theories and misperceptions about the Zika virus and outbreak were widely believed in Brazil and beyond.[31] A University of Pennsylvania survey found that 35 percent of Americans believed that genetically modified mosquitoes were responsible for the spread of Zika.[32] Another study found that almost one in five Americans believed in at least one Zika-related conspiracy theory.[33]

Misinformation about the disease continued to spread despite efforts by governments and public health organizations to correct it. In fact, government actions, like health officials in several areas of Brazil banning a pesticide used for mosquito control, fed a conspiracy that it was tied to the microcephaly cases despite no supporting evidence. By acting on fear-based rumors, officials only fueled conspiracies that a pesticide, not Zika, was responsible for the rash of microcephaly cases.[34]

Your Role

Lastly, there is your role. Even though this chapter is about how public health workers communicate to the public (you), it should not be a one-way relationship. It is your responsibility to be informed, to protect yourself and those around you. So, when you follow an ongoing outbreak, try to be engaged using these techniques:

- **Questioning.** Questioning is the root of science. Don't rely on just one source; try to get information from multiple channels.
- **Fact-check.** Assess the sources you are getting your information from. A WhatsApp group, your uncle's Facebook page, or your roommate's social media thread may not be the best sources for information, unless one of them happens to be an expert in the pathogen causing the outbreak.
- **Spread accurate information.** Before sharing information, consider where that information came from. Is the source trustworthy? Did you investigate that fact? Sharing misinformation is dangerous and can harm people.
- **Things change.** Remember that in an outbreak, particularly one with a new pathogen, knowledge and understanding of how to stop the spread of disease will evolve over time; the pathogen itself may also evolve.

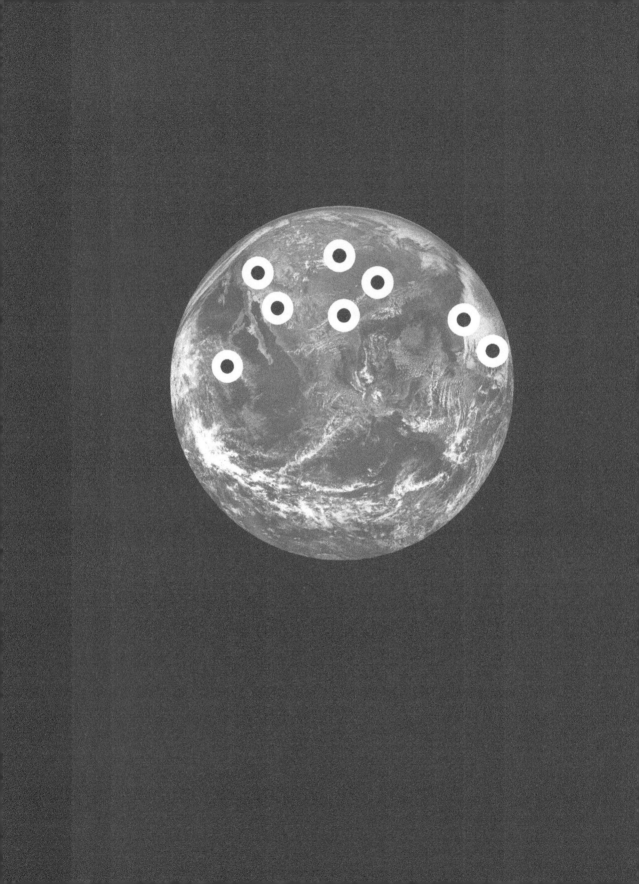

STAFFING AND TRAINING

Meet the People behind Outbreak Response

Outbreak prevention, detection, response, and recovery is possible because of the incredible people involved. A large number of people from a vast array of fields are involved in the range of activities associated with detecting and responding to outbreaks—from community volunteers and local health workers to epidemiologists, clinicians, and logistics experts from international organizations. These individuals come from epidemiology, environmental, public health, animal health, entomology, virology, security, laboratories, communication, and government sectors. In large outbreaks, the response may involve every sector of society. Almost every outbreak, though, requires individuals to participate in the response who normally have other responsibilities. Facilities and teams need to be staffed, and those staff need to be trained. In this chapter we provide only a snapshot of the massive workforce required for an outbreak response and the training they go through to prepare for outbreaks.

Staffing

The response efforts and facilities involved in preparing for and managing outbreaks require sufficient and competent staff. Human resource requirements for outbreaks should be clearly defined in preparedness plans, identifying the personnel required, specifying their responsibilities, and mapping operational hierarchies and reporting structures. Specific guidance should be provided for staffing operational facilities key to outbreak response, such as clinics, hospitals, community health centers, isolation and quarantine facilities, laboratories, and emergency operation centers, to ensure they can effectively serve their purpose. Organizers should also consider the human resource demands

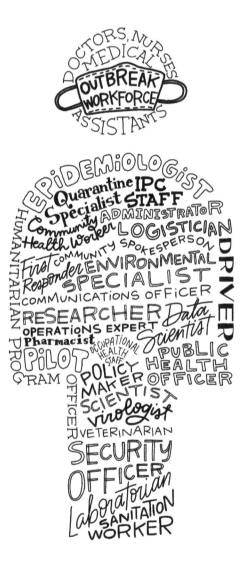

involved not just in response efforts, but also required to maintain essential services. Clearly, different outbreaks require different types of experts, so there needs to be a decent amount of flexibility built into all plans. For example, some outbreaks may require deep expertise from veterinarians, while others may need ventilation experts or contact tracers. Key considerations for outbreak staffing include[1]

- identifying networks of professionals who can be mobilized if and when a need arises;
- providing incentives and other means of support for staff;
- ensuring sufficient PPE and access to occupational health services should staff experience work-place exposure and/or become ill; and
- offering ongoing education for professionals to ensure they are up to date on current best practices.[2]

Planning for Staff Shortages

Mobilizing and retaining a health workforce during something as emotionally and physically exhausting as outbreak response poses many challenges.

Illness, burnout, inadequate compensation, and overwhelming workload can lead to staffing shortages. Outbreak response cannot happen without a workforce.

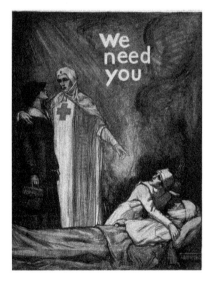

Because of this, outbreak plans should outline contingency plans for potential staffing shortages. This can include cross-training, expanding scope of practice, and mobilizing staff from other specializations with training in health and infection control and/or emergency response. Recruiting and training volunteers can also help. Establishing mutual aid agreements and requesting staff support from relief agencies and organizations are other methods to manage potential staff shortages. Officials also need to consider which roles will need to be backfilled. Surge response during a public health emergency often pulls people from their normal jobs to take on special roles during the outbreak. Officials will need to identify existing or new personnel who can temporarily fill those original roles until emergency responders can return at the end of an outbreak.

American Red Cross Poster, 1912. Courtesy of the NLM.

Grant Relevant Credentials to Responders

Rapidly securing appropriate credentials and legal documents for trained personnel involved in a public health response is essential.[3] An expedited legal credentialing process can include obtaining visas and establishing valid legal status for responders who are traveling across international borders or credentialing responders traveling across jurisdictions within a country.[4] Granting credentials can also include expanding the scope of practice for relevant personnel in response to a public health event.

Relaxing or waiving regulations can help offset workforce deficits during a public health response and address increases in disease burden in hospitals and clinics. The process of granting credentials often includes:

- registering the basic and credential information of each worker;
- granting emergency credentials based on the responder's certifications and education;
- re-verification by periodically verifying responder information; and
- assigning emergency identification badges in accordance with credential levels.[5]

Expanding Credentials in an Emergency

In late 2020 and early 2021, as COVID-19 vaccines were becoming available, decision makers and planners tried to think about how best to rapidly vaccinate as many people as possible in as many locations as possible. One way to do this would be to expand the number of people permitted to distribute a vaccine beyond physicians, nurses, and pharmacists. This included allowing emergency first responders and dentists to deliver vaccines.[6] Many jurisdictions also allowed final-year medical students or retired physicians to support vaccination efforts. Most thought this decision made a lot of sense. Dentists, for example, receive ample training and experience in giving injections, and were keen to help.

Long-Term Staffing Plan

In addition to planning for immediate staff demands during a typical emergency response, it is just as important to plan for long-term staffing needs and resource allocation. In long-lasting outbreaks or global health crises, organizers need to consider the possibility that human resource demands change as response efforts shift to long-term response and operations. Many of the strategies used for adapting to staff shortages can be used to ensure sufficient staff capacity and needs for a long-term response. These include additional workforce recruitment and training, long-term staff compensation, reserving resources, or adjusting geographic staff distribution.[7] To support calculations for the number of health care workers necessary as part of a longer-term staffing plan, the WHO publishes an Excel-driven tool, the Health Workforce Estimator (HWFE).[8]

Training

Due to all the different activities involved in outbreak detection and response, from disease surveillance and epidemiological investigation to clinical treatment, laboratory analysis, and security, there is a massive human workforce. These people all need to be trained. Depending on the topic and skill level required, this could be an hour-long online workshop or an eight-year professional degree program. National and local governments and INGOS and NGOs run in-person and virtual training programs around the world for the different areas of expertise required during a public health event.

Training for Proper PPE Donning and Doffing
in Preparation for West Africa Ebola Response

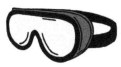

As Ebola spread throughout West Africa in 2014, clinicians from around the world were getting ready to deploy and help their colleagues in Liberia, Guinea, and Sierra Leone. Treating Ebola patients, though, is complicated and requires wearing extensive PPE. Médecins Sans Frontières set up a two-day course in Brussels for healthcare workers heading to West Africa to treat Ebola patients. After attending the training, US CDC officials then set up a US-based version of the course, conducted in Alabama. The training course taught healthcare workers how to stay safe while treating patients. This included covering how to put on and take off (donning and doffing) PPE, best practices for disinfection, how to deal with medical waste, and personal safety. In all, approximately 570 people attended the course in Alabama supported by the US CDC.[9]

Expanding Contact-Tracing Workforces during COVID-19

Contact tracing was a central part of many countries' early response strategies to the COVID-19 pandemic. Many nations in South Asia and sub-Saharan Africa had strong networks of community health workers and experience tracing polio, HIV, or tuberculosis (TB), and were able to rapidly mobilize their preexisting and trained workforces. However, other countries struggled to implement contact-tracing programs at the scale required.[10]

Several countries, including Israel, Sri Lanka, Australia, the Philippines, Ukraine, and Spain, used military, defense, and police forces to support contact-tracing efforts. Other countries bolstered public health contact-tracing teams with cadres of volunteers. Around the world, from Nepal to Germany, college students, teachers, librarians, gardeners, traffic wardens, and community clubs worked as contact tracers in their communities.

Field Epidemiology Training Program in Action

2012 MERS-CoV in Jordan

Field epidemiology training programs (FETP), along with field epidemiology laboratory training programs and field epidemiology training programs for veterinarians, support national and subnational workforce development to lead public health surveillance and outbreak detection, response, and containment.[11] Public health professionals learn in both the classroom and the field to apply epidemiological concepts and skills.

Originally modeled after the US CDC's Epidemic Intelligence Service (EIS) program, individual countries manage their own FETPs so trainings can be tailored to meet country needs, and now more than eighty-seven such programs train public health workforces across more than 165 countries and territories.[12]

In 2012, the Jordan Field Epidemiology Training Program (J-FETP) played a key role in investigating the origin of the MERS-CoV outbreak in Jordan. Middle East respiratory syndrome coronavirus (MERS-CoV) is a coronavirus that affects the respiratory system. This zoonotic virus was first isolated and identified in Saudi Arabia in September 2012.[13] Earlier that year, in April 2012, a cluster of cases of severe respiratory disease of unknown origin occurred in an intensive care unit (ICU) in a hospital in Jordan.[14] At the time of the outbreak, public health authorities were unable to identify the illness and classified it as suspected pneumonia.

The discovery of MERS-CoV months later, in September 2012, prompted a retrospective analysis of stored samples from the April outbreak in Jordan. The J-FETP, involved in the initial April outbreak, conducted the retrospective serologic and epidemiologic studies.[15] The samples were tested and came back as positive for MERS-CoV.

In collaboration with the Jordan Ministry of Health, the Eastern Mediterranean Public Health Network (EMPHNET), and the US CDC, J-FETP worked on retrospectively investigating the April 2012 outbreak to determine whether the surviving cases had MERS-CoV antibodies and to identify unsuspected cases.

As part of the larger Jordan MERS-CoV team, the J-FETP team conducted interviews and collected serological samples from the surviving case-patients, household contacts, hospital staff, and Ministry of Health field workers. During this retrospective investigation, they obtained 124 samples and interviews. Their investigation identified seven previously unconfirmed cases of MERS-CoV from the April 2012 outbreak.[16]

Training Rapid Response Teams

In 2018, the WHO, along with support staff from the US CDC, Brazil MOH, and Portugal MOH, hosted forty-two Angolan response personnel in a week-long training session in Luanda to support Angola's strategic priority to enhance its capacity for Ebola response.[17] Training included lectures and exercises covering disease surveillance, risk assessment, infection prevention and control, contact tracing, risk communication, and safe burial.[18]

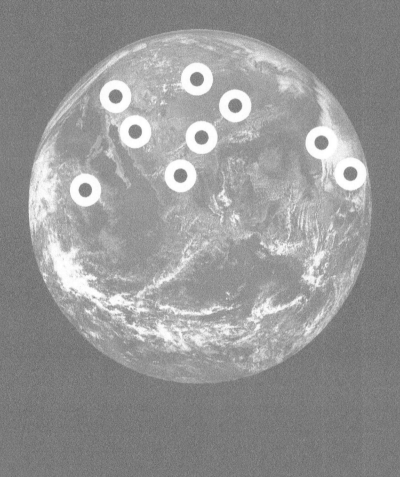

DISEASE PREVENTION AND MITIGATION

Stop the Spread

There are a number of public health tools and strategies available to public health responders to prevent an outbreak from occurring, and if it does, to mitigate the spread of disease. Prevention and control measures target the different ways susceptible and infectious people interact. The point is to either prevent people who are susceptible from becoming infectious, or infectious people from then infecting those who are susceptible. The susceptible population can be reduced through public health measures like vaccination, and reducing the interactions between infectious and susceptible populations (physical distancing) can slow an epidemic.

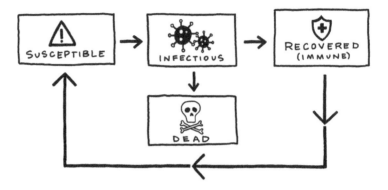

Nonpharmaceutical Interventions (NPIs)

Nonpharmaceutical interventions (NPIs) are often the first step in controlling an outbreak. Proper hygiene, use of PPE, and physical distancing (isolation, quarantine, temporary closures, etc.) can help limit the spread of disease early on in an outbreak, protecting both members of the community and the health workers caring for sick patients.

The Anti-Handshake Society

On the podcast *No Such Thing as a Fish*, guest Ella Al-Shamahi's fact was that an anti-handshake society was formed in Baku, Azerbaijan, in response to fears of a cholera outbreak in 1894.[1] Society membership was six roubles and members wore pins to identify themselves. If a member made the mistake of shaking hands, they were fined three roubles.[2]

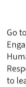

Go to the Community Engagement and Humanitarian Response chapter to learn more about humanitarian efforts during an outbreak.

Water, Sanitation, and Hygiene (WASH)

Good hygiene can be a simple but powerful tool in preventing and stemming many kinds of outbreaks. Water, sanitation, and hygiene (WASH) facilities are essential to the provision of safe health care. This includes potable water, sanitation, health care–waste management, and hygiene and environmental-cleaning infrastructure and services.[3] WASH strategies are critical to mitigating the spread of an outbreak as well as preventing the emergence of other kinds of infectious disease, including those with pandemic potential. Hygiene promotion is a good disease mitigation practice at all times to improve overall population health. WASH principles and distribution of essential hygiene items are often invoked for the kinds of infectious disease outbreaks that occur as the result of natural disasters and other humanitarian crises, particularly diarrheal diseases. Health and humanitarian officials can aid response by promoting good, evidenced-based hygiene practices and ensuring that access to the resources needed for that hygiene are available to everyone. Hygiene-promotion specifics vary depending on the pathogen and the impacted population, but core hygiene principles apply across pathogens, such as proper handwashing techniques (soap and clean water) and decontamination of water through use of chlorine tablets or filtering.

WASH services are also important in health facilities, allowing health workers to maintain proper infection prevention and control (IPC) measures and to model safe WASH practices to their patients and communities. Outside of health facilities, water sanitation infrastructure is crucial in making sure households have access to potable water for drinking and cleaning, and are not at risk of exposure to sewage and possible disease.

Read about what can happen when water treatment systems fail in the "WASH Rapid Response Teams Fight Cholera in Yemen" case study.

Personal Protective Equipment (PPE)

PPE such as gloves, masks, gowns, goggles, and biohazard suits serve two purposes: 1. Protecting yourself from a pathogen 2. Preventing the spread of a disease if you are infected.

An adequate supply and correct use of PPE is particularly important to protect health care workers and other individuals likely to be exposed to a pathogen.[4] For health care workers, this is crucial to ensuring that they can safely continue to deliver clinical care to the infected. Clinical and public health professionals should be trained on the appropriate use of PPE, including the specific donning and doffing processes needed.

See the Staffing and Training chapter for a case study on donning and doffing PPE.

CASE STUDY

PPE during the 2014–2016 West Africa Ebola Outbreak

Health care workers were subjected to a risk of contracting Ebola virus disease (EVD) twenty-one to thirty-two times higher than that of the general population during the 2014 through 2016 West Africa EVD outbreak.[5] Every health care worker was vital to the containment effort; there were fewer than 0.1 physicians for every ten thousand people in Guinea, Sierra Leone, and Liberia. In the absence of a vaccine, the correct use of PPE proved to be critical in limiting the transmission of EVD from patients to health care workers.[6] However, unclear protocols, improper donning and doffing, and limited supply of PPE compromised the effectiveness of the PPE in protecting health care workers from contracting EVD.

Because EVD is transmitted when infected bodily fluids come into contact with the mucous membranes or broken skin of an uninfected person, the PPE required for the EVD outbreak focused on barrier protection.[7] This involved a scrub suit, rubber boots and boot covers, disposable gloves, a disposable gown or coverall, a face mask, a face shield or goggles, a head and neck covering or hood, and a disposable waterproof apron.[8] The pieces of this set of PPE are meant to overlap

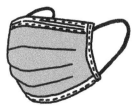

Read more about training EVD responders in correct donning and doffing in the "Training for Proper PPE Donning and Doffing in Preparation for West Africa Ebola Response" case study.

and not leave any skin exposed in order to protect the individual from highly infectious bodily fluids.[9]

PPE is effective in protecting health care workers when used properly. However, improper donning greatly increases the likelihood of EVD patients' bodily fluids coming into contact with health care workers' skin and mucous membranes, and incorrect doffing exposes health care workers directly to the infectious fluids on the surface of used PPE.

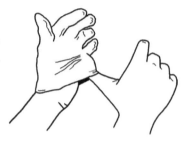

Even the most cautious health care workers can make mistakes in doffing due to complicated protocols, exhaustion, and insufficient oversight.[10] Protocols implemented by Médecins Sans Frontières stressed that during doffing, an observer should audibly walk the health care worker through each step of PPE removal, regardless of how many times the health care worker has been through the process, and alert them if they were contaminating themselves or breaking procedure. Furthermore, donning and doffing areas were to be physically separated to prevent exposure of infectious fluids to health care workers whose PPE was not fully secured.[11]

Equipment shortages posed a significant problem. Complete PPE kits were scarce or inaccessible in many areas of West Africa. In Sergeant Kollie Town, Liberia, for example, hospitals faced severe shortages of protective equipment as basic as rubber gloves. With health care workers unprotected and rapidly contracting EVD, many hospitals were forced to shut down. Not only did this leave EVD patients without care, but it also left patients with other illnesses such as dysentery, typhoid, and malaria deprived of medical attention.

Physical Distancing

In some outbreak settings, physical distancing measures are a valuable public health tool to reduce disease transmission and prevent associated illness and death. Physical distancing reduces the frequency of contact between people, thereby minimizing the risk for transmission. Typically, physical distancing measures are useful when disease transmission occurs from person to person, including transmission by people who are asymptomatic, meaning they do

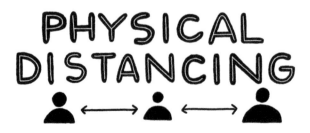

not appear visibly unwell. These measures can be particularly helpful where there is no population immunity, and a vaccine or treatment does not exist.[12]

Physical distancing policies can range from individual physical distancing (e.g., isolation or quarantine of infectious cases, stay-at-home recommendations for cases and/or contacts) to large-scale community physical distancing (e.g., closure of educational institutions, workplace closures, measures for special populations, mass gathering cancellations).[13]

Ultimately, because disease transmission is not homogeneous, physical distancing measures must be implemented and calibrated to the disease and community context.[14] Health officials conduct risk assessments to determine which physical distancing measures should be instated to limit disease spread. Officials must clearly communicate the policy for physical distancing measures to have a socially accepted and positive effect on the community.[15]

See the Risk chapter to learn about risk assessments.

Quarantine across History

Quarantine has been around for hundreds of years. Merchant cities across Europe implemented various forms of quarantine to stop the spread of the Black Death, the bubonic plague that killed one-third of Europe's population.[16]

In 1377, the Republic of Ragusa, what is now the city of Dubrovnik in Croatia, enacted the first quarantine legislation.[17] Visitors were required to spend thirty days on Lokrum, an island off the coast of the city. Violation of quarantine could result in having your nose or ears cut off, or torture.[18] Throughout the late fourteenth century, city-states like Venice, Genoa, and Marseilles also implemented similar laws, requiring ships to anchor outside the city for a period of forty days, a *quarantino*, the origin of the term quarantine. In the fifteenth and sixteenth centuries, these port cities began building *lazarettos*, dedicated quarantine buildings to house arrivals before they were allowed to enter cities.[19]

CASE STUDY

Quarantine during MERS Outbreak in South Korea

In May 2015, South Korea declared its first case of MERS-CoV (also known as MERS or Middle East respiratory syndrome coronavirus), a respiratory disease caused by a coronavirus in the same family as SARS and COVID-19, with a case fatality rate (CFR) of approximately 35 percent.[20] The index case was a man who had recently returned from a business trip to four countries in the Middle East, including Saudi Arabia where MERS is endemic. Upon his return to South Korea he sought care at two hospitals, the first from May 15 to 17, the second between May 22 and 28. The patient did not clearly articulate his symptoms nor his travel history, which limited the ability of medical professionals to correctly diagnose him and he was not isolated from other hospital patients until May 30.[21] The rather significant gap between his arrival in the

> ### Quick Reference: Isolation versus Quarantine
> **Isolation** is for people who are already sick. **Quarantine** is for people are not sick, but may have been exposed, to monitor whether they develop the disease.

country and his diagnosis facilitated the spread of MERS among those that had interacted with him during the patient process, and the disease spread quickly throughout hospitals around Seoul.[22]

In order to curb further spread of the disease, the South Korea government issued cohort quarantines starting on June 1 for individuals that may have been exposed in the same setting or at similar times in the same hospitalization area as patient zero. Cohort quarantines are when groups of people are quarantined because of their confirmed or potential exposure to a positive case. The large-scale quarantine was facilitated by the fact that many of the individuals in the quarantine cohort were already confined to the hospital. The quarantine cohort included patients who waited or were treated in the same room as patient zero. Clinicians who were exposed to the infected patient were placed in home-based quarantine with restricted interaction with family members until the incubation period for the disease had passed. Unexposed clinicians equipped with appropriate PPE were kept within the hospital to help treat and care for those that were under quarantine. Between the individuals under hospital quarantine and those subjected to home-based quarantine, approximately 6,700 people made up the quarantine cohorts during the height of the outbreak.[23]

The quarantine proved to be effective at limiting the spread of MERS in South Korea. The government enforced the quarantines with the support of police to make sure that people were abiding by the quarantine set in place. Officials would call people under home-based quarantine twice a day. If there was no answer, the police would be sent to the home to investigate. Anyone found to be breaking the quarantine or lying about their potential contact with infected patients was penalized, facing up to two years in prison or a fine of approximately US$18,000.[24] A more passive way that the government tracked quarantine compliance was through the monitoring of cell phones to identify if someone had left the location of where they were supposed to be staying.[25] There was one notable violation of the quarantine, which was a man who had left the country after being in contact with someone who was found positive with MERS. The man went to China, where he was later diagnosed as positive with MERS, creating an opportunity for international spread of the disease.

The quarantine in Korea lasted for roughly two months. When it was lifted the government announced the outbreak was over. By the time the outbreak came to an end, there had been overall 186 laboratory-confirmed cases and 38 deaths.[26]

Medical Countermeasures (MCMs)

Medical countermeasures (MCMs) typically include vaccines, antiviral drugs, antibiotics, and other medicines used to prevent or treat the health effects of a pathogen. MCMs are developed through extensive research in public and private laboratories and undergo highly regulated trials. Once an MCM is in use, officials and scientists continue to monitor its effectiveness and long-term safety. Monitoring processes help track how MCMs protect different demographic groups, defend against possible new strains or variants of disease, and help identify their potential use for other diseases. Public health officials and regulatory agencies typically establish a system that allows the public and medical providers to report any adverse health consequences.[27] It is critical to track any adverse health events to ensure that the benefits MCMs provide continue to outweigh any health costs.

MCMs need to be used appropriately; inappropriate use can not only be ineffective, it can directly contribute to the development of antimicrobial resistance.

Drug-Resistant Tuberculosis

Tuberculosis (TB) remains one of the world's leading infectious disease killers, particularly in low- and middle-income countries. It is estimated that nearly a quarter of the global population is infected with TB, and 5 percent of those cases are drug-resistant (DR).[28] Incidence of DR-TB, cases that are resistant to one or more first-line TB medications, is rising around the world. Deaths from DR-TB account for close to one-third of all antimicrobial resistance (AMR)-related deaths.[29] Multidrug-resistant tuberculosis (MDR-TB) is resistant to rifampicin (RMP) and isoniazid (INH), the two key first-line TB medications. DR and MDR-TB cases are significantly more costly and logistically complicated to treat as there are fewer medication options. The options that remain are longer, more toxic, and more expensive treatment regimes.[30] Yet another form of antimicrobial resistance has also developed in some TB cases, referred to extensively drug-resistant TB (XDR-TB), where MDR-TB cases are also resistant to second line drugs, including injectables and fluoroquinolone. Compared to 85 percent treatment success for standard cases of TB, MDR-TB treatment success can range from 48 percent to 64 percent, and 20 to 40 percent for XDR-TB.[31]

Vaccines

Vaccines are one of humankind's greatest scientific achievements. They can prevent outbreaks from happening entirely, and if an outbreak occurs, their timely and thorough distribution can slow transmission and minimize the severity of disease. For example, ring vaccination is a strategy where health officials vaccinate close contacts of confirmed cases. It was a key measure used during

The first vaccine was invented for smallpox in 1796. See "Smallpox and the Origins of Vaccination" on page 51 to learn more.

Go to the Community Engagement and Humanitarian Response chapter to learn more about the importance of mobilizing local public health advocates.

See the Governance chapter to learn about vaccination policies, including prioritizing distribution and issuing vaccine mandates.

See the Security chapter to learn how health and security personnel work together to protect PODs.

the elimination of smallpox, as well as during more recent outbreaks, like EVD and mpox.

Typically, vaccines are produced in lots; manufacturers are required to test each lot to ensure all vaccines are safe, pure, and potent.[32] Health officials continuously monitor various vaccine-related data to inform public health program planning, delivery, and performance.[33] Real-time data on their availability, effectiveness, and use can help ensure safe and equitable vaccine distribution and promote vaccine uptake. Transparent information about vaccine side effects and their benefits, along with concerted public health campaigns, can encourage vaccine confidence and increase vaccination rates, avoiding resurgence of vaccine-preventable diseases.[34]

There are a number of strategies used for immunization campaigns, from behavior and education efforts to distribution and logistics approaches. Vaccine confidence, when people trust that vaccines are safe and effective, is essential for uptake and community cooperation for both preventing an outbreak from happening and slowing it should one occur. Identifying trusted members of the community to help share information about vaccines and combat misinformation, offering financial incentives, getting recommendations by health

Points of Dispensing (PODS)

Points of dispensing, often called PODS, are locations from which vaccines and other MCMs can be rapidly distributed or administered to a target population. In organizing an effective delivery of MCMS, health officials consider both the number and location of POD sites.

Officials consider population density, infrastructure availability, use and need estimates, and broader community context to determine the number of PODs needed.[35] When selecting POD sites, emergency response organizers consider the following information:

- **General site information**: size, environment free of hazards, proximity to medical facilities, accessibility (major roads, public transportation), handicap accessibility, garbage and waste disposal options
- **Site exterior conditions**: number of entrances and exits, parking considerations, loading docks, sufficient lighting, capacity to hold a large number of people under cover out of poor weather conditions
- **Site interior conditions**: sufficient lighting, adequate number of restrooms and water dispensers, outlets, secure storage area, separate rooms for health assessments, large waiting assembly areas
- **Equipment availability**: refrigeration to hold MCMs, generators, material handling equipment, adequate number of chairs and tables
- **Security status**: minimize harm to POD staff, materials and attendees

Many potential sites that may meet this criterion include public schools, universities, arenas, military bases, community recreation centers, and polling places.[36]

providers, and hosting immunization events at schools, workplaces, and other easily accessible locations are all methods used to prevent and mitigate outbreaks. In some situations, there may be standing policies or emergency declarations requiring vaccination to attend school, work in a certain job, or travel.

Infection Prevention and Control (IPC)

Infection prevention and control (IPC) is a scientific, evidence-based approach to protecting patients and health workers from avoidable infections.[37] IPC standards are established at national, subnational, and facility levels and can be general or disease specific. IPC guidelines include standard precautions, transmission-based precautions, and clinical device management and aseptic techniques, such as hand hygiene, injection safety, PPE use, disinfection protocols, and waste management, to reduce the risk of antimicrobial resistance (AMR) and health care–associated infections (HAI).[38] IPC programming is present in health care settings, including clinics, ambulances, and community health programs. Many IPC measures assist in preventing the spread of both endemic and emergent infectious diseases. Agencies update IPC guidelines to ensure that they remain relevant, such as during the management of a novel infectious disease or after scientific understanding of an existing pathogen changes.[39]

Health officials carry out site visits and IPC assessments at health facilities to ensure they are practicing safe clinical management, adhering to standard IPC precautions, and capable of rapidly identifying highly infectious patients and initiating the appropriate isolation and testing.[40]

In 2015, amid the Ebola outbreak in Liberia, IPC training efforts consisted of a ring approach, an intensive, short-term strategy where teams are rapidly mobilized to support implementation of IPC measures specifically in health care facilities and communities with active transmission.[41] Employees at sites with increased risk of exposure to an Ebola patient received focused IPC training on rapid triage, isolation, and referral. An appropriately targeted ring IPC approach might be an effective strategy to focus IPC support in response to clusters of disease.

A ring approach is also a vaccination strategy! Go to the "Vaccine" subsection of this chapter to learn more.

Sanitation and Decontamination

Sanitation and decontamination are important elements of infection prevention and control. When done effectively, they can help limit pathogen transmission by reducing the burden of a pathogen in an environment. Decontamination refers to physical and chemical processes that kill or remove infectious microorganisms from premises and surfaces.[42]

Not all sanitation methods work against all pathogens. For example, additional sanitization of water sources and restroom facilities is needed during a cholera outbreak, whereas a mosquito-borne-disease response would focus on

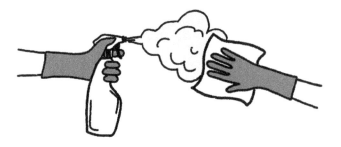

vector control. Choosing the right disinfectant and cleaning method is crucial for actually getting rid of the infectious agent. In general, there are five groups of disinfectants: soaps and detergents, oxidizing agents, alkalis, acids, and aldehydes. In addition to disinfection, pasteurization and the use of ultraviolet light are other techniques for eliminating bacteria and viruses. Responders identify which disinfectants and processes to use based on the properties of the pathogen in question, such as the cellular structure. When a novel pathogen emerges, responders follow best general practices for decontamination while researchers work to identify the infectious agent and which disinfectants and cleaning measures it is susceptible to.

General IPC measures for sanitation and decontamination combined with proper disposal of waste are carried out as routine practices outside of an outbreak to prevent one from happening, particularly in areas with high levels of risk for the spread of disease, like health care, animal, and food preparation facilities, as well as dense public areas and public transportation vehicles. During an outbreak, a variety of structures and areas may require enhanced decontamination, including surfaces in busy workspaces, transportation vehicles (ambulances, buses, trains, planes, ferries, etc.), and any other areas or items that could have been exposed to the pathogen. Some buildings, like health care facilities, are at increased risk given the higher number of sick individuals present. Similarly, areas with heavy traffic and dense interaction, like public transportation, require frequent cleaning given the high chance for disease transmission when so many people can be exposed to an infectious person or surface. During an outbreak, shops, schools, and office places may implement enhanced sanitization practices to help prevent the spread of disease within their communities. Cleaning and disinfection of equipment, materials, and premises used for animals and food processing can also help prevent or mitigate the spread of disease between animals and to humans, as well as contamination of animal and other food products, helping to stabilize and protect animal agriculture, the food supply, the economy, public health, and the environment.[43]

Materials used for cleaning need to be sanitized or disposed of safely to prevent spread of the pathogen they came into contact with. In some cases, equipment or supplies may be unable to be cleaned or disinfected, in which case they need to be disposed of appropriately.

CASE STUDY

Sanitation and Decontamination to Stop Norovirus Outbreak

Norovirus, or the "vomiting bug," is the most common cause of gastroenteritis, causing diarrhea, vomiting, and severe stomach pain.[44] It is highly infectious, able to spread from person to person directly or via contaminated surfaces, food, or water.

Proper hand sanitation and decontamination are the most effective ways to stop its spread. A chlorine bleach solution is an effective cleaning tool to disinfect surfaces.[45]

Between April and June 2022, more than two hundred rafters and backpackers in the Grand Canyon were infected with norovirus.[46] Rafting outfitters saw the disease spread quickly within groups where people were in close quarters, practiced limited hand hygiene, used communal toilets, and ingested contaminated water while going through rapids.[47] The US CDC and National Park Service advised proper handwashing with soap and water, improved symptom screening before backcountry trips, isolation of ill passengers, and regular disinfection of water spigots.

Safe Treatment, Management, and Disposal of Waste

The amount of medical and laboratory waste increases during an outbreak, and can sometimes even be a source of infection. Health care–related waste must be properly managed, transported, and disposed of to prevent unintended health and environmental consequences.[48] Potentially hazardous waste can take many forms, including infected blood; human or animal tissue, cultures, or specimens; liquid wastes; sharps; and other materials contaminated by blood, body fluids, and other infectious waste.[49]

Health care personnel practice safe waste management through appropriate waste storage, decontamination, and disposal, following regulations that protect the safety of both health personnel and the environment. Medical and laboratory waste is typically most dangerous at the point of time it is generated. Therefore, risk is generally greater for health care personnel and people involved in the collection, transport, and disposal of medical waste rather than the general public. Waste should be carefully contained as close to the point of generation (think a sharps box for disposing a needle used for a blood draw) as possible before being treated to make it safer for further handling and disposal. Waste treatment can involve different approaches, such as sterilization by heat, chemical disinfection, or disinfection by steam, followed by waste disposal via inactivation or incineration. The materials and equipment required for personnel to safely and effectively carry out their responsibilities depend on the management and disposal strategies implemented, and the selected treatment strategy depends on the infectious agent, local capacity (resource availability, technical expertise, disposal site size, etc.), and regulations. Major barriers to effective waste treatment, management, and safe disposal include inadequate infrastructure (e.g., no running water), insufficient resources (e.g., lack of PPE or safe storage containers), inadequate training, and poor regulation and enforcement of safe practices.[50]

ANIMAL CARCASSES, LITTER, AND ANIMAL PRODUCTS

A zoonotic outbreak may result in hazardous waste, including infected carcasses, litter and other byproducts. These can be potentially infectious environmental hazards that can create further opportunity for transmitting infectious pathogens, either as fomites, as carrion, or as a substrate for insect vectors. The World Organisation for Animal Health (WOAH) and the United Nations Food and Agriculture Organization (FAO) provide guidance on proper disposal of carcasses, animal products (feathers, hair, etc.) and animal litter (bedding, excrement, feed, etc.) to protect against specific zoonotic diseases, like foot-and-mouth or avian influenza.[51]

Managing the Deceased

Outbreaks that result in human deaths require thoughtful consideration of the logistical, health, and cultural elements of moving human remains and carrying out burial practices. It is a critical duty of health personnel to ensure safe, respectful, and dignified burials for individuals who have died during outbreaks. Proper burial practices, particularly for those infected with diseases like Ebola, Marburg fever, and Lassa fever that remain contagious after death, can help stop the spread of infectious disease postmortem from the deceased and among persons in contact with the body, like family and health workers.[52] Postmortem infection typically occurs when family members, friends, or community members of the infected deceased perform cultural or religious ceremonies that involve touching a body that still contains high levels of viral loads.[53] Infectious diseases that can spread post mortem also require special attention by those performing autopsies.

Tasks for the management of human bodies typically involve:

- **Body retrieval and storage**: Bodies should be stored in climate-controlled environments, such as cold storage, and placed in body bags to allow time for autopsy or identification.
- **Identification**: Identity is confirmed by visual recognition and additional information.

- **Transport**: Staff in appropriate PPE transport the body/bodies using an approved transportation route.
- **Operational communication**: Clear communication among levels of government, between emergency response officials, and with the media is vital.
- **Communication and support for families**: Respect for the bereaved must be ensured.
- **Burial**: Remains should be released to relatives of the deceased for safe and dignified burial when possible.[54]

Consider Issuing Burial or Cremation Restrictions

During outbreaks where postmortem infection or spread of disease among mourners is highly likely, governments may choose to issue restrictions for infection control, such as limiting the size of funeral gatherings, mandating the use of PPE for all individuals (health workers, bereaved, etc.) involved in the funeral processes, and completing burial or cremation quickly after death as part of infection prevention.[55]

The intention of any restrictions should be to stop transmission; protect those involved with the handling of human remains, including health care workers, funeral workers, and any other individuals, family, friends, or professionals, involved in the burial or cremation of a deceased patient; and not place an unreasonable burden on the affected communities and families.

Safe and Dignified Burials

The passing and burial of a loved one is a sensitive issue that must be handled in a psychologically safe and respectful manner. As such, conducting safe burial practices relies not only on clear infection control protocols, but also on respect, communication, and collaboration.

Once health officials are notified of a death tied to a specific infectious disease, whether in a hospital or home, they deploy a trained burial team to initiate the established processes for conducting safe and dignified burials.[56]

BURIAL OPERATIONS

Health personnel tasked with handling the deceased follow standard operating procedures (SOPs) developed by national health agencies and international health organizations that clearly outline tasks—from the notification of a reported death to conclusion of a burial and return to the public health office.[57] This includes team composition, the list of required equipment, transport and burial etiquette, and protocols for disinfection of reusable equipment and disposal of contaminated supplies. SOPs for burials will be disease-specific, as the appropriate behavior to prevent and limit spread of a disease from the dead body and/or between individuals involved in the burial will be dependent on the mode of transmission. SOPs also will often be context-specific to reflect the

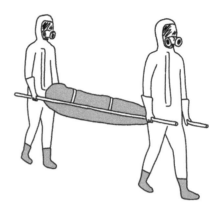

cultural and religious practices of the affected community and other factors unique to the outbreak.[58] With diseases where postmortem transmission is a concern, as well as with highly infectious diseases where transmission among the living at a gathering is possible, burial teams will supply the family with PPE and enforce relevant public health guidance, such as limiting gathering sizes and encouraging hand hygiene, while respecting time for prayers and other traditions.

IDENTIFY POTENTIAL BURIAL SITES

When an outbreak has high morbidity, health officials may need to identify burial sites to accommodate the increased number of deceased persons. Burial sites are chosen based on soil conditions, available area, site-use agreements with the communities, and distance from water sources.[59] When choosing a location, cultural factors should be considered, such as whether the remains must be buried facing a certain direction or if there is a preference for burying bodies individually.

PROTECTING AND EQUIPPING BURIAL TEAMS

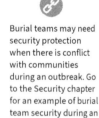

Burial teams may need security protection when there is conflict with communities during an outbreak. Go to the Security chapter for an example of burial team security during an Ebola outbreak.

Not all infectious disease outbreaks require an extensive infection control burial response with a lengthy list of equipment. However, while handling the remains of individuals who have died from highly infectious diseases like hemorrhagic fevers, burial teams are equipped with specific supplies to protect themselves.

PPE: Masks, gloves, protective gowns, fluid repellent trousers, and proper footwear. In some cases, burial teams may also need to bring extra PPE to supply to the friends and family of the deceased.

Body bags: Puncture and leak-resistant bags that can fully contain any bloodborne pathogens

Hand hygiene materials: Alcohol-based hand rubs or clean running water with soap

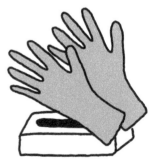

Disinfectants: Disinfectant for the body and the deceased's belongings

Swabs: Test swabs to collect samples from the deceased to test for the cause of death

Waste management materials: Two infectious waste bags—one for belongings or materials that need to be disinfected, and one for belongings or materials that should be disposed of

Vehicles: Ideally, the burial teams should have two vehicles—one that provides transportation for the burial team and the other for the deceased's body

Radio equipment and telecommunications equipment: Means of communicating with their base office and with security personnel[60]

COORDINATING AND COMMUNICATING WITH THE COMMUNITY

As an outbreak unfolds and fatalities grow, ongoing communication with the community must be a priority. Health workers should clearly and frequently communicate with leaders and members of the community to help stop the spread of misinformation, provide information about how bodies are being managed, explain the need for adapted burial practices to reduce potential infection, and alleviate fears. Involving community leaders and family members in the decision-making around body preparation and burial practices can help build trust.[61] Burial and cremation processes can be sensitive for families, and if not handled with respect, can result in resistance or even conflict against health workers.

For more information, see the Communicating with the Public chapter.

Food Safety

Food and water safety involve critical everyday functions to ensure that people are not harmed by the food and water they consume. Foodborne illness is a growing public health problem; there are more than 550 million annual cases of diarrheal disease annually worldwide.[62] *Salmonella*, *campylobacter*, and *E. coli* are examples of pathogens that regularly impact food safety. Thus, controlling hazards, pests, and other agents likely to contaminate food and water sources is an essential part of outbreak prevention.

To prevent outbreaks, food producers and the entire chain of services that process, prepare, and deliver food from farms and factories to consumers must adhere to a variety of national and subnational food safety regulations; if the food is shipped across international borders, additional principles often apply.

Food and waterborne outbreaks can occur if an animal has a zoonotic disease, food (animal or plant) products are contaminated during production, processing or delivery; an infectious agent enters the water supply; or environmental contamination is caused by sewage leaks. To manage a food or waterborne outbreak, health authorities identify the source of the outbreak and contain it to limit further spread. This could be done through decontamination or removal of a food product from the market. Foodborne outbreaks can be caught through routine surveillance or direct reports from members of the food industry or general public.[63] Once a foodborne outbreak is detected, national food safety emergency response plans outline the steps for investigation, risk assessment, mitigation, collaboration with partners in the food industry, and ongoing communication with the general public about exposure risks and prevention efforts.

Food Safety in Germany during *Escherichia coli* Outbreak

In early May 2011, a highly virulent strain of *E. coli* in Germany triggered the deadliest *E. coli* infection outbreak to date.[64] Infection spread rapidly around the country with more than one hundred cases of gastroenteritis reported each day during the first two weeks of the outbreak.[65] The O104:H4 strain produces a toxin that targets internal organs, leading to bloody diarrhea and potentially hemolytic-uremic syndrome (HUS), a complication that can cause kidney failure and red blood cell destruction.[66]

The outbreak continued to spread as German officials tried to identify the source of the outbreak, complicated by the lengthy ten-day incubation period of the bacteria.[67] On May 26, 2011, German authorities announced that researchers had located *E. coli* bacteria in four cucumbers imported from Spain and declared them as the source of the outbreak, despite other epidemiological evidence suggesting tomatoes and lettuce.[68] In response, grocery stores began removing Spain-imported cucumbers from their shelves and Spanish farms suffered severe economic hardship, losing around seven to eight million euros per day.[69]

German public health officials later retracted their statement claiming Spanish cucumbers caused the outbreak when additional testing revealed a lack of evidence. Through epidemiological investigation, the Robert Koch Institute revealed that people who ate bean sprouts were nine times more likely to be infected with *E. coli* than people who had not, confirming that sprouts were the source of the outbreak.[70] This claim was backed by the German Federal Institute for Risk Assessment under the Federal Ministry of Food, Agriculture and Consumer Protection.[71] The contaminated sprouts originated from a farm in Northern

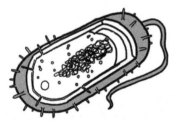

ESCHERICHIA COLI (E. COLI)

Germany that had used sprout seeds imported from Egypt.[72] Officials shut down the farm and lifted the warnings against cucumbers, tomatoes, and lettuce.[73]

Germany declared the outbreak over on July 26.[74] Even with the outbreak over, the government faced widespread criticism for their slow identification of the source and the incorrect claim that Spanish cucumbers were the cause of the outbreak. The European Commission estimated that Spain lost upward of 350 million euros in the first two weeks of the outbreak as a result of that claim.[75] Additionally, German officials were criticized for not testing sprouts initially as they are a common food associated with foodborne illnesses.[76] Cases were also found in several other European countries throughout the outbreak period due to travel to and from Germany.[77] In total, the outbreak caused over 3,100 confirmed cases and 53 deaths.[78]

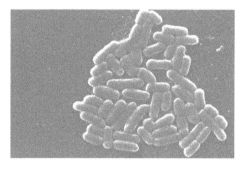

Escherichia coli bacteria. Photo Credit: Janice Haney Carr; CDC PHIL

The severity of the outbreak led to improved surveillance measures to prevent another *E. coli* outbreak, including carrying out increased research on foodborne threats and preparedness activities.[79]

Modify Food Production or Preparation Processes

An outbreak may necessitate that food producers and handlers modify their production and transport processes to protect public health. If an outbreak is caused by contamination during some stage of production, processing, and distribution, health officials work with food producers to identify the source and implement immediate control efforts. Contamination can happen anywhere along the chain from producers and commercial processors to food preparers and consumers. Touchpoints include food production, processing, transportation, handling, and preparation; processes at any point in this chain may need to be modified to prevent further contamination or the survival and spread of pathogens already present in food products.[80] Such modification is key in preventing an infectious contaminant from entering the human population and in controlling a foodborne disease outbreak that has already started.

The exact measures taken will depend on the offending pathogen, but general control measures include initiating or refreshing training on general practices of safe food handling; emphasizing proper hygiene and sanitation practices, such as hand washing and cleaning and sanitizing of surfaces and equipment used for food processing, transporting, and preparation; informing the public how to modify its food handling and preparation, such as by cooking food to a certain temperature; and follow-up by health officials to ensure that modified processes have been implemented and are effective.[81]

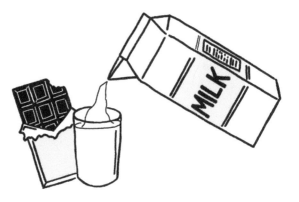

Tracing a Listeria Outbreak to Chocolate Milk in Ontario, Canada

Listeriosis is a bacterial infection primarily transmitted through the ingestion of contaminated foods. Between November 2015 and June 2016, thirty-four Ontario residents, most of whom frequented the same grocery store chain, contracted listeriosis. Of these patients, 94 percent (thirty-two) were hospitalized, and 12 percent (four) died.

To trace the outbreak, Public Health Ontario collaborated with local, provincial, and federal public health and food safety partners.[82] Public health professionals completed a national listeriosis questionnaire, conducted case interviews, reviewed purchase records from cases' shopper loyalty card programs, and collected food samples. One of the working hypotheses was that the outbreak was connected to an ongoing listeriosis outbreak tied to leafy greens in the United States and to a food manufacturer of coleslaw that supplied several of the venues at which six case-patients had eaten. After further laboratory analysis of food samples using pulsed-field gel electrophoresis (PFGE) and whole-genome sequencing, researchers isolated the strain associated with the Ontario listeria outbreak in pasteurized chocolate milk. On June 5, health officials recalled all chocolate milk from the brand processed at the facility where the bacteria were identified. Interestingly, no white milk samples were positive for the bacteria.

Milk had initially been ruled out as a source during the first wave of the outbreak given that exposure to pasteurized milk was only reported by 60 percent of case patients in the outbreak's first wave (as compared with 76 percent of controls). With the new laboratory results however, investigators re-interviewed case-patients from the second wave and found that 75 percent of case-patients reported consuming the suspected contaminated brand of chocolate milk.

Through environmental sampling at the manufacturing plant, investigators ultimately traced the contamination to post-pasteurization equipment dedicated to chocolate milk. Presence of the outbreak strain was confirmed within a post-pasteurization pump used solely for chocolate milk and on nonfood contact surfaces. Contamination was speculated to have occurred due to a specific maintenance event or poor equipment design. Prior to resuming chocolate milk production, the manufacturer replaced the contaminated equipment and implemented corrective food safety and hygiene measures to prevent recurrence.[83]

Mad Cow Disease

Bovine spongiform encephalopathy (BSE), more commonly referred to as mad cow disease, is a member of a family of diseases called transmissible spongiform encephalopathies (TSEs), which degrade mammals' central nervous systems as a result of the accumulation of abnormal, infectious proteins called prions. There are two types of BSE—classical BSE, caused by cattle ingesting prion-contaminated feed, and atypical BSE, which occurs spontaneously in cattle populations.[84]

Classical BSE was first identified in Britain in 1986.[85] Over two years, 421 cattle were diagnosed with BSE. Around the country other animals, including pet cats and antelope in zoos, died from TSEs after being fed with pet food containing cattle by-products and commercial cattle feed.[86] In 1992, it was estimated that three out of every one thousand cows in Britain had BSE.[87] Investigators discovered that cattle were infected with BSE after being fed meat-and-bone meal containing remains from either scrapie infected sheep remains, or cattle remains infected with spontaneous BSE. By 1993, 120,000 cattle had been diagnosed with BSE. However, throughout the early nineties the British government insisted that BSE was not a threat to humans.

The first documented case of variant Creutzfeldt-Jakob disease (vCJD), the human form of BSE, occurred in May 1995, when a nineteen-year-old and two other people in Britain died from the new condition.[88] In response, 4.5 million cattle were culled during 1996.[89] This triggered an investigation into the connection between BSE and vCJD when humans ingest BSE-infected meat.

In March 1996, the British health secretary acknowledged that human cases of vCJD were the result of infected cattle consumption. In response to the BSE outbreak and vCJD cases, the European Union banned the export of British beef for ten years between 1996 and 2006, and several other countries around the world restricted the import of beef products and live cattle.[90] A little over a year later, in July 1997, twenty-one vCJD cases

Learn about another transmissible spongiform encephalopathy (TSE)—Kuru—in the "Anthropologists in Outbreaks" case study.

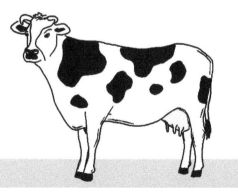

had been identified, and by 1999, there had been forty cases of vCJD and five deaths. In the 2000s, cases of BSE and vCJD began appearing in other countries around the world, including Japan, the US, and Canada. By January 2004, 143 people in Britain had developed vCJD, and at least 180,000 cattle had BSE.

During the British BSE and vCJD outbreak, a total of 178 people died. The BSE and vCJD outbreak led to agriculture and food agencies around the world implementing heightened restrictions on cattle used for human consumption, stricter testing measures, and more extensive livestock feed regulation.

Remove Implicated Foods from Market

Once a food safety issue is identified, it may be necessary to remove implicated foods and other food products (like bulk ingredients used in processing marketed foods) from the supply chain.[92] This is often referred to as a recall, which is defined as "the action to remove food from the market at any stage of the food chain, including that possessed by consumers."[93] Recalls can protect public health by rapidly removing unsafe food products from the market and keeping consumers informed of risk.

CASE STUDY

Bad [Chocolate] Eggs

Salmonella Outbreak in Chocolate Eggs Due to Contaminated Milk

In April and May 2022, 270 cases of salmonella were linked to several chocolate products including chocolate Easter eggs across fourteen European countries, Canada, and the US. The outbreak was characterized by an unusually high proportion of hospitalized children. The European Center for Disease Prevention and Control (ECDC) reported that 86.3 percent of the cases were among children aged ten or younger, and for all cases in Europe with information available, 41.3 percent of those children were hospitalized.[94] Health officials traced the infections to specific chocolate products using epidemiological studies, laboratory testing, and patient interviews. ECDC investigators matched the salmonella strain to infected samples detected at a Ferrero plant in Belgium in December 2021. Despite hygiene measures and increased salmonella testing, they identified a step during buttermilk processing as the point of contamination. The food safety agency in Belgium shut down the factory in April following inspection and confirmation of the link between the continental outbreak and the specific plant.[95] The ECDC issued food safety warnings and the chocolate company issued a full recall of the potentially contaminated products.

Codex Alimentarius

The FAO and WHO publish the *Codex Alimentarius*, a document that describes a recommended code of practice to ensure food hygiene.[91] It identifies essential principles of food hygiene applicable throughout the food chain (from primary production through to the final consumer) to ensure that food is safe and suitable for human consumption. To achieve this, it recommends a Hazard Analysis and Critical Control Point System approach. The guide explains how food producers and processers can assure food safety, principles that apply whether or not there is an outbreak:

- Hygiene during the primary production process
- Facilities designed to help ensure hygiene
- Control of food hazards in the course of operations

- Maintenance and sanitization
- Personnel hygiene
- Transportation
- Training
- Consumer awareness

Closing Food Premises

An outbreak of foodborne illness may necessitate the temporary closure of premises that provide food, including wholesale and retail markets, restaurants and other eateries, catering companies, and any other outlet that provides or sells the implicated ingredient in some form, until the root source of the outbreak is resolved.[96] The decision to close food premises should follow local regulations and outline the necessary steps for reopening, such as disinfection protocols, implicated product destruction, relevant environmental testing, and a timeline for reinspection.

Chemical and Radiation Safety

Chemicals and radiation are both critical threats to public health, and key capacities for health security and pandemic preparedness and response are having detailed chemical and radiation event response plans that spell out procedures, roles and responsibilities, and response protocols for the release of chemical or radiologic agents.

Preparing for and responding to chemical and radiologic events requires specific planning and training. International organizations have created guidelines for countries to develop their own safety and response protocols. The Organization for the Prohibition of Chemical Weapons (OPCW) maintains guidelines for the medical management of people who have been exposed to chemical agents.[97] A consortia of international organizations, including the WHO and the International Atomic Energy Agency (IAEA), have published guidelines for preparedness and response for a nuclear or radiological emergency.[98] Any event with either of these types of hazards would trigger international assistance from global experts at these organizations.

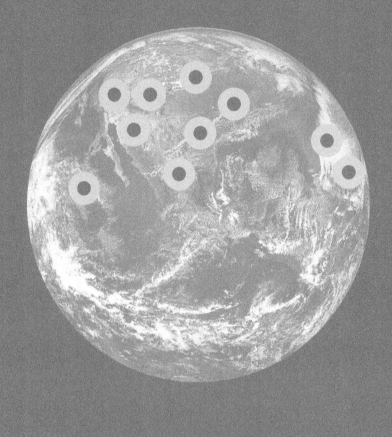

10

TREATING PATIENTS

Taking Care of People

Infectious diseases cause people to get sick and those people need to be cared for. An astute health worker is often the first person to identify that an outbreak is occurring and sound the public health alarm. The cascade of investigative events that follows helps identify other infected people early and get them treated before they spread the disease further. Sometimes though, it is not possible to capture a disease before it spreads, and health systems need to be ready to respond to a larger outbreak. This requires a coordinated response between government officials, private sector businesses, NGOs, and other actors involved in providing health services to mobilize surge personnel, medical supplies and equipment and to designate temporary care facilities.

In this chapter, we review the steps health officials and workers take to diagnose, manage, and treat cases during an infectious disease outbreak.

Diagnose Cases

Learn more about case definitions in the Epidemiology chapter.

To figure out what disease is causing an illness and determine the appropriate course of treatment, a sick person must first be diagnosed. Case diagnosis can be clinical or through laboratory confirmation. Following established case definitions, health professionals can diagnose probable and suspect cases based on a person's clinical features—their signs, symptoms, and history.[1] Case diagnosis through laboratory techniques requires testing biological samples to confirm a case. Health workers will collect biological sample(s) from the sick person and send it to a lab for testing.

See the Laboratories and Lab Analysis chapter for information on sample collection, transport, and testing!

Differential Diagnoses

Diagnoses may be uncertain, particularly early in an outbreak or when the cause of illness is a new disease. The early signs and symptoms of many infectious diseases can be similar to one another, necessitating a process by which health care providers can distinguish the etiology of a patient's illness. They do this by forming differential diagnoses, a list of possible diagnoses that could explain a patient's signs and symptoms based on information gathered during the initial clinical assessment, primarily through history taking and physical examination.[2]

Differential diagnoses are then used to determine clinicians' next steps, such as requesting laboratory tests (e.g., blood tests, viral cultures) or diagnostic imaging (e.g., chest x-rays, CT scans), as well as implementing preliminary treatment and possible IPC measures like isolation. The specific diagnostic approach they use is done to help them to rule out or confirm conditions on their list. As more information is gathered through laboratory testing and further epidemiological investigation, the list of differential diagnoses may narrow until a definitive diagnosis is made. Differential diagnoses are also sometimes progressed through trial and error with treatments (e.g., if a patient doesn't respond to antimalarial drugs, take malaria off the list). However, health care providers exercise caution when using a trial and error approach with antibiotics or other drugs where resistance can develop. In these cases, when the resources are available, health care providers work with laboratory technicians to test for antimicrobial resistance before prescribing drugs.

Learn more about antimicrobial resistance in the Laboratories and Lab Analysis chapter.

> ### Quick Reference: Differential Diagnosis for a Patient with a Cough and Fever
>
> A patient presents with a cough and a fever—the list of differential diagnoses may include an upper respiratory tract infection, bacterial pneumonia, or tuberculosis. The differential diagnoses inform which investigations may need to be carried out, such as blood cultures, a throat swab, and a chest x-ray.

Diagnostic Tests

Diagnostic tests aid both epidemiological investigation and clinical management. Tests can be laboratory-based, requiring trained personnel and specialized equipment, or point of care (POC), which are designed to be simple and quick; they can even be conducted by members of the general public. Diagnostic tests for biological agents identify the presence of a pathogen's DNA, RNA, or antigens; other tests may detect a host's particular antibodies suggesting prior exposure.

Health workers, laboratorians, and any organizations involved in distributing or conducting tests follow disease-specific diagnostic protocols. They outline which tests should be used (lab versus POC; antigen versus antibody, etc.), when tests should be used, who they should be used on to facilitate rapid diagnosis and to prevent misinterpretation, and what clinical or nonpharmaceutical steps should be taken depending on the results. Guidance is especially important when testing resources are limited and specific groups should be targeted for testing. However, for new infectious diseases, laboratory-based and POC diagnostics to assess the presence of a pathogen in a patient sample are not yet available. Ruling out differential diagnoses for which tests are available and adhering to the provided case definitions will help guide clinicians.

Go to the Epidemiology chapter to learn about the rest of the steps involved in outbreak investigation.

In November 2022, a person in Maricopa County, Arizona, USA, was diagnosed with what looked like locally acquired dengue fever. This raised concern, as previous cases of dengue in the county had been tied to travel, while this case seemed to be tied to a person who was bitten by a mosquito in Arizona. County health officials became worried that others in the area might have also been exposed, so the county public health department provided residents with mosquito prevention kits. They also went door to door conducting rapid testing of the population.[3]

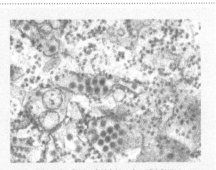

Dengue virus. Credit: Frederick Murphy; CDC PHIL

Based on clinical diagnosis and the results of diagnostic tests, medical personnel report suspected and identified cases to the relevant disease monitoring system. Health facility records, medical reports, and other clinical data are key sources for indicator-based surveillance that can capture signs of an outbreak. Epidemiologists investigating a potential outbreak will review and confirm clinical diagnoses by conducting additional questioning, reviewing clinical records, and conducting additional diagnostic testing.

Manage and Treat Cases

Once diagnosed, a sick person receives treatment. When treatment is ineffective or unknown (either because no treatment exists yet for the disease in question or if it is a never-before-seen disease), health care providers can help manage symptoms and provide palliative care. Clinicians follow standardized guidance for case management and treatment based on the best available information about the disease and observed symptoms. Clinical guidelines are "systematically developed statements to assist practitioner and patient decisions about appropriate health care for specific clinical circumstances."[4] Guidance may also cover recommended observation periods and infection prevention and control.[5] For new and emerging diseases, it is expected that guidance will be updated as the outbreak progresses to reflect new understandings, based on scientific evidence of how a pathogen impacts the human body and can be treated.

See the Logistics chapter to learn about procuring durable and consumable medical equipment and supplies.

Although patient care is adapted to the circumstances and nature of the particular outbreak, health care providers continue to rely on their fundamental training in history taking, clinical examination, development of differential diagnoses, implementation of treatment plans, and medical record keeping.

Health Care Outbreak Operations

An infectious disease outbreak could involve five people, or five million. The scale of the response—the number of personnel involved and the amount of supplies, equipment, and facilities needed—depends on the size and severity of the outbreak.

Providing health care during an outbreak is part of a coordinated medical response that may involve local, regional, national, and international health authorities and responders. They work together to standardize treatment and IPC guidelines, mobilize surge staff and resources, and identify and stock designated treatment, isolation and quarantine, and points of dispensing facilities. Further, to provide safe and reliable health services, these facilities, vehicles, and equipment need to be cleaned and disinfected frequently and have consistent access to power and clean water.

To avoid spreading disease among patients, health facility staff, and visitors, health centers continue to follow routine health and safety precautions and establish public health and IPC measures tailored to the outbreak. These policies can be individual-specific or facility wide, such as isolating or quarantining certain patients, reducing visitors, shifting some services to telehealth and other digital platforms, changing facility flow, and enforcing physical distancing and use of PPE. For large-scale outbreaks, health officials may group patients with the same infectious disease in designated wards to limit spread to the rest of the health facility.[6] During outbreaks of highly dangerous pathogens, infected cases may be treated at specialized health facilities with personnel trained in biosafety and equipped with appropriate equipment and facilities like negative pressure isolation rooms.

To learn more, see the "Ensuring Biosafety and Biosecurity" section in the Laboratories and Lab Analysis chapter.

Operational Coordination and Communication

It is important to activate national public health emergency management mechanisms across ministries to provide a coordinated response.[7] Interdisciplinary and cross-sector coordination and communication between health care organizations, other response disciplines, nongovernmental organizations, and government agencies involved in treating sick people during an outbreak is integral to managing a cohesive medical response. The private sector also plays an important role and should be included in response planning prior to an outbreak given how many medical assets are privately owned and managed. Real-time information exchange among response partners in the health care system helps to track burden of disease, availability of supplies, and medical needs, and to adjust the surge response accordingly. At the end of an outbreak, or when surge operations are no longer required for a long-term response, authorities initiate a demobilization process. This involves incrementally decreasing surge staffing, equipment, and temporary facilities, and beginning the process of restocking stockpiles used for the emergency response.

See the Governance chapter for more on decision making and the coordination involved in multisector disease response.

See the "Declare When the Outbreak Is Over" section in the Declarations and Notifications chapter.

See the Staffing and Training chapter for a case study example of expanding scope of practice to respond to outbreaks.

Staffing

When possible, doctors, nurses, and other care providers managing the treatment efforts of an outbreak should be locally or nationally based. When staff capacity is overwhelmed, affected localities may choose to expand scope of practice and request surge assistance from other sectors, like emergency medical technicians or military health personnel, or even from other countries, international NGOs like IFRC or MSF, or regional health organizations. Health authorities need to ensure that health care staff have access to appropriate tools for the assessment, testing, and treatment of patients, as well as adequate PPE to protect themselves.

See the Governance chapter to learn more about requesting assistance.

Medical Surge

Medical surge is the provision of adequate medical attention during public health events that exceed the normal operating capacity of medical infrastructure.[8] Health officials assess the nature and scope of the public health event and mobilize surge personnel and additional care facilities, resources, and financing to meet the needs of the response.[9] This can involve approving the use of national stockpiles of medicines, supplies, and equipment or requesting assistance from other countries or international organizations. The specifics of initiating surge response are often contained in a jurisdiction's emergency operations plans, ideally developed by authorities in advance of an outbreak.

CASE STUDY

Refurbishing Ventilators by a Local Energy Company

during the COVID-19 Pandemic

Ventilators are a vital piece of medical equipment for certain patients infected with COVID-19. Severe cases of COVID-19 can experience hypoxemia, an abnormally low concentration of oxygen in the blood that inhibits the lungs' ability to transfer oxygen into arterial blood, making it nearly impossible to breathe.[10] Ventilators can save some patients' life by helping pump oxygen into their lungs.

During the COVID-19 pandemic there was significant concern globally about countries' supplies of ventilators, particularly as early clinical guidance relied heavily on ventilator use. In some hospitals in the US, patients were having to share ventilators, and states turned to their emergency stockpiles to ensure they had adequate ventilators for their residents.[11] The California state stockpile contained more than 4,200 ventilators. However, upward of one thousand of those did not work.[12] In fact, many had been in storage since the Health Surge Capacity Initiative to stockpile medicines and equipment was dismantled in 2011 with no funds allocated to the maintenance of the already procured supplies.[13] The original manufacturers informed the California state government that they would need a month to fix two hundred ventilators.

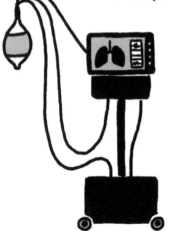

So the California governor reached out to Bloom Energy, a private green-energy fuel cell company, to ask for help to restore the critical equipment.[14] A Bloom engineer downloaded the ventilators' service manual and taught himself how to dismantle and rebuild it in one day.[15] Other company employees learned how to refurbish the ventilators, and soon after, Bloom Energy repurposed their manufacturing facility and fixed two hundred ventilators in three days. Bloom ended up retooling approximately one thousand ventilators for California.[16] The company continued to leverage its expertise and adaptive capacity to meet the need for ventilators around the country; for example, it used its Delaware plant to refurbish one hundred ventilators for that state.[17]

For more information, see the Communicating with the Public chapter.

Access to Services

Health authorities often must determine which health services are essential and which can be delayed or reassigned to areas with lower disease burden.[18] Routine health and emergency services remain important parts of a community's health even when an outbreak is occurring. However, health care systems can be overwhelmed during medical surges, decreasing access to basic care. Additionally, fear of contracting disease may dissuade people from seeking important health services. The reduction in access to and use of health services can directly increase mortality from outbreaks and indirectly increase preventable and treatable health conditions.[19] As such, it is important that authorities commit resources and personnel to maintaining routine services. Health authorities should also be clearly and consistently communicating with the public to keep them informed on health service availability and details on how to use services during the emergency situation.

Reduction in Health Services Utilization during Ebola, West Africa, 2014–2016

The indirect effects of outbreaks on general health services is substantial—as a result of both strained systems unable to perform routine and emergency services due to staffing, supply, and financial shortages and reduced use because of patient fear of contracting the disease from a medical center. In 2014–15, during the Ebola epidemic in West Africa, morbidity and mortality in other preventable diseases increased due to a reduction in health services utilization. Antenatal care visits, use of children's health services, child vaccination, and surgeries all decreased.[20] Additionally, many pregnant women had no option but to give birth at home. With an already high rate of death during childbirth in West Africa, home births were dangerous for the mother and baby.[21] More people died from car crashes, childbirth, and other challenges during Ebola because hospitals were shut down.[22]

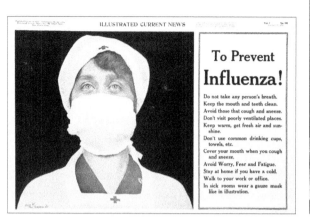

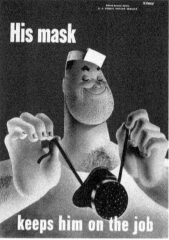

Courtesy of the NLM.

Supporting and Protecting Health Care Providers

Health care workers are critical members of an infectious disease outbreak response. They clinically identify cases, generate differential diagnoses, request and at times perform diagnostic tests, and initiate treatment based on the results of testing and clinical guidance. They do all of this while continuing to provide regular care for non-outbreak-related conditions to keep populations healthy. In order to perform these essential tasks, their health, professional needs, and safety must be assured throughout a response.

The nature of their job places health care providers at high risk for pathogen exposure and infection, as well as possible physical violence and psychological stress from fatigue, stigma, and burnout.[23] Without health responders, effective outbreak response is not possible, and when they leave their jobs due to illness, burnout, or threats of violence, it weakens the health system and negatively impacts the community.[24] Leadership in health facilities and/or on the outbreak response team can support the health and uphold the security of responders in multiple ways:

- Provide adequate PPE
- Establish IPC measures in health facilities
- Ensure health workers have access to relevant vaccinations
- Provide access to mental health and counseling resources
- Notify health care staff if they have been exposed in the workplace
- Allow sick staff to stay home and provide them with appropriate support
- Maintain an effective communication mechanism between responders and leadership throughout the outbreak and into the recovery period[25]

See the Emergency Operations and Logistics chapter to learn more about transporting or evacuating patients and health care personnel.

Political and civil unrest and violent conflict hinder outbreak response efforts and contribute to the spread of infectious disease. In some situations, patients and health care personnel will need to be transported or evacuated from dangerous environments. To protect health responders, coordination with security professionals is a high priority during outbreak response planning and operations.[26]

See the Security chapter for more information on protecting health workers.

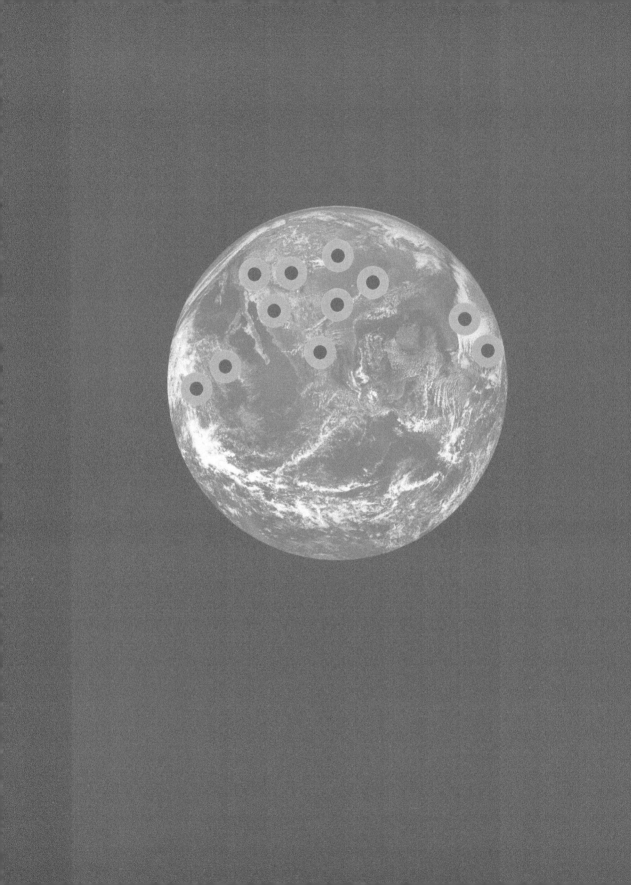

11

SECURITY
Keeping the Peace

Outbreaks can be scary. People become frightened for their own health and well-being, as well as that of their families and community. Populations may push for, or against, access to care or medical countermeasures. There may be disruptions in supply chains for goods and food. Certain mitigation activities, like quarantines, may lead to civil unrest.[1] The public may lose trust in their governments and become unruly, especially when people are scared or feel their civil liberties are being infringed upon.

Therefore, security—and keeping the peace—may be critical components of outbreak response, as decision makers try to balance the needs of individuals with the needs of society. Doing so in a way that helps a situation, and doesn't make it worse, can be complicated.

Coordinate with the Security Sector and Law Enforcement

Coordination between public health and law enforcement agencies is critical to help contain the spread of a disease while maintaining public order.[2] Security and law enforcement professionals are tasked with balancing the needs to uphold the rule of law, promote the common good, and safeguard individual liberties.[3]

Local and national public safety agencies should be prepared to support public health efforts (if asked) and manage additional challenges created by the outbreak, all while managing regular service demands and possibly operating under resource constraints.[4] As security personnel and law enforcement are in close contact with communities, they may be at a heightened risk of disease exposure and sickness. Thus, they must be prepared to perform their increased workload with a diminished workforce.

During an outbreak, law enforcement agencies may be asked to perform additional duties:

- **Enforce new restrictions and regulations**: Police may be required to implement new quarantine, travel, and curfew restrictions critical to preventing the spread of infectious diseases.
- **Contact trace:** Police investigation resources may be needed to aid in contact tracing.
- **Maintain public order**: Police may be called on to manage crowds.
- **Secure public health resources and institutions**: Law enforcement or private security may be needed to help protect health care personnel, facilities, medical countermeasures, or other critical resources.
- **Assist with public messaging**: Law enforcement agencies can also play a critical role in disseminating and promoting information about local or national public health measures to the population.[5]

Public health and law enforcement are critical partners, but this partnership may not always be easy. During an outbreak, these entities need to figure out how law enforcement should enforce public health measures without damaging public confidence.[6] Overall effective coordination and communication between law enforcement and public health agencies, as well as the ability for both groups to adapt to changing situations in communities, can dramatically affect the success of outbreak management efforts.

Law enforcement and security personnel need to be trained on how to respond appropriately and safely during an outbreak to standard cases as well as to outbreak-related civil unrest. They need to understand how a disease spreads and who may be particularly vulnerable to infection in order to protect themselves and the people they are serving.

Toronto Police during SARS

In spring of 2003, SARS spread from Guangdong Province in China to countries around the world—including Canada—through the infection of travelers staying at a Hong Kong hotel.[7] On March 26, 2003, with about two dozen cases of SARS in Toronto, a declaration of emergency was issued by the premier of Ontario. This declaration prompted the Toronto police to stand up its Police Command Center. Over the subsequent weeks, the Toronto police worked with the rest of the provincial government to acquire information about the outbreak, enforce quarantines, help track cases, and communicate with the public.[8]

Civil Unrest at the Start of the West Africa Ebola Outbreak

In August 2014, Ebola was spreading through Liberia. Almost one thousand people had been infected in the country by that point. In the capital city of Monrovia, in the neighborhood of West Point, government officials had converted a local school into a holding center for Ebola patients without informing local residents. Residents were enraged and broke into the school, taking supplies, including blood-soaked mattresses.[9] In the third week of August, with rising cases and unrest, the president announced a curfew in Monrovia and quarantined the neighborhood of West Point. The residents of West Point became more angry. They were given no advanced notice, were unable to secure food, and felt like they were being left to die. Crowds tried to get past checkpoints. Soldiers assigned to maintain the quarantine opened fire and a teenage boy died.[10] The lockdown of neighborhoods and criminalization of public gatherings during the Ebola outbreak of 2014 created resentment and confrontation with the police that ultimately harmed containment efforts.

Identify and Address Social Disturbances

Disease outbreaks may have unpredictable social effects, depending on existing social conditions and outbreak management measures implemented during the crisis. These disturbances may be a direct or indirect result of the outbreak, outbreak management policies, or changes in economic conditions due to the disease. Interpersonal dynamics may also be altered in the face of an outbreak. Evidence shows that during disasters, including disease outbreaks, rates of domestic violence increase.[11] Economic pressures may increase violence both within and outside the home. Supply chain disruptions may lead to hoarding of supplies.[12]

Government officials need to plan for these types of social disturbances when managing the outbreak response. Officials, working with civil society organizations, must monitor social conditions, plan for the possibility of these events, and direct response efforts accordingly.

Increase in Domestic Violence during the COVID-19 Pandemic

When people around the world went into lockdown for the COVID-19 pandemic, individuals were forced to spend more time—under significant stress—with people from their households. The number of domestic violence incidents spiked by 25 to 33 percent around the world.[13] The National Commission on

COVID-19 and Criminal Justice found increases in domestic violence in the US alone spiked by more than 8 percent.[14] At the same time, victims were constrained from safely reaching out for help; the number of calls to some domestic violence hotlines dropped by more than 50 percent.[15] The United Nations labeled violence against women the "shadow pandemic."[16]

The Montreal Vaccine Riot of 1885

Violence over Smallpox Vaccine Mandate

A smallpox outbreak was spreading through the Canadian city of Montreal in the summer of 1885, leading to almost four thousand cases by end of September. Health officials tried to control the outbreak but faced resistance from a population that was concerned about the safety of the smallpox vaccine. Sanitary police used force to remove people from locations where they could not isolate—often

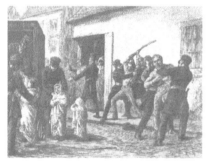

Drawing by Robert Harris, titled "Incident of the small-pox epidemic, Montréal."

poor, overcrowded homes. By the end of September, a decision was made to mandate vaccination. Protesters responded by attacking the health office building and then going through the city smashing windows at pharmacies, homes of public health officials, and the police station. Shots were fired by the protesters at the police station, which were answered by police firing into the air. After that night, police and sanitation officers were armed while they tried to enforce the vaccine mandate. The rioters quieted down after the first night of violence; eventually the population was sufficiently vaccinated, and the outbreak subsided. After this outbreak, the protesters and public health officials pivoted to focus on legislation and regulations for future vaccine requirements.[17]

Provide Security for Patients, Health Care Workers, and Health Facilities

Experience has shown that part of outbreak response is providing proper protection for patients, health care workers, and health care facilities. Although violence against health care services violates international and humanitarian law, medical providers, facilities, and even patients still have been documented as coming under attack. In fact, health workers are more likely to be victims of violence and physical and verbal abuse than police officers.[18] This may occur more often in fragile emergency settings, but can—and has—happened in highly developed, otherwise stable environments.[19]

Attacks on health care providers and patients may keep people from accessing necessary care, displace populations, and even disrupt critical supplies like water and electricity.[20] To counter such threats and protect patients, health care workers, and facilities, governments can strengthen policies and legislation, train and provide security forces when appropriate, and ensure facilities have emergency procedures in place.[21] Successful protection of health care workers against these violent attacks is vital to both their safety and to the eventual containment of the outbreak, but underlying political turmoil can complicate security efforts.[22]

Comprehensive protection of health care workers requires thorough understanding of the concerns of the community, ideally enabling officials to mitigate the concerns that provoke attacks, as well as to implement approaches to security that do not incite fear and suspicion.[23]

CASE STUDY

Violence against Health Care Workers
during the 2018–2020 DRC Ebola Outbreak

The world's second deadliest and second largest Ebola virus disease (EVD) outbreak occurred in the Democratic Republic of Congo (DRC), lasting nearly two years from 2018 to 2020. The outbreak originated in the northeastern region of the DRC, where long-standing armed conflict between insurgent groups, government forces, and United Nations peacekeeping forces dramatically impacted outbreak control efforts. Frontline health workers responding to the outbreak operated in an exceptionally dangerous environment, facing both a deadly virus, which had a fatality rate of 66 percent during the outbreak, and an active conflict zone. Over the course of the outbreak, there were at least 420 targeted attacks on EVD-response health facilities, killing an estimated eleven health care workers and patients, and injuring eighty-six others.[24]

Protecting health care workers, patients, and EVD facilities proved to be a significant challenge over the course of the two-year outbreak; they were routinely subjected to targeted violence from organized armed groups and

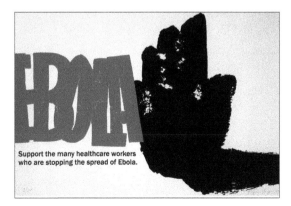

Support the many healthcare workers who are stopping the spread of Ebola.

Poster supporting healthcare workers during Ebola outbreak. Courtesy of the National Library of Medicine community members, often resulting in fatalities, injuries, destroyed facilities and equipment, furthering the spread of the disease. Many attacks were rooted in long-standing suspicion and distrust of the national government and foreign organizations and, by extension, health workers and their operational facilities. Mistrust was further fueled by rumors that EVD was either a fictitious scam or an intentional infection caused by the DRC government and/or international governments for political or economic gain.

Nations like the US protected their public health responders by restricting their physical presence, learning early on that international workers attracted violent attacks. In August 2018, four health care workers from the US CDC and USAID were sent to the northeastern city of Beni. A few days later, an organized armed group attacked the DRC military base where the US workers had traveled.[25] The health care workers were evacuated, and the US CDC then limited personnel responding to the EVD outbreak to two thousand miles away from the epicenter, in Kinshasa and later in Goma.[26]

By June 2019, at least 174 attacks on health care workers or EVD facilities had occurred. At least five of them were fatal.[27] One of the most widely reported attacks was the murder of a WHO epidemiologist at Butembo University Hospital in North Kivu on April 19, 2019.[28] Two other health care workers were injured in the attack. After the attack, about two hundred doctors and one thousand nurses working in hospitals and health centers in Butembo threatened to strike if the government did not improve security within one week.[29]

Subsequent efforts taken by the UN and DRC government to protect health care workers, patients, and treatment centers had an adverse effect. In May 2019, the United Nations Organization Mission in the Democratic Republic of Congo (MONUSCO) deployed approximately eighteen thousand armed personnel to protect EVD response efforts in the DRC.[30] However, given the association of uniformed security personnel with the DRC government, there was an increase in the already high frequency of violent attacks on health care workers and centers.

Several international organizations refused protection from MONUSCO's peacekeeping forces and DRC security personnel to maintain neutral status, including the Red Cross and Médecins Sans Frontières. In February 2019, an MSF Ebola treatment facility in Katwa was attacked and set on fire. Only a few days later, another MSF treatment unit was attacked and partially burned down in the city of Butembo. MSF evacuated health care workers and patients and was forced to suspend activities at the centers. After the attacks, the international president of MSF criticized the use of a heavy security presence in the DRC Ebola response, saying that it caused health care workers to be seen as "the enemy."[31] The Red Cross also had to limit their activity after multiple attacks where Red Cross health care workers were injured by community members while performing burials of EVD victims.[32] The WHO and UNICEF also pulled Ebola responders due to threats of violent protests.

In spite of the tremendous challenges, and due to the courageous efforts by responders, the outbreak was eventually controlled.

Provide Security at Points of Dispensing (PODs)

It is a logistical challenge to figure out how to deliver critical supplies like MCMs, diagnostic tests, or protective equipment like masks to many people in a short period of time. Yet getting these things to the population that needs them makes all the difference in an outbreak response. Policy planners have been working on different types of distribution protocols for decades, including using fast food drive throughs, engaging the postal service, or even pre-positioning certain drugs with households.[33]

One of the tools for getting these lifesaving supplies to the population is through PODs—points of dispensing. PODs are areas where health care personnel, support staff, and the public can gather in potentially large numbers. Imagine, though, a situation in which the population knows it may have been exposed to a deadly virus, and the MCM at the POD may be the only thing that saves them. People will be frightened and maybe desperate to get a drug or vaccine for themselves or their families. Public health professionals will not be able to manage this alone. They will need robust security.

Read more about PODs in the Disease Prevention and Mitigation chapter.

Providing proper security for PODs is critical to maintaining the full operation of POD sites and thus helping manage public health crises efficiently.[34] Public health and public safety agencies must work in advance to coordinate how best to manage the security of the facility, the people, and the MCMs without sacrificing the efficiency and effectiveness of POD operations.[35]

There are a number of key security requirements for PODs:[36]

- **Management of points of entry and exit**: POD security should assist at entry and exit points to ensure the orderly movement of people and vehicles and prevent unauthorized access to the PODs.
- **Crowd control**: POD security should help manage the flow of people both throughout the facility and around the POD.
- **Routine security checks**: Security personnel should establish guidelines for and conduct regular POD security checks.
- **Physical security**: POD security should ensure the physical protection of all personnel, equipment, supplies (including medications), vehicles, and buildings.

Protecting the Postal Service when Responding to Bioterrorism

At the end of December 2009, President Obama issued Executive Order 13527, establishing the National US Postal Service Medical Countermeasures dispensing model. The idea was that in the event of a biological attack against the US, the postal service could be used to rapidly deliver drugs to households across the country. This would be particularly important for countering attacks by agents that can be treated after exposure. For example, you can take antibiotics after exposure to anthrax: Ciprofloxacin is approved for post-exposure prophylaxis (PEP) to "reduce the incidence or progression of disease following exposure to aerosolized *Bacillus anthracis*."[37]

Now imagine the situation where an anthrax attack has occurred in a city. Millions of people may have been exposed. The population is told to please return to their homes and wait for postal service workers to deliver the post-exposure drug they and their families need to keep them from becoming sick or dying. In order to avoid chaos and a complete breakdown in civil society at first glimpse of the mail delivery truck to come down the street, this model relied on pairing the postal service workers with law enforcement.[38] Local police would be charged with protecting not only the postal carriers but also the stockpile of medication stored in the mail delivery truck.

Provide Security for Burial Teams

Read more about burial teams in the "Managing the Deceased" section of the Disease Prevention and Mitigation chapter.

Providing proper security for burial teams in outbreak settings helps control and manage the spread of infectious diseases and helps ensure the safety of public health personnel. As burial processes can offer a high risk for postmortem disease transmission for specific infectious diseases, burial teams must have the full capability to perform their proper duties. Disturbance of a safe burial can place the burial team, support staff, and any other individuals present at risk of contracting a possibly deadly infectious disease. Security is especially important in fragile zones characterized by conflict, unrest, or mistrust in government or health providers.

Implementing safeguards to protect burial teams is essential for conducting safe burial practices and stopping the spread of infectious diseases. To perform safe burials, the burial team should "seek security clearances of the site before proceeding" with the recovery of dead bodies and the burials.[39] If the retrieval of the body or the burial is in a region with a history of conflict or violence against health care workers, it is best to include security personnel on the burial team. Before proceeding with burial practices, team managers should set security protocols indicating evacuation and security plans for the

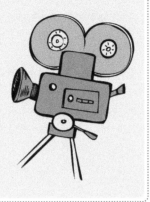
burial team's various locations, take the shortest route to minimize chances of attack while driving to and from burial sites, and make sure the burial team is aware of local conflict.[40]

Ensure Laboratory Biosecurity

While most of us in the world want to do everything we can to stay away from dangerous pathogens, some bad actors want to get their hands on them for nefarious purposes. To protect against this, facilities that store or work with dangerous pathogens need to have security measures in place—both infrastructure (locks and gates) and security personnel (guards) to keep scary pathogens away from dangerous people.

Consider Issuing and Enforcing Curfew Restrictions

Officials may need to consider implementing curfews during an outbreak as part of broader mitigation efforts. Issuing a curfew can minimize spread of an infectious disease between individuals by limiting mobility and interactions with members outside of a household that could result in transmission. Curfews can also help control any civil unrest resulting from the outbreak.[43]

Curfews can, however, have harmful impacts on public trust, economics, and mental health. Curfews require strong coordination between health officials and law enforcement to ensure that they are issued and enforced properly. Messaging should come from the relevant high-level governing official, supported by guidance from public health officials and disease data. The announcement should define which activities are and are not permitted during the period of the curfew, and exactly how long it will last. The public should also be notified of any public health efforts that will be carried out during the curfew, including case identifications by health care workers, door-to-door education efforts, burials, or other relevant public health activities depending on the type of infectious disease.[44]

Strategies to enforce curfews should focus on community empowerment and engagement, employing practices that build trust and solidarity. Law enforcement responsible for enforcing curfews should be adequately trained in safe health practices and equipped with appropriate PPE.

CASE STUDY

Use of Curfews to Help Mitigate the Spread of Ebola in Sierra Leone

In the fall of 2014, Ebola was spreading through Guinea, Liberia, and Sierra Leone. By September 2014, approximately five hundred people had died just within Sierra Leone. The government of Sierra Leone was struggling to contain the spread of the virus and, as a mitigation effort, decided to impose a curfew for three days, from September nineteenth to the twenty-first. The decision was met with mixed reactions—some doubted whether it would have any impact and feared it would contribute to a further deterioration of trust in government.[45]

Approximately thirty thousand volunteers came together to support the curfew.[46] Community activists and leaders in civil society worked with law enforcement to help enforce it. Simultaneously, health workers went door-to-door searching for cases, including patients hesitant to seek out medical resources. Other volunteers distributed sanitation supplies, such as bars of soap, and information about prevention to help further limit the spread of the disease.[47]

The minister of health in Sierra Leone, Abubakarr Fofanah, reported that about 80 percent of homes were visited in the three days.[48] From those visits, 130 new cases were found, 39 more suspected cases were discovered, and 100 bodies were buried to prevent further spread.[49] Some volunteers, though, felt that the curfew and consequent home visits only highlighted the lack of health capacities of the government, and decreased trust held by some Sierra Leoneans since no cures or treatments were offered.[50]

Cases continued to rise, particularly in the northeast region of the country, and on June fifth, the president of Sierra Leone declared another curfew and restriction of movement from 6 p.m. to 6 a.m. for two districts, Kambia and Port Loko.[51] This curfew lasted twenty-one days. Military officials patrolled during the curfew to make sure that no travel occurred between regions and monitored the population to prevent unsafe burials. Restaurants and other businesses stayed open during the day, but they had to check every person for a fever upon entrance as a safeguard.[52]

This second curfew was not deemed very effective, particularly in regard to preventing unsafe burials. The population did not understand the reason for the rules of curfew and the limitations on burials, and thus there was significant noncompliance.

Consider Enforcing Border Closures

During certain outbreak situations, a government may decide to close borders to mitigate the spread of disease. The decision to close the borders is often driven by a mix of public health, trade, and political factors. Enforcing the border closure, however, is left to the security sector. This may include border agents, military, or law enforcement professionals, tasked with ensuring individuals are prevented from entering a jurisdiction or country while respecting human rights.

Learn more about how governments issue border restrictions and closures in the Governance chapter.

CASE STUDY

Border Closures during COVID-19

Throughout the COVID-19 pandemic, different countries at different times utilized some form of border closures to prevent the spread of disease. Sometimes countries completely closed their borders to any individuals, including citizens. Sometimes they insisted that people coming into the country first spend time in a quarantine facility. Regardless of the action, security and law enforcement personnel were utilized to enforce the policies. Whether it was border control agents banning access to a border crossing, or law enforcement monitoring quarantined travelers, security personnel were essential to ensuring travelers obeyed the—often changing—rules.

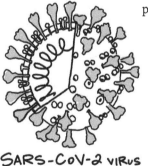

SARS-CoV-2 VIRUS

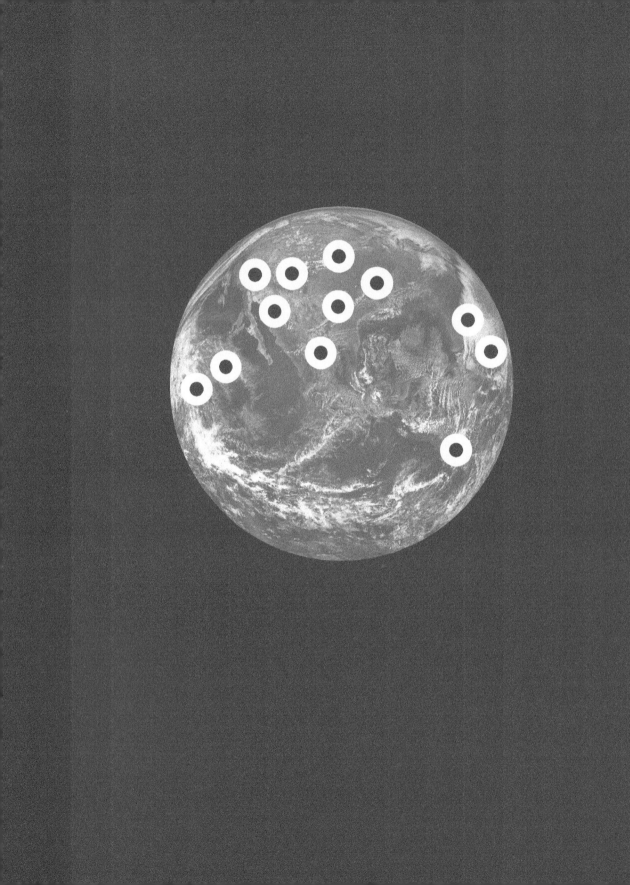

MONEY

Finding It, Giving It Out, and Keeping the Economy from Collapsing

Money is important.

It is really important.

It is hard to prepare for and respond to an outbreak without money.

Figuring out how to successfully budget for outbreaks that may or may not happen, finding emergency funding for response, getting money to the people who need it in an outbreak, and making sure the economy is resilient and can bounce back are all critical parts of outbreak preparedness and response.

Budget for Outbreaks

Long before an outbreak happens, governments need to think about how to budget for ongoing public health activities, like surveillance, as well as how to fund emergency situations. Daily preparedness and detection efforts are integrated into normal budgetary processes. Emergency funding, however, takes many different forms. In some jurisdictions, an emergency fund is established that can be triggered by public health emergency declarations.

See the Declarations and Notifications chapter for more information on public health emergency declarations.

Federal Funding for the Response to Outbreaks in the US: 2000 to 2016

Different public health events in the US have led to very different federal funding levels. Before COVID-19, the US mounted nationwide response efforts to several disease events:

- In 2000, over $2.4 million was provided in public assistance grants and another $2.4 million in emergency work for West Nile virus.
- In 2009, Congress granted $6.15 billion to fight the H1N1 pandemic.
- In 2014, Congress approved $1.1 billion for the domestic response to Ebola.
- In 2016, $1.1 billion was approved for the Zika virus response.[1]

Identify Legal Framework for Emergency Funding

There are a multitude of pathways for obtaining rapid, secure, and adequate funding for an outbreak response. These pathways are often defined by a legal framework that identifies requirements for funding eligibility that may vary depending on the nature and geographical spread of the threat.

For example, in the US, there are multiple legal frameworks for accessing emergency federal funds for a public health emergency. Some funds are linked to a Presidential Emergency Declaration under the Stafford Act. Other funding sources become available if the Secretary of Health and Human Services issues a public health emergency declaration.

Explore Fundraising Options and Request Resources

Regardless of how well-prepared and resourced a country or region is, it is rare that they are sufficiently equipped to contain an outbreak without some type of international assistance. Global fundraising and requests for assistance may be necessary for adequate response efforts to an outbreak. Factors such as size of the outbreak event, time since the first case was reported, geographical characteristics of the region, and national capacity for disaster response inform the need for and type of fundraising and resource requests.[2]

Specific response activities that may rely on global support include the procurement of PPE, medical countermeasures, diagnostics, and vaccines; research and development of medical technology; and deployment of medical and public health workers.

Funding can come bilaterally from other nations, philanthropic organizations, international organizations like the World Bank, or regional development banks. New funding mechanisms for preparedness and response to outbreaks are being set up at development banks to facilitate more rapid disbursement of funds and other resources.

Financing Options

Multiple sectors will require additional funding to sustain surge capacity and resources during an outbreak response. Governments, multilateral development banks, NGOs, and international organizations may all play a role.

Governments

During an outbreak response, public financial management systems are responsible for ensuring funding for health care resources (e.g., PPE, vaccines), supporting vulnerable populations, and maintaining essential services. The International Monetary Fund (IMF) outlines five traditional sources of emergency government funding to maintain essential services during an outbreak: contingency appropriations, emergency spending provisions, expenditure reprioritization through reallocations and virements, supplementary budgets, and external grants.[3] Accessing these resources may require approval from legislatures.

Multilateral Development Banks

Low- and middle-income countries (LMICs) may require additional external assistance from multilateral development banks (MDBs), such as the World Bank, the Inter-American Development Bank, the African Development Bank, and the Asian Development Bank, to compensate for reduced investment and increased expenditures. MDBs disbursed billions of dollars collectively over the course of the COVID-19 pandemic, nearly doubling their support in the health care sectors and continuing support for agriculture, education, social, and other sectors. Despite these increases, these loans only made up 0.5 percent of LMIC combined global GDP for 2020, indicating that the primary burden of financial support remains with governments themselves.[4]

A financial intermediary fund (FIF) for pandemic prevention, preparedness, and response (PPR) was approved by the World Bank board of directors on June 30, 2022.[5] This new mechanism, now called the Pandemic Fund, is designed to pool international funding for PPR capacity improvements in LMICs.

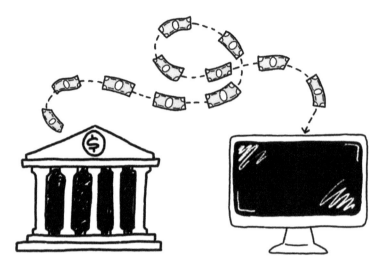

International Organizations

International organizations, particularly the WHO and its constituent country offices, can distribute vital health care–specific support. Funding for the WHO primarily comes from governments (both assessed and voluntary contributions), MDBs, and high-impact philanthropists. Many donate directly to the WHO Contingency Fund for Emergency (CFE), which rapidly allocates resources to respond to disease outbreaks and health emergencies across the world. As a readily available source of money, CFE can "provide funding during a critical gap—from the moment the need for an emergency response is identified, to the point at which resources from other financing mechanisms begin to flow."[6] The WHO and its country offices use this funding to purchase and distribute equipment and vaccines, improve laboratory capacity, and distribute information.[7]

Assess Ability to Rapidly Transfer Funds

Once a government identifies how and where to secure funding, it must then figure out how to rapidly transfer funds to organizations and first responders. In certain contexts, pre-existing infrastructures may be utilized to support these efforts.

Cash transfer can be of vital importance but is more useful in some sectors than others. For example, cash transfer has been found to be useful in addressing malnutrition caused by disease outbreak, but malnutrition due to environmental factors may not be addressed so easily.[8] Determining who most needs the financial assistance, whether organizations or individuals, is a necessary step in determining the ability to transfer funds.

Ensure Response Workers Are Compensated

When an outbreak begins, personnel must be deployed. These critical front-line responders serve important functions to meet the needs of their community and keep the threat in check.

Examples of response workers in an outbreak include health care practitioners and technicians (doctors, nurses, etc.), health care support workers (pharmacy aides, medical assistants, etc.), direct care workers (nursing assistants, personal care aides, etc.), and health service workers (housekeepers, janitors, etc.).[9] These individuals must be fairly and adequately compensated for their service. In an outbreak that touches all sectors of society, essential personnel might also include those deployed to maintain energy sources and other critical infrastructure, grocery store workers, food delivery personnel, law enforcement, and others deemed essential to support the community.

Not only do all essential workers and first responders need to be compensated, but additionally, eligible workers should receive a compensation and benefits package that covers remuneration and motivation for high-risk assignments, and compensation in case of death. Liability insurance for those required to act outside the scope of licensing or other authorization may also be required. Other forms of compensation for these responders can include psychological support, child care, and job security.[10]

Payments should be provided transparently and responsibly. Incentives vary based on the country, paying institution, and workers in question. Across scenarios and settings, the secure transfer of funds to responders promotes trust and encourages efficacy in the response to the outbreak.[11]

CASE STUDY

Digitization of Payments to Ebola Response Workers in Sierra Leone

In August 2014, in the midst of the West Africa Ebola outbreak, health workers in Sierra Leone at a government-run hospital went on strike to protest their working conditions and pay.

On July 29, 2014, Sheik Humarr Khan, a leader of the Ebola response, died at the treatment center in Kailahun. His death highlighted the magnitude of the threat of EVD and raised questions about the safety of the treatment facilities. Just weeks later, a WHO-deployed epidemiologist and three individuals at a hotel where foreign medical teams were staying became infected. Moreover, the US CDC reported that health care workers in Sierra Leone were at one hundred times greater risk for contracting EVD compared to the general population.[12]

Health care workers felt unsafe at work and were further frustrated by slow, inadequate compensation. In response, the United Nations Development Programme (UNDP) partnered with the government to implement digital technology to pay these workers. This enabled more effective management of the outbreak due to improved relations with frontline responders.

Before the Ebola crisis, cash payments to health workers were slow, inaccurate, and vulnerable to interception. Notably, two e-transfer service providers were already operating in the Sierra Leone cities of Freetown, Makeni, Kenema, and Bo. The UNDP, with support from partners including the UN Mission for the Ebola Emergency Response, set up a new payment program to address these issues with an awareness of existing in-country resources. Through collaboration with existing e-transfer providers and the Central Bank of Sierra Leone (representing all commercial banks in the country), Sierra Leone created a robust private sector payment platform. This initiative represented an attempt to improve relations with responders and end the strikes.[13] E-transfer providers fully digitized more than twenty-one thousand payments to workers, largely through mobile money deliveries.[14]

The lack of network coverage and service provider capacity in (often rural) program areas made full e-transfers challenging. Instead, providers used their services to facilitate offline payments at a series of pay points. This better payment system helped to end the strikes, in turn enabling Sierra Leone to better contain EVD by treating the infected and saving lives.[15]

Compensate Impacted Populations

Funding and economic support can assist populations impacted by disease outbreaks. Outbreaks can lead to large costs at many levels of society.[16] Public health responses involve coordinated compensation to individuals or groups of people in order to target these economic burdens. When workers are directly infected with disease, productivity loss can be substantial. Additionally, public health measures to combat the spread of outbreaks such as isolation, quarantine, and social distancing can also yield loss of earnings for individuals subject to these interventions.[17]

Cash-based assistance can provide financial support that is both flexible and dignified.[18] Relative to other forms of assistance, cash assistance allows recipients more control over how to prioritize their needs. Providing cash also reduces logistical requirements involved in shipping goods, making it a potentially faster form of providing access to essential goods where they are already available and generating economic exchange within communities.

Cash assistance can be provided in several ways: direct physical cash, vouchers, or mobile and account transfers.[19] While there are many benefits to providing direct cash assistance over other forms, providers should remain aware of the financial market context, particularly in volatile situations.[20] Rapid inflation during a crisis, for instance, might reduce the impact of pre-established assistance amounts. Careful planning and consideration of context can help mitigate unintended negative consequences.

CASE STUDY

CARES Act

Getting Funds to the Public

Over the course of the first several months of 2020, the first cases of SARS-CoV-2 arrived in the US, COVID-19 was declared a national emergency, stay-at-home orders were implemented across the country, and 22 million Americans filed for unemployment.[21] Businesses shuttered, wages were lost, and an additional 17.1 million people faced food insecurity.[22]

In response, the US Congress passed the Coronavirus Aid, Relief, and Economic Security Act (CARES Act) to provide financial relief to the US population. This legislation targeted critical infrastructure, small businesses, and low income and furloughed individuals. It included $367 billion in loans and grants for small businesses and $500 billion in loans to corporations who agreed to not take part in stock buybacks for one year. In addition, airlines received $32 billion and the health care industry $130 billion in direct payouts. State and local governments received $150 billion in aid.

Individual citizens making less than $75,000 received direct payments of $1,200 per adult and $500 per dependent, with gradually reduced amounts for those with larger incomes. Unemployment payments were also increased by $600 per week. This massive stimulus package cost over $2.3 trillion, making it the largest in US history.[23]

CASE STUDY

Mobile Cash Technology in Togo

In December 2020, *Wired* ran a story describing how Togo was using satellite data to distribute funds to vulnerable populations in response to COVID-19.[24] Many governments around the world delivered direct payments to vulnerable populations in order to support people economically through lockdowns and other physical distancing measures. In the US, people received checks in the mail or through direct deposit. The small nation of Togo disbursed payments through a mobile cash technology, using machine learning algorithms that identified signs of poverty, such as the use of inferior roofing material, through satellite photos. Payments were instantaneous, once individuals were confirmed to have an informal occupation or live in a poor area.

Assess Impacts to Regional, National, and International Financial Systems

Disease outbreaks can have financial impacts at the regional, national, and international scale, including reduced labor supply, trade, per capita income, and investment, as well as unemployment, migration away from outbreak sites, and prices of necessities increased across multiple countries in a region.[25] The selection of economic indicators utilized to assess impact on regional, national, or international financial systems depends on the structure of the economy examined, the duration of the problem, and the mode of comparison.

Some common measures used to assess economic impact include:

- **Gross Domestic Product (GDP)**: GDP can help track economic growth, compare economic conditions in one region to another, and reveal which industries may be growing while others decay.[26]
- **Exports, imports and overall trade balance**: These may change in response to disease outbreak and response measures.
- **Remittances**: Comparing pre- and post-outbreak levels of remittances may provide indication of income changes to families.
- **Foreign direct investment**: This is particularly important in less developed nations.

The primary utility of these measures comes through comparison. One may consider comparing values before and after a disease outbreak or comparing numbers in the region of outbreak to an economically similar region that is not currently undergoing a disease outbreak.

Assess Impacts to Local Banks and Economic Systems

Outbreaks, particularly prolonged outbreaks, can threaten global economies and local economic systems. Well-designed fiscal, monetary, and financial-sector policies, though, may lessen the economic risks of pandemics.[27]

Long periods of lockdown have negative impacts on economic growth, although researchers are still trying to understand how different levels of lockdown impact GDP.[28] Travel restrictions are another type of policy measure that may be instituted during disease outbreaks. Nations are working to estimate how these types of policies affect their economies, so they can develop strategies for recovery. Disease outbreaks often impact the tourism sector, which negatively impacts economies that are dependent on that industry for economic growth. Yet these economic impacts are not yet fully understood. Additional analyses of the economic effects of a pandemic are needed to fully understand repercussions on trade, travel, business revenue, and the financial cost of response and recovery.[29]

Other financial systems indicators such as interest rates, commodities, prices, and capital flows are also being evaluated to determine local and wider-scale economic impacts. Pandemic recovery efforts should include targeted efforts to restore local and regional economies in the short, medium, and long term.[30]

Address Shocks to the Financial System

Morbidity and mortality, combined with behavioral changes by consumers trying to avoid disease, may contribute to multisectoral economic shocks.[31] Travel restrictions and fears of infection reduce tourism.[32] Border control measures affecting goods can slow or inhibit trade.[33] Reduced productivity can lead to increased unemployment and lost wages. In-person working conditions may become unsafe, forcing businesses to close and reducing domestic manufacturing and overall economic productivity.[34] Regionally, interruptions in the supply chain and lost income can destabilize sectors like agriculture, generating food insecurity.

Together, these factors may translate to reduced tax revenue while government expenditures rise to meet response needs, leading to budget deficits. Outbreaks may also reduce GDP growth by disincentivizing foreign direct investment (FDI) and reducing productivity. If left unchecked, decreased investment, declining productivity, and rising prices will exacerbate economic distress. Which means that banks and financial systems must anticipate economic interventions early in an outbreak.

> Guinea, Liberia, and Sierra Leone faced between 1.8 and 5.1 percent reductions in GDP growth due to short term effects from the 2014 to 2016 Ebola outbreak.[35]

Respond to Outbreak-Related Shocks

Given the impact of outbreaks on economies, governments have several pathways they may follow to mitigate the economic impact of large-scale disease event. These include:

Central Governments (Fiscal Policy): Because of the outsized impact of outbreaks on tourism, countries with large tourism industries may need to consider distribution of stimulus packages.[36] Access to credit plays an important role in allowing countries to apply nonpharmaceutical interventions without jeopardizing their economies.

Banks (**Monetary Policy**): Regulations put into place after the 2008 financial crisis require large banks to have more liquidity available as demand for dollars rise, which can help contribute to economic stability during an outbreak. Some large economies have used expansionary monetary policy in response to outbreaks, but it is unclear how responsive markets are to these types of interventions.[37]

International Financial System: MDBs can be a source of financial support by providing emergency loans to countries. Nations may take advantage of these loans or Special Drawing Rights- an international reserve asset maintained by the International Monetary Fund transactions, which allow governments to establish a line of credit so they can pay for things like medical countermeasures.[38]

Revitalize Local Economies

Recovery from an outbreak must include addressing any negative impacts on local economies, with a focus on revitalization. Investments may be required in multiple sectors of the economy in order to provide widespread benefits and pull an entire region out of economic distress. This may come in the form of short-term or longer-term projects, some of which may resemble traditional development projects. Governments have helped revitalize agricultural programs through provision of seed, livestock, and farming supplies; utilized cash handouts to populations; made short-term loans more available; launched tourism campaigns; provided housing assistance; and enhanced unemployment benefits.

Governments facing a disease outbreak of any kind have a long and challenging road ahead of them. Even after resolution of the outbreak, vulnerable populations are likely to have experienced a multitude of adverse economic effects. Interventions should address current financial straits, and then ideally provide support for future growth. Furthermore, recovery plans must be structured with resilience against future outbreaks in mind.

Economic Impact of 2001 Foot and Mouth Disease Outbreak
The 2001 outbreak of foot and mouth disease in the UK resulted in estimated costs of £2.06 billion, which covered compensation for livestock destruction, infrastructure disinfection, and appropriate disposal of animal carcasses.[39]

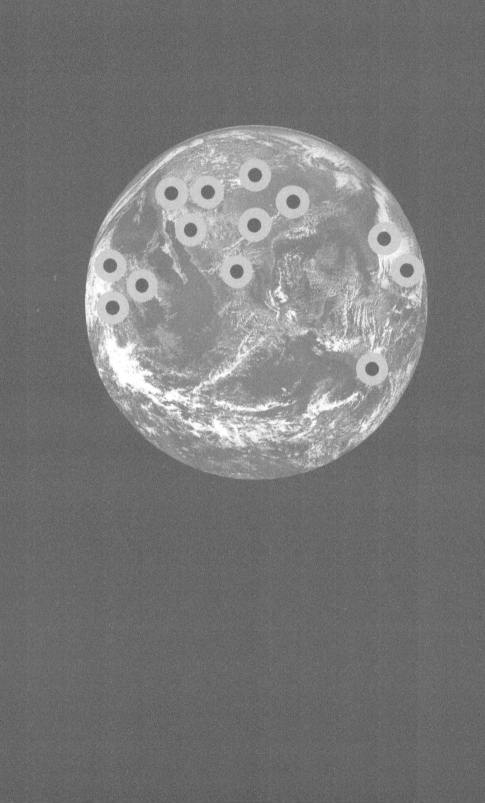

GOVERNANCE

Who Is in Charge and How?

Governance in an outbreak relies on a web of agreements, policies, plans, and guidelines. There are often multiple entities "in charge," depending on the event, location, and spread. Governance for outbreaks includes a collection of international and regional agreements between countries. Countries then create national policies, strategies, and regulations, which then need to be implemented at the local level through specific guidelines. It can get complicated fast, especially when trying to figure out who is in charge of what. In this chapter we review some of the main international and regional agreements, as well as policies often in place to govern disease.

International Agreements

Regional Agreements

National policies, strategies, & regulations

Subnational policies, & local implementation guidelines

LEVELS OF GOVERNANCE

Global Governance

There are a series of international agreements and organizations that all contribute to global governance of outbreaks. International organizations like the WHO and the rest of the UN system each play a role in providing assistance to populations experiencing outbreaks.

The WHO might provide technical guidance on best practices in disease control. The World Food Programme (WFP) might provide logistical assistance. Gavi, the Vaccine Alliance, may assist with the acquisition and delivery of necessary vaccines. WOAH may assist with containing disease spread in animals. In complex outbreaks, almost every part of the UN is engaged, as well as other international organizations, global financing institutions, and country consortia, like the G7 and G20.

International Public Health Treaties

There are more than fifty multilateral international agreements, some binding, some nonbinding, that attempt to govern different areas of outbreaks. Below are some of the key agreements related to outbreaks.

International Health Regulations

See the Declarations and Notifications chapter for more information on PHEICs.

The International Health Regulations (IHR) is a global treaty concluded under the auspices of the World Health Organization. The IHR is an evolution of the International Sanitary Conferences and was significantly revised following the SARS outbreak of 2002–2003. It was adopted by the World Health Assembly in 2005 and entered into force in 2007. The revised agreement governs how to detect, assess, report, and respond to any public health emergencies of international concern (PHEIC). It creates obligations for reporting potential emergencies to the World Health Organization and building and maintaining public health infrastructure to identify and conduct an initial response to an outbreak (including building and sustaining laboratory and epidemiologic capacity at all levels of government); it provides for communication from countries to the WHO; and it defines expected global cooperation in responding to an event. Over time, the interpretation of what it means to have the capacity to detect, assess, report, and respond to public health emergencies has evolved, and the list now includes activities to prevent disease emergence in the first place, and the capacity for health care in addition to public health.

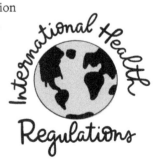

Public Health Emergencies of International Concern (PHEIC)

Through the IHR process, countries report potential PHEICs, which are then assessed by the WHO in Geneva to decide if the event meets the criteria of a PHEIC. To help make that determination, the IHR calls for an Emergency Committee of global experts that provides recommendations to the director general of the WHO on whether a declaration should be made, and makes evidence-based travel and trade recommendations associated with the outbreak. Once an event is declared, the Emergency Committee meets every three months to assess whether an event is still an emergency or if it has resolved.

Between 2005 and 2022, there were seven declared PHEICs:

2009 **Influenza A (H1N1).** A new strain of flu was identified in North America (Mexico and the United States), and in June 2009, it was declared a pandemic as it spread around the world. STATUS: RESOLVED, 2010

2014 **Polio.** Despite massive efforts to dramatically reduce the number of global polio cases from tens of thousands to just a handful of cases, patient counts began to increase around 2013, mostly due to polio circulating in ungoverned regions of the world. Polio was declared a PHEIC in May of 2014, in part to encourage additional efforts by national governments responsible for some of these areas of conflict to increase efforts to find cases and stop the spread. STATUS IN MARCH 2024: ONGOING

2014 **Ebola West Africa.** Ebola virus disease emerged in Guinea in December 2013 and spread across Guinea, Liberia, and Sierra Leone, eventually leading to more than twenty-two thousand cases and eleven thousand deaths, and requiring a previously unprecedented global response. The WHO declared it a PHEIC in early August of 2014. STATUS: RESOLVED, MARCH 2016

2016 **Zika virus disease.** Zika virus spread to the Americas in 2015 and the arbovirus was becoming linked to congenital defects. WHO made the declaration of Zika as a PHEIC in February 2016 even before the full linkages between the virus and microcephaly (babies born with small/deformed heads) was understood. STATUS: RESOLVED, NOVEMBER 2016

2019 **Ebola Democratic Republic of Congo (DRC).** DRC had a history of small Ebola outbreaks, but in 2018, the virus emerged in a region of the country engaged in active conflict, making the response to the outbreak extraordinarily complicated. WHO did not initially consider this outbreak a PHEIC, but eventually made the PHEIC declaration in July of 2019. STATUS: RESOLVED, JUNE 2020

2020 **COVID-19.** In late January of 2020, the WHO declared the outbreak of a novel coronavirus a PHEIC. At the time, the majority of cases were still in China, but cases were rapidly starting to be identified around the world. STATUS: RESOLVED, MAY 2023

2022 **Mpox.** In 2022, mpox, which had been slowly spreading through Nigeria for years, started to emerge in Europe and North America. Cases spread primarily though populations of men who have sex with men, leading to a campaign to get vaccines to this community and antivirals available to identified cases. The WHO declared mpox a PHEIC in late July of 2022. STATUS: RESOLVED, MAY 2023

What's in a Name?

Throughout history, new pathogens have often been named for the geographic location they were first found. Ebola virus disease is named after the Ebola river, where it was first identified in humans. Lyme disease is named after Lyme, Connecticut, where an outbreak was first seen. Ebola Zaire and Ebola Sudan are strains named after countries where they were first seen. MERS stands for Middle East respiratory syndrome—indicating the region in the world where it was first identified. Nipah virus is named after a village in Malaysia where it was first documented to emerge in humans.

It was convenient and made naming things easy. The problem was, though, that the names led to stigma and economic loses. No one wants to plan a cruise on the Ebola river. The names sometimes provoked attacks against particular ethnic communities.

In 2015, WHO issued best practices for naming new diseases, specifically recommending against inclusion of geographic locations, individual names, species, occupational references, or words that might incite public fear," like "fatal."[1]

The naming convention grandfathered in existing disease names, but in 2022, scientists and communities around the world petitioned the WHO to change the name of "Monkeypox," claiming it led to racism and stigma. In November 2022, the virus was officially renamed mpox.

Nagoya Protocol of the Convention on Biological Diversity

The Nagoya Protocol on Access to Genetic Resources and the Fair and Equitable Sharing of Benefits Rising from Their Utilization of the Convention of Biological Diversity (also known as the Nagoya Protocol of the CBD) is an international agreement adopted in 2010. The Nagoya Protocol addresses genetic resources, such as plants or animals, in countries, and for the purpose of outbreaks, is often applied to pathogens. It states that countries own the genetic resources within their borders and anyone who wants access to those resources needs permission from the country (prior informed consent), and has to have a contract in place that spells out mutually agreed upon terms that balance access to the material with equitable sharing of benefits from the material.

For outbreaks, the Nagoya Protocol means that if researchers want access to a pathogen causing an outbreak in one country, they need to get consent from the country of origin and develop terms so that, for example, if the researcher develops a vaccine, the country receives royalties. The benefit to the country may also be nonmonetary, such as acknowledgments, joint publications, or joint research efforts.

Biological Weapons Convention (BWC)

The Biological and Toxins Weapons Convention (BWC) was the first treaty to ban an entire class of weapons. It bans the development, production, acquisition, transfer, and stockpiling of biological and toxin weapons. (Regarding use, the preamble directs readers to the Geneva Protocol of 1925, which bans the use of the weapon.) The language in the treaty most relevant to outbreaks is Article VII and X.

Article X is about cooperation and assistance, noting that States Parties "have the right to participate in the fullest possible exchange of equipment, materials and information for peaceful purposes."[2] Member States work with each other to build capacity around things like disease surveillance or research collaborations.

Article VII says that nations should come to the aid of other nations if they have been exposed to a violation of the treaty. This means that if a biological weapon is used in one country, the other countries that are party to the BWC are obliged to help with the response. Because it can be hard to differentiate a deliberate use of a biological weapon from a naturally occurring event, in practice this article means that nations should have the capacity for preparedness and response to outbreaks. It also means that there should be a global system in place to assist with preparedness and response efforts.[3]

United Nations Secretary General's Mechanism for the Investigation of Alleged Use of Chemical or Biological Weapons (UNSGM)

The Biological Weapons Convention notes that if there is an alleged use event, the allegations can be taken to the United Nations Secretary General. Approved by a UN General Assembly Resolution in the 1980s, the United Nations Secretary General (UNSG) has a mechanisms that allows him or her to investigate allegations of biological or chemical weapons use events.[4] Once an allegation and request for an investigation is made, the UNSG then decides whether to mount a fact-finding team to the site(s) of the alleged incident(s). The members of the team may represent diverse geographic areas as well as expertise.

The results of a fact-finding mission are reported back to all member states of the UN. These findings can then contribute to any attribution assessment that may be made.

Investigating Chemical Weapons Use in Syria Using the UNSGM

The UNSGM had only been used about a dozen times since its creation in the 1980s, including four times during the Iran/Iraq war. In subsequent years, the Chemical Weapons Convention was adopted, and with it the creation of the Organization for the Prohibition of Chemical Weapons (OPCW) in 1997. Part of the OPCW mission is to respond to the use or alleged use of chemical weapons, including conducting a formal investigation. Through a Resolution adopted by the General Assembly, the UN established an agreement of cooperation between the UN and OPCW to "closely cooperate with the Secretary-General in cases of the alleged use of chemical weapons."[5] In 2011, the UN entered into a Memorandum of Understanding with the WHO, in which the WHO agreed that upon the Secretary General receiving a report on alleged use, the WHO would assist in the health aspects of an investigation.[6] These two agreements were operationalized when the UNSGM was activated in March 2013 to investigate alleged chemical weapons use in Syria.

A fact-finding mission was organized, led by Professor Ake Sellstrom from Sweden, with a team from the OPCW and WHO. The investigative team presented its findings in September 2013, confirming that chemical weapons had been used against a civilian population.

Diplomatic Relations

Outbreaks often lead to social, economic, and political consequences in addition to health outcomes. The impacts of outbreaks may require joint global cooperation, cohesion, and multilateralism to protect international systems and preserve order.[7] Strong diplomatic relations between nations can enable multiple perspectives to come together to shape and manage the global policy environment for health.[8]

Outbreaks cause far-reaching issues beyond just the health sectors, creating a need for international assistance and partnerships. Health diplomacy, guided by international laws, norms, agreements, and donor assistance, can help mobilize global stakeholders to manage the crisis collaboratively with the necessary resources and humanitarian aid. Yet developing intergovernmental cooperation between regional, national, and international stakeholders requires investment in the institutions and capacity that support these partnerships.[9] Ultimately diplomatic relations help build a common position on disease outbreaks and allow countries to share best practices, pool technical and resource capacities, and ensure peace and stability.[10]

Consulate Affairs Repatriated Americans Stranded Overseas

at the Start of the COVID-19 Pandemic

COVID-19 emerged and began to spread around the world in the spring of 2020, leading to a string of rapid travel restrictions and policies from airlines, cancelling international flights. In March 2020, the US State Department issued a worldwide alert telling Americans not to travel and advising those overseas to return immediately.[11] Many Americans were still abroad and in some countries, such as Peru, no commercial flights were available—the government of Peru had banned all flights in and out of the country.

The State Department set up a repatriation task force. They chartered airlines and set up repatriation flights from Peru. They established partnerships with the military, police, and the foreign ministry to secure safe travel for Americans throughout the country to get to regional airports. They set up communication channels between Americans in Peru and the US embassy. The consular affairs team fielded more than ten thousand emails and calls from Americans, providing information on who needed to be prioritized for flights back to the US. These efforts, though, required diplomatic engagement, as the government of Peru wanted assurances that Peruvian citizens in the US would be allowed to travel home before allowing American citizens to leave Peru.[12] Some claimed the government of Peru was holding the Americans hostage in order to ensure safe passage of Peruvians out of the US. Peru pushed back and called it a matter of reciprocity. Through active negotiations and diplomacy, by March 23, five hundred Americans had been flown back to the US.[13] By June, more than eight thousand Americans had been repatriated just from Peru.[14]

Regional Governance

Coordination with Neighboring Nations

Agreements between and among countries to coordinate on the activities needed to prepare for and respond to an outbreak can help facilitate improved detection, control, and overall response capacity. Such agreements facilitate any number of activities that can advance outbreak preparedness and response, particularly as diseases spread across borders. More and more regions are establishing regional organizations, or regional centers for disease control, to formally coordinate outbreak preparedness and response. Even where such entities do not exist, neighboring nations are creating agreements and setting up communication avenues for response.

During the preparedness phase, cross-border agreements, data sharing agreements, and plans for sharing assets like laboratory capacity or epidemiologic response teams can be created or updated. Agreements may be considered between countries that share a border, region, or continent; countries between which there is significant air traffic; and countries around the globe that may assist outbreak response in a variety of ways. The establishment or updating of agreements may continue during an outbreak, and agreements may be modified after an outbreak based on lessons learned.

Examples of key activities that cross-border agreements can be used to support include:

See the "Surveillance" section of the Epidemiology chapter to learn more.

Surveillance: Cross-border biosurveillance can enable improved biological intelligence. Agreed-upon cross-border surveillance systems at points of entry (or another mechanism of regularly sharing data and information between neighboring countries) supports regional disease surveillance.[15]

See the Staffing and Training chapter and the Emergency Operations and Logistics chapter for more information.

Personnel deployment: Legal and regulatory processes and logistical plans can allow for rapid cross-border deployment and receipt of public health and medical personnel. Regional/international collaboration assists countries in overcoming the legal, logistical, and regulatory challenges to deployment and receipt of such personnel.[16] Visas, licensing, and customs duties are all items for consideration during this planning process.

See the Data chapter and the "Data and Specimen Sharing Policies" section later in this chapter for more information on countries' policies on data and sample sharing.

Information sharing: Surveillance, epidemiology, and emergency response information relevant to outbreaks should be shared internationally, according to the World Health Organization.[17] Countries should consider the kind of data and information they will be required to share, and the mechanisms for doing so, such that prompt sharing can occur during an emergency.

Sample sharing: International transport of biological samples may be necessary if in-country laboratory testing resources are insufficient. Other countries may also wish to sequence and otherwise analyze pathogen samples to support epidemiological investigation and medical countermeasure development. Agreements between and among countries and international laboratories for this purpose can be worked out in advance. Material transfer agreements ensure the movement of samples is mutually agreed upon between the provider and recipient.[18]

Medical countermeasure sharing: Some countries may wish to send or receive medical countermeasures to other countries to assist with outbreak response. While the availability of specific countermeasures for a given emerging disease may be limited or nonexistent, countries may still wish to work out good-faith agreements for these countermeasures in advance of their development; they may also determine mechanisms for sharing available generic drugs and medical supplies with countries in need.

Migration: The continued movement of people (legally or illegally) during an outbreak requires consideration, including for such elements as point of entry capacity development and border health risk mitigation such as through strengthened surveillance. Organizations such as the International Organization for Migration can provide guidance for planning, developing, coordinating, and exercising standard operating procedures and other supportive activities to protect migrants and official personnel operating at points of entry.[19]

While bilateral agreements between countries and the WHO have become common to facilitate activities like information sharing, regional coordination among groups of countries lags.[20] Improved regional health security strengthening may be achieved through the promulgation and maintenance of regional cross-border agreements.

Travel and Border Restrictions

In public health crises, countries may resort to travel restrictions or full or partial closure of their borders to prevent disease introduction and transmission, though there is ongoing research on the effectiveness of border closures in mitigating the spread of disease, and such effectiveness measurements are correlated with types of disease transmission.[21]

Under the International Health Regulations, states that implement health measures interfering with international traffic, such as travel bans, are required to notify the WHO within forty-eight hours and provide a rationale based on scientific evidence or guidance from the WHO (Art. 43).[22] Travel restrictions that meet the threshold for reporting under Article 43 include, but are not limited to:

- Complete border closures
- Trade and travel bans (universal or applied to specific countries)
- Refusal of visas
- Inspection of baggage or cargo, especially involving the refusal and/or delay of entry of goods and other items for more than twenty-four hours
- Refusal of entry/departure for more than twenty-four hours (such as mandatory quarantine periods)[23]

There are social, economic, and humanitarian challenges and costs created by travel restrictions that need to be weighed against the potential effectiveness of mitigating disease spread. Border closures go against human mobility rights and may create discrimination and stigmatization of people from affected countries.[24] Travel restrictions can also interfere with the outbreak response by inhibiting the flow of supplies and medical personnel and causing economic damage.[25] Without major economic or humanitarian intervention, they can also cause shortages in food, energy, and other essential resources.[26]

See the Security chapter for more information about enforcing border closures.

Additional travel regulations, such as vaccination prerequisites, entry/exit screening, and personal protective equipment requirements may be put in place during a response. Many countries will post travel regulations on a government website managed by their ministry of foreign affairs and/or health. Countries or international organizations may also produce lists of travel restrictions that apply directly to citizens or all travelers. Tracking these measures is important to manage the response and ensure travelers are informed about regulations.

Yellow Cards

International travelers may be familiar with the WHO's International Certificate of Vaccination or Prophylaxis, also referred to as the Yellow Card. The Yellow Card is a paper form that lists an individual's vaccines. This form is used to document whether an individual has received a yellow fever vaccine, which is required for entry into certain countries.

Unfortunately, because this is a paper card, it is easy to create forgeries. Some nations have started working on more secure digital versions, but these have yet to be adopted by the global community.

CASE STUDY

Travel Restrictions during Omicron

Countries have applied travel regulations of varying intensity in response to SARS, Ebola, and COVID-19. During the SARS-CoV-2 pandemic, nearly every country in the world implemented some form of border closure.[27]

When the Omicron variant of SARS-CoV-2 emerged in November 2021, governments around the world quickly took measures to restrict travel in order to slow the spread of the variant. Over a three-week period, more than 220 national-level policies were issued. Initially, many countries established entry bans and flight suspensions from southern Africa, the region that was first to alert the world to the new variant but not the first region to have cases. Regardless, policies continued to target this region, even as the Omicron variant was identified around the world. Over the course of several weeks, most nations rolled out more nuanced travel restrictions, including enhanced screening, but there was little coordination on testing, quarantine, or other travel restrictions between countries.[28]

Trade Restrictions

Restricting trade is another tool sometimes used to prevent or delay the spread of disease, one governed by the International Health Regulations as well as international agreements under the Food and Agriculture Organization (FAO) and the World Trade Organization (WTO). Trade restrictions may be related to food products, agriculture, or possibly contaminated goods. Nations also have, in the past, restricted the export of items they deemed critical to their own response or national security, such as food, energy, personal protective equipment, or medical countermeasures produced within their borders, although such actions are often admonished.[29]

While the WTO typically prohibits export restrictions, it allows exceptions for measures taken to protect human health.[30] Countries that do decide to implement trade restrictions are obligated to provide the WHO "within 48 hours of implementation, the public health rationale and relevant scientific information for the measures implemented."[31] Both the WTO and WHO require that any trade restrictions issued be "targeted, temporary, and transparent."[32]

CASE STUDY

Anthrax Spread through Drums

In 2006, a Scottish man became sick with anthrax. It turns out he was exposed to bacteria from a contaminated animal hide drum that had been imported from West Africa.[33] In 2007, a drum maker in Connecticut developed cutaneous anthrax from contaminated goat hides that had been imported from Guinea. One of his children also developed anthrax, most likely from cross contamination of their home.[34] And in 2009, a woman developed gastrointestinal anthrax in New Hampshire after participating in a drumming circle.

CASE STUDY

Mpox in the US, circa 2003

In 2003, small mammals from West Africa, including Gambian rats, were imported into the US as part of what was an extremely extensive trade of exotic pets. The small mammals were imported to Texas and happened to be infected with mpox. The rats shared cages and bedding in the US with domesticated prairie dogs. The prairie dogs, which also became infected with mpox, were then sold to households throughout the Midwest before they showed any signs of illness. The infected pet prairie dogs eventually infected forty-seven humans across six states.[35]

National and Subnational Governance

There are many decision makers in an outbreak and depending on the jurisdictional authorities of a geographic area, governance of an outbreak may be split between global, national, subnational (like state level), and local leaders. This can make for an extremely confusing landscape and difficulties understanding who is in charge.

Before an outbreak, national and local preparation plans should be formulated with government and community representatives and other key stakeholders. These plans should be integrated into general national health emergency response planning, indicate priorities regarding the allocation of finite resources, and include relevant information for clinical health services such as:

- mapping of resources;
- a comprehensive list of practitioners (including mental health) trained and locally available to offer appropriate advice and to participate in a response to an infectious disease outbreak (ideally the list should address competencies, areas of expertise, gaps in resources, etc.);
- communication plans; and
- an appropriate, realistic training plan for personnel.[36]

During the outbreak, interventions should be guided by careful planning and prompt evaluation of the local context. Collaborations should be intersectional, bringing together health and non-health agencies to deliver needed services.

Create Interagency Committees

The creation of a governmental interagency committee is crucial to the effective, timely, and coordinated multisectoral response to a public health event.

The interagency coordinating committee should include officials across all relevant ministries, agencies, and departments that contribute to the prevention, detection, and response to public health emergencies. Examples of stakeholders that should be represented on the interagency coordinating committee include the directorates of health services, directorates of veterinary services, the food safety agency, disaster management authorities, humanitarian response agencies, environmental protection authorities, regulatory bodies, national reference laboratories (human and animal), and the public health emergency operations center. The committee should not be formed ad hoc at the outset of an emerging event but rather meet regularly, such as on a monthly or quarterly basis, in order to be most effective at mitigating and rapidly responding to new threats.

Routine activities that can be performed by the interagency coordinating committee include:

- sharing information on each sector's risk monitoring;
- reviewing stocks of equipment for event investigation and response; and
- providing recommendations on ongoing or emerging events of potential public health importance.

It is important to note that the information sharing that forms the core of the interagency coordinating committee's mandate and purpose should be multidirectional, with all stakeholders receiving mutual benefit to advance their own sectoral priorities.[37]

Identify and Address Legislative Gaps

A country's response to an outbreak is influenced by legislation, regulations, and administrative requirements at the national, state/province, and/or local level. With this in mind, it is critical to identify which policies and expectations are pertinent to the threat at hand, and what entities have authority, as well as the limits of that authority.

Regular assessment of legislation pertaining to public health risks and emergencies is critical to the prevention and management of disease outbreaks. The assessment of public health legislation, though, can be a challenging project and requires the examination of existing legal codes, interviews with key stakeholders, and consultation with local legal experts. A wide variety of gaps may exist at every level of governance. Furthermore, legislative overlap may exist such that multiple institutions may be given responsibility for the same task. These overlaps and gaps may lead to confusion, inefficiency, and delays during emergent conditions.

Manage Potential Clashes in National Policy

Infectious disease outbreaks create unique policy challenges between different levels of government agencies that require coordinated responses.[38] Health officials must prioritize national interests so that the security of individuals and communities directly and indirectly affected by the disease outbreak is maintained. Although national governments serve the primary role in outbreak preparedness and response policy, local and subnational governments are on the frontline of response implementation. Given the territorial nature of outbreaks, local authorities are often best suited to understand and respond to the unique challenges created in their community, even when jurisdictional authority for decision making lies with a state or national government.[39] Thus, thorough and ongoing communication and coordination between governmental levels are required to manage clashes in policy and best protect communities' public health and security.

Throughout different phases of the outbreak, officials may switch between decentralized and centralized models of governance.[40] Decentralized models serve best in the initial and recovery phases of outbreaks when more localized and tailored policy responses are required. Broad-reaching centralized policy responses may be most effective during outbreak peaks when expedited executive policy can help create a more effective general response.

Expand Access to Medical Countermeasures

A country's ability to expand access to drugs and vaccines during a disease outbreak is critical to advance medical responses and protect populations. Increasing access to drugs, devices, personal protective equipment (PPE), and vaccines can occur by states issuing emergency use orders, expanded market authorizations, and other rapid regulatory pathways designed to increase access to necessary products during an emergency. Expansion to access, though, may require boosting manufacturing, transport, and storage infrastructure to support the production, delivery, and distribution of health resources to populations. This can be particularly challenging if maintaining a cold chain is required. Supply chain management is also necessary to ensure the materials needed for adequate storage and handling of these supplies can be accessed.

If drug and vaccine products do not yet have market authorizations, governments can consider granting preliminary emergency authorization while ensuring that any medical countermeasures utilized for the outbreak response meet expedited regulatory requirements. Some countries have designated departments or agencies with dedicated, established evaluation processes to issue emergency market authorizations for new drugs. The European Medicines Agency (EMA) can grant "conditional marketing authorization" during public health emergencies, such as pandemics, to support the development of medicines that address unmet medical needs. In this context, less comprehensive clinical data than normally required for a product in the regulatory process is needed because the immediate availability of the product could be immensely beneficial.[41] Similarly, the US Food and Drug Administration (FDA) has the Emergency Use Authorization (EUA) authority to facilitate the availability and use of medical countermeasures needed during public health emergencies. The FDA can utilize the EUA to allow use of unapproved medical products given certain statutory criteria have been met and there are no adequate, approved, and available alternatives.[42]

The World Health Organization (WHO) Emergency Use Listing Procedure (EUL) "is a risk-based procedure for assessing and listing unlicensed vaccines, therapeutics and in vitro diagnostics with the ultimate aim of expediting the availability of these products to people affected by a public health emergency."[43] The WHO EUL aims to help UN agencies and member states determine if specific new products designed and created to mitigate effects from disease outbreaks are adequate for widespread use and uptake. The WHO EUL is based on evaluations of a product's quality, safety, efficacy, and performance data; ultimately, in the context of a public health emergency of international concern (PHEIC) and given uncertainties, the benefits of the product must outweigh any foreseeable risks in order for the EUL criteria to be met.

Global Equitable Distribution of COVID-19 MCMs

At the beginning of the COVID-19 pandemic, the WHO launched a partnership called the ACT-Accelerator (ACT-A) to coordinate a global effort to develop tools to fight the disease.[44] One large focus of ACT-A was to support equitable distribution of therapeutics and vaccines, and ACT-A specifically created a vaccine introduction toolbox to expand drug access within countries.[45] The toolbox was in line with the detailed WHO publication *Guidance on Developing a National Deployment and Vaccination Plan for COVID-19 Vaccines*, which is about how national strategies can be created to roll out and increase access to vaccines.[46] Key messages from this guidance included the primary need for countries to have national regulatory authorities to use risk-based approaches through regulatory pathways to assess vaccines. Sadly, ACT-A was unable to ensure the full, equitable distribution of COVID-19 vaccine around the world.

Data and Specimen Sharing Policies

During an outbreak, data and pathogen samples can provide critical insight into the threat and guide an appropriate, effective response. Sharing this data, though, can become complicated. Therefore, countries must develop policies that are aligned with their national implementation of the CBD and Nagoya in order to have secure, straight-forward, and efficient movement of information and samples internationally and domestically.[47]

See the section in this chapter about the Nagoya Protocol for more information.

Clinical, epidemiological, laboratory, diagnostic, genetic, and vaccination data are some of the types of information that may be shared in an outbreak.[48] Policies should provide stipulations on appropriate rationales for sharing information and logistical needs for transferring data. These regulations on sharing of data and specimens should also be flexible and updated regularly.

There are many challenges associated with rapid sharing of data and specimens:

- Data protection including consent for individual patient data and country-specific legislation
- Tension between rapid sharing and accuracy and the risk of misinformation
- Political and cultural issues

- Reciprocity among nations and/or individuals
- Poor systems for knowledge curation
- Issues with academic journal publication
- Inadequate time and/or resources[49]

Policies should be developed and updated with these challenges in mind, prioritizing consistent and clear regulatory frameworks, improved communication among stakeholders, and sociocultural awareness. Emergency response teams should remain apprised of changes in policies and practices that affect data and specimen sharing. This will ensure that movement of information and samples aligns with the current legal framework and that they reach their intended recipients safely and promptly.

SHARING GENETIC SEQUENCE DATA

To learn more about what GSD is and how it is used, go to the Laboratories and Lab Analysis chapter.

See the "GISAID" case study in the Outbreak Data chapter.

Genetic sequence data (GSD) is now an essential part of disease surveillance, pathogen research, and epidemiological investigations.[50] Rapid, ethical, and equitable sharing of GSD with the international community enables researchers and scientists around the globe to collaborate more effectively to characterize a causative agent, understand its spread, and develop diagnostics, treatments, and vaccines.[51] While data that describe the genetic sequence of a pathogen can be a valuable tool for understanding and controlling infectious disease outbreaks, it is essential that the data is collected, analyzed, and shared following appropriate data governance practices.[52] Tenets of good GSD governance include transparency, accountability, appropriate recognition, patient privacy, and mutual benefit.[53]

To reach national and international stakeholders, sequence data can be uploaded to online databases such as GenBank, ENA, DDBJ, or GISAID depending on the pathogen and the interests of data ownership. Among others, these stakeholders may include epidemiologists studying transmission dynamics, health officials looking to make decisions for their own countries, and law enforcement agencies working on attribution investigations.

Information sharing among health care providers, health officials, security professionals, environmental experts, and laboratories is needed to pool such information and make it available for public health benefit. The data governance surrounding GSD collection, use, and publication is still developing as new technology and uses emerge, and new concerns around privacy arise.[54]

Determine Policy on Mandatory Screenings and/or Testing

Screening and/or testing for disease is a fundamental tool in public health and preventive medicine, and can be critical for outbreak response. Sometimes public health officials may wish to institute a mandatory screening or testing program, but this may be challenging when it threatens civil liberties.[55]

Policies on mandatory screenings and/or testing should be integrated into the emergency response plan to inform protocols. Collecting surveillance information is generally mandatory and ethically acceptable on the grounds of public interest. Compulsory testing should be utilized as a last resort and in a manner as unobtrusive as possible. Testing should be transparent, fair, and nondiscriminatory as well.[56] These policies should be flexible, allowing for adjustment to the unique scenario of an outbreak. They should acknowledge the needs of the community and the individual, providing criteria and guidelines for promoting health among all. They should describe when mandatory screenings and testing are appropriate and how they can safely and effectively be implemented.

Informed consent prior to testing or screening presents an opportunity for individuals to maintain their autonomy and foster a collaborative relationship between citizens and health professionals. The policy on mandatory screenings and/or testing should outline an appropriate protocol for this approach, acknowledging when informed consent is acceptable, how a patient would be informed, if and how their decision would be documented, and what the next steps would be.[57]

Determine Vaccination Policies

PRIORITIZATION

In an outbreak, it is often the case that the availability of a medical countermeasure does not equal demand. There are seldom enough drugs or vaccines for all the people who need to access them. Because of this, nations and even subnational entities develop processes and policies to prioritize access to vaccines and other medical countermeasures when there is limited supply. Normally, the policy for how such a process works is established well in advance of an event. The decision making itself, though, will be informed by the specific pathogen of concern's mode of transmission and virulence, the clinical progression of disease, and other factors as they become more well-understood. Prioritization policies are often designed to protect the most vulnerable members of a population, reduce disease spread to protect the greatest number of people, protect workers key to the outbreak response and critical infrastructure, minimize years of life lost, maximize the quality of life years saved, or safeguard national security.[58]

Groups selected as high priority may include:

- health care workers
- emergency service workers
- infrastructure/essential workers
- people of specific age groups (depending on disease threat)

- people with preexisting conditions (that may make them more vulnerable)
- socially vulnerable groups (e.g., homeless people, prisoners)
- groups that amplify the spread of contagious disease (e.g., school-age children)

Furthermore, prioritization should take into consideration the rate of expected adverse effects.[59]

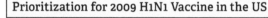

See the Declarations and Notifications chapter for more information about PHEIC and pandemic declarations.

CASE STUDY

Prioritization for 2009 H1N1 Vaccine in the US

In the summer of 2009, H1N1 influenza was circulating around the world and had been declared both a PHEIC and a pandemic by the WHO. A vaccine was developed, but it was initially in limited supply. The US CDC Advisory Committee on Immunization Practices (ACIP)—a panel of medical and public health experts—met in late July 2009 to identify who would receive the vaccine first. Prioritization groups were as follows:

- **Pregnant women**: at higher risk of complications
- **Household contacts and caregivers of children under six months**: infants were at higher risk of complications and were not eligible for vaccines
- **Health care workers and emergency medical service personnel**: to combat absenteeism and to ensure these workers didn't pass the virus to vulnerable populations
- **Children and young adults six months to twenty-four years of age**: due to spread in schools and daycares, and the living conditions of young adults
- **Adults age twenty-five to sixty-four with underlying health conditions**: due to higher risk of medical complication from influenza[60]

Interestingly, older adults (over sixty-five) were not prioritized for vaccine as their risk of infection was less than in younger age groups. This may have been due to partial immunity cause by exposure to similar influenza strains earlier in life.

DISTRIBUTION

It is not enough to just have a vaccine or other medical countermeasure. It has to be distributed to the people that need it. Governments at all levels create plans to distribute vaccines in an outbreak once they are available.[61] The scale of distribution is dependent on the type of outbreak; a pandemic response will require mass vaccination efforts, whereas an outbreak that is local or regional or containable through strategies like ring vaccination will require more targeted efforts. For vaccines requiring refrigeration, distribution strategies must take into consideration the need for a strong cold chain from shipment to administration.[62] To accomplish this, governments must coordinate between local public health officials, vaccine manufacturers, nonprofits, community leaders, private health care systems and pharmacies, and private sector logistics companies.[63] This can become extraordinarily complicated, but is a critical part of response.

Getting the vaccine to the people is just one step. Getting the people to take the vaccine is another. Policies and plans must be established to promote vaccine uptake among the populations at risk. Vaccination campaigns should provide information to combat vaccine hesitancy, counter mis- and disinformation, and ensure adequate uptake and coverage.[64]

REQUIREMENTS

Once vaccines are available in surplus, governments, as well as other organizations, may institute proof-of-vaccination requirements for entry in public spaces, transportation, schools, workplaces, and other venues of potential transmission. Countries may also institute vaccine requirements for international travelers. Vaccination and other risk prevention requirements are regular practice for diseases such as yellow fever, poliomyelitis, and measles.[65]

Reverse Previously Issued Restrictions—Always Adapting

Previously issued restrictions may be reversed following a phased approach while an outbreak is still ongoing or once an outbreak has been declared over. This includes rollback of restrictions on travel, trade, curfew, business hours or openings, gathering sizes, and burials, among other measures.[66]

The appropriate authority should issue a statement about lifting the restrictions, making clear whether all restrictions are reversed or only some. Announcements on lifting restrictions should be made using various communication sources to ensure that the public is aware of the changes and possible nuances. In the case of a gradual reversal of previously issued restrictions, clear guidance should be provided to health workers, the private sector, and the public on the phasing of the process, timeline, key indicators, behavior guidance, and any remaining restrictions.

Rollback of measures requires coordination among the different government structures involved in monitoring and enforcing restrictions, as well as collaboration with those impacted by the restrictions, in order to balance effective public health response and individual rights. Reversing restrictions might also require legal actions, official declarations, or orders depending on the authority that issued the initial restriction. Governments may choose to publish official guidance for strategies on lifting restrictions.

Reversing restrictions must be based on evidence and science-based decision making, similar to the decisions to impose restrictions in the first place.

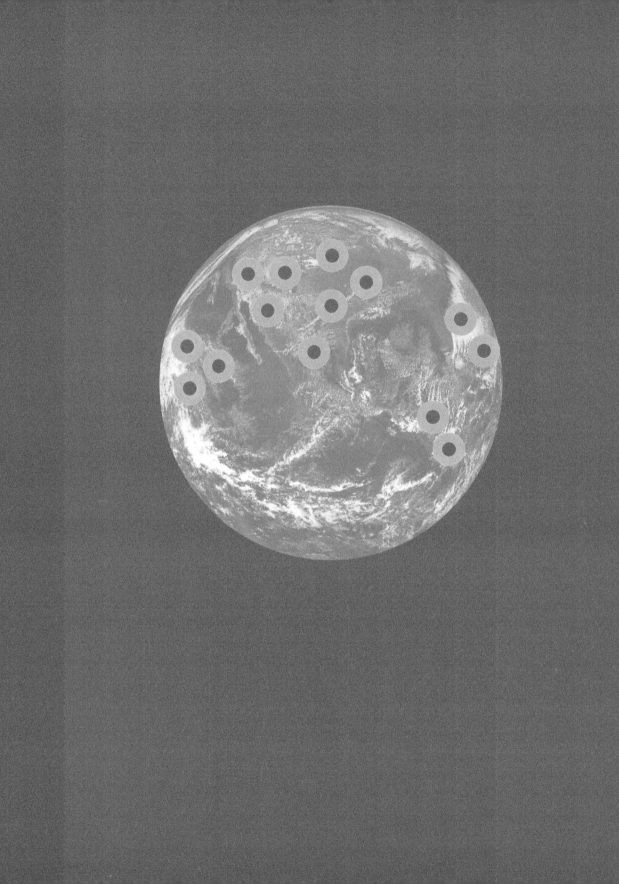

14

ANIMAL HEALTH AND SAFETY

Tackling Zoonotic Outbreaks

Just like humans, animals get sick. Sometimes the diseases that impact or live inside animals can "crossover" or "jump" species. These are zoonoses, or zoonotic diseases: illnesses caused by viruses, bacteria, and fungi that can spread between animals and humans. An estimated 60 percent of known human infections are zoonotic, and more than 75 percent of emerging diseases are transmitted from animals.[1] By preventing and mitigating the emergence and occurrence of zoonotic diseases, we can avoid the ripple effects they can have on public health, the environment, trade, food supply, and the economy and protect animal and human health.

Humans have interacted with and used animals for companionship, transportation, sustenance, and materials to make clothing, shelters, tools, and medicines for thousands of years. The proximity of humans and animals, whether they are pets, livestock, or wild animals, creates opportunities for infectious disease to spread. These opportunities have only risen as humans and animals come into increasingly close contact as a result of urbanization, deforestation, climate change, and advanced transportation.

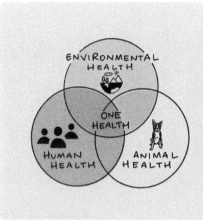

One Health

Human, animal, and environmental health are interdependent. One Health is an approach to disease surveillance, detection, response, and recovery that recognizes this interconnected relationship and reacts accordingly. It means coordinating, communicating, and collaborating across the numerous sectors involved in human, animal, and environmental health. A One Health approach to outbreak management is important because it allows health personnel to see things from different perspectives, prevent outbreaks from occurring, and design more holistic responses when they do happen.

See the Declarations and Notifications chapter for more information about PHEIC and pandemic declarations.

Zoonotic diseases have been around as long as humans have. Some zoonoses exist endemically in regions or occur seasonally, like Q-fever, brucellosis, Lyme disease, rabies, anthrax, Rift Valley fever, and zoonotic TB. New diseases can also develop; emerging zoonotic diseases include H1N1, Middle East respiratory syndrome (MERS-CoV), highly pathogenic avian influenza (HPAI), Zika, and Ebola virus disease (EVD). Some diseases can start as zoonotic and mutate into human-only strains. Many zoonotic diseases are also categorized as vector-borne—meaning the pathogen is transmitted to a human via a vector, such as a mosquito or tick. Examples of this include Lyme disease, West Nile virus, leishmaniasis, and Crimean-Congo hemorrhagic fever. These diseases can cause severe short-term infections or long-term chronic morbidity.

In this chapter, we discuss the animal health and safety measures taken to limit the spread of emerging, reemerging, and endemic zoonotic diseases, and what is done when a zoonotic illness is detected.

CASE STUDY

Rift Valley Fever

Rift Valley fever (RVF) is a zoonotic viral disease that primarily affects livestock like cattle, buffalo, sheep, goats, and camels in sub-Saharan Africa, but it can spread to humans via contact with an infected animal or a bite from a mosquito carrying the virus. The transmission cycle of the virus is a favorite example of public health experts to demonstrate the interconnectedness of environmental, animal, and human factors that can trigger an outbreak.

In a regular enzootic cycle, *Aedes* mosquitoes serve as the primary reservoir and vector for RVF, infecting mostly wild animals. However, during exceptionally high periods of rainfall and flooding (like during the weather phenomenon El Niño) *Aedes* mosquito eggs hatch early and across wider areas because of the

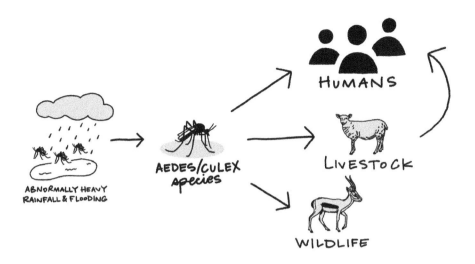

AEDES/CULEX *species*

ABNORMALLY HEAVY RAINFALL & FLOODING

HUMANS

LIVESTOCK

WILDLIFE

floodplains. The infected *Aedes* are then able to spread the virus to livestock herds, where it is amplified among livestock and to other mosquito species like *Culex*. Humans working or living near infected livestock are then more likely to be exposed to either a sick animal or an infected mosquito and get sick.

RVF outbreaks are preventable through sustained animal vaccination. Vaccinated animals cannot become infected, thus cannot transmit the virus to a mosquito, which cannot then transmit it to a human. Scientists have also developed early warning systems to track rainfall patterns to predict outbreaks, allowing health officials to put prevention measures in place and respond early.

CASE STUDY

Canary in a Coalmine? Try Flamingo in the Bronx Zoo

West Nile virus (WNV) is a mosquito-borne disease without treatment or vaccination. While most people infected with WNV do not develop symptoms, 1 in 5 may develop a febrile illness, and 1 in 150 may develop a severe condition—encephalitis, inflammation of the brain.[2]

WNV arrived in the US in 1999. Late that summer, crows began dying around New York City, raising the concern of chief pathologist at the Bronx Zoo, Tracey McNamara. Then three flamingos in the Bronx Zoo suddenly died, followed by a snowy owl, a bald eagle, and some cormorants.[3] When McNamara examined the birds, she found that they had encephalitis, brain hemorrhages, and heart lesions, suggesting they were killed by the same viral infection as the crows.[4]

Around the same time in Queens, health officials were struggling to identify the etiology of encephalitis cases in several elderly patients. On September 3, the US CDC declared an outbreak of St. Louis encephalitis in NYC. Given the timing and similarity of human and animal cases, McNamara encouraged the US CDC to reexamine the human cases for a possible connection but

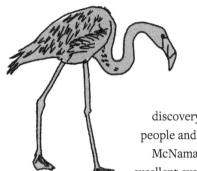

was dismissed.[5] Ultimately, support and additional testing from the US Army Medical Research Institute of Infectious Disease and the National Veterinary Services Laboratory revealed that the deaths of crows and Bronx Zoo birds and the human encephalitis cases were related, leading to the discovery of WNV in NYC, an outbreak that infected at least fifty-nine people and killed seven.[6]

McNamara's effort and the eventual discovery of WNV in NYC is an excellent example of the importance of a One Health approach to outbreak preparedness and response, as well as the value of animal health events as sentinels for potential human public health events.

Myths and Zoonoses

Some of the most enduring monsters of folklore and popular culture—vampires, werewolves, and zombies—were inspired by infectious diseases. Diseases are frightening, especially when there appears to be no explanation or there are no cures, and so people turn to the supernatural.

Bram Stoker's mother's stories from the 1832 deadly cholera outbreak in Sligo, Ireland, inspired him as he wrote *Dracula*.[7] Rabies in particular, transmitted through the bite of an infected animal, is suspected to be the disease behind many supernatural creatures, vampires and werewolves included. In fact, "during the period when dramatic tales of vampires were first emerging from Eastern Europe, a major epidemic of rabies in dogs, wolves, and other wild animals was recorded in the same region between 1721–1728."[8]

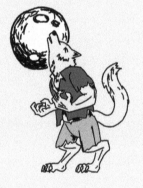

Zoonotic Disease Surveillance

Surveillance of domestic animals, livestock, and wildlife is the "systematic ongoing collection, collation, and analysis of information related to animal health and the timely dissemination of information so that action can be taken."[9]

When a surveillance system captures a potentially zoonotic disease, the cascade of events, from conducting an epidemiological investigation to collecting samples and processing them in a lab, follow similar steps to those outlined in the "Epidemiology" and "Laboratories and Lab Analysis" chapters for human-only outbreaks. The main differences are that the origin of the outbreak is an animal, so samples need to be taken from animals; the environment for laboratory testing and mitigation measures involve animal populations; and animal professionals like veterinarians, animal scientists, and animal and livestock decision makers will play key roles in the response. Surveillance of wildlife presents different challenges and is more resource intensive—yet is extremely important to capturing emerging infectious diseases.

Animal disease surveillance systems are fed by various sources, including disease reporting to the relevant national animal authority, surveys, inspections, wildlife data, clinical data from veterinarians, and laboratory reports. When a disease has zoonotic origins, animal authorities coordinate with the relevant health authorities to design a joint response and ensure effective communication and data sharing. Vector surveillance is another essential tool to track disease probability and occurrence using geospatial data, climate and seasonal information, animal population density data, and vector risk assessments.

WOAH's *Terrestrial Animal Health Code*

The World Organisation for Animal Health (WOAH), founded as the Office International des Epizooties (OIE), publishes the *Terrestrial Animal Health Code*, a resource of animal health standards intended for use by veterinary authorities to enable early detection, reporting, and control of pathogens in terrestrial animals and the prevention of their spread via international trade.[10] It also presents case definitions, diagnostic methods, vaccination recommendations, and surveillance guidelines for a long list of specific infectious diseases of concern, such as anthrax, foot and mouth disease, and avian influenza, as well as guidance on collecting wildlife surveillance data.

Preventing Zoonotic Outbreaks

Most zoonotic diseases transmit via direct or indirect contact with animals or their byproducts.[11] Direct physical contact includes touching, holding, kissing, or being bitten or scratched by an infected animal. Indirect transmission occurs through contact with a surface, material, or object that is contaminated by an infected animal's bodily fluids, like saliva, blood, urine, mucus, or feces. Zoonotic diseases can also be transmitted through droplets or aerosols coming directly from the infected animal or by inhaling particulates from its waste.

Based on the different modes of transmission, certain measures for preventing zoonotic outbreaks are disease specific, but there are several general best practices for reducing risk and controlling possible disease emergence or spread.

- Vaccinate domestic animals, livestock and wild animals
- Establish vector control programs
- Practice personal hygiene and use appropriate PPE around animals
- Sanitize animal infrastructure frequently

- Follow established national and international guidelines for safe and appropriate animal import, export, and care in agricultural and food production sectors
- Provide information on risk reduction practices (define at-risk populations, diseases currently circulating, and proper hygiene, and avoid touching and eating wild animals)

VACCINATE DOMESTIC ANIMALS, LIVESTOCK, AND WILD ANIMALS

Vaccinating animals is an essential preventive measure to reduce the risk of disease occurrence in animal and human populations given our close contact with them as pets, resources, and neighbors. Livestock animals are the key income and food source for many farmers and workers involved in the food processing sector, constituting 40 percent of the total value of global agriculture and supporting the livelihoods of roughly 1.3 billion people.[12] Many people also share their homes with animals. In the US, an estimated 70 percent of the population has cats and/or dogs, and more than thirty-six million families have "non-traditional pets," such as rodents, rabbits, ferrets, birds, reptiles, amphibians, and fish.[13] Vaccination protects both the animals and the humans around them. Animal vaccination can occur systematically through routine vaccination programs and established veterinary systems, or through an emergency campaign during an outbreak as a control measure.[14]

CASE STUDY

Flavored Vaccines

In an effort to eliminate rabies in wild animals like raccoons, foxes, coyotes, and skunks, the US Department of Agriculture is scattering millions of tasty (if you're an animal) fishmeal-coated oral rabies vaccine (ORV) baits via helicopter and plane over the wilderness areas of sixteen states.[15] When a raccoon, for example, bites into one of these "rabioli" packets, the sachet containing the vaccine inside the bait bursts, and the animal swallows the vaccine. ORV is a proven tool used in the US, Canada, and Europe for decades to vaccinate wild animal populations, limiting the need for previous wildlife rabies control measures like hunting, trapping, and poisoning.[16] By targeting wild animals, experts hope to reduce rabies disease rates and thus prevent infection of domestic animals and humans.

Rabies is fatal in over 99 percent of cases in both animals and humans if left untreated.[17] The rabies virus is transmitted through the saliva of an infected animal, usually via bite, and impacts the nervous system. Vaccinating an animal against rabies allows it to develop an immunity to the disease, meaning it can no longer contract or spread the disease.

Plague is another zoonotic disease found in wild animals in the Western region of the North America. It primarily affects rodents, like prairie dogs, ground squirrels, and chipmunks. In seven US states, biologists are using drones to drop peanut butter pellets laced with an oral sylvatic plague vaccine (SPV) onto prairie dog colonies.[18] The brightly colored, peanut butter–flavored treat inoculates prairie dogs against the sylvatic plague.

Plague, caused by the *Yersinia pestis* bacterium, can spread to other wildlife, livestock, and humans. While it is treatable in humans, it can decimate rodent populations, severely impacting the ecosystem and food chain when keystone species, like prairie dogs, disappear.[19]

Plague in Madagascar

Plague is endemic to Madagascar. The country contains 75 percent of global plague cases.[20] Around four hundred cases are diagnosed per year, most of them bubonic plague, and they usually occur between September and April.[21] However in 2017, between August and November health personnel noticed a sharp increase in cases, suggesting an outbreak. They found that the majority of cases were pneumonic plague, a form of the disease that develops when bubonic plague is left untreated and spreads through respiratory transmission from human to human, making it much more contagious than bubonic plague, which is contracted through an infected flea bite.[22] Over the course of the outbreak, there were 2,417 cases and 209 deaths.[23]

Plague infection can be treated with antibiotics and patients often make a full recovery if treatment begins in the early stages.[24] During a plague outbreak, health responders use both curative and prophylactic antibiotics; curative are used to treat those who are already infected, and prophylactic prevent others from becoming infected.[25]

Rabid Politics

Exposure to rabies is not limited to deep wilderness. We live side-by-side with wild animals even in urban and semi-urban cities. In spring 2022, a fox bit nine people over a series of days on the grounds of Capitol Hill in Washington, DC. The fox was eventually captured and humanely euthanized, testing positive for rabies.[26] The victims sought medical attention and received postexposure prophylaxis (PEP), a series of four shots.

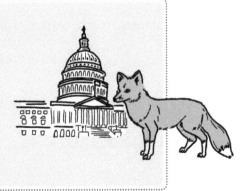

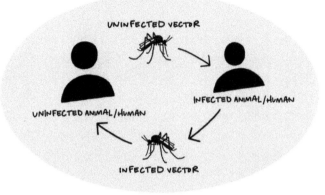

VECTOR CONTROL

Vectors are arthropods, like mosquitoes, fleas, and ticks, that can spread disease from other animals to humans, or between humans. Vector-borne diseases like malaria, dengue, Zika, chikungunya, yellow fever, leishmaniasis, Chagas disease, and West Nile virus are illnesses caused by bacteria, viruses, or parasites transmitted by vectors; they make up more than 17 percent of the global infectious disease burden.[27] Many of these diseases do not have vaccines or cures yet, so vector control is the best option for preventing and mitigating disease. Vector control methods limit people's exposure to vectors by targeting specific habitats and behaviors of vector species. This can be through

Aedes, Anopheles, and *Culex*: Meet the Mosquitoes behind Disease

There are more than three thousand species of mosquito.

They have different climate and ecological preferences and associated behaviors, such as feeding sources, resting locations and times, and egg laying locations. Some feed at night, others at dusk and dawn. Some feed and rest indoors, others outdoors, some do both. Some spread disease, others do not.

Aedes, *Culex*, and *Anopheles* mosquitoes are the ones that most commonly spread germs—parasites or viruses.

- *Aedes* are the mosquitoes behind Zika, dengue, chikungunya, and yellow fever. *Aedes* bite during the day and sometimes during dawn and dusk. They lay their eggs on small water surfaces of small natural and artificial water-holding receptacles (like tree holes and flower pot saucers).

- *Anopheles* is the malaria mosquito. *Anopheles* primarily bite humans and other mammals at dusk and dawn. They lay their eggs on the surfaces of natural bodies of water, like ponds, marshes, and swamps.

- *Culex* is the primary transmission vector for West Nile virus. While *Culex* usually bite birds, they will also bite humans. They feed at night as well as dusk and dawn. *Culex* lay their eggs on stagnant water surfaces of natural and man-made containers (bird baths, flower pots, pools, gutters, ditches, septic system water, etc.).[28]

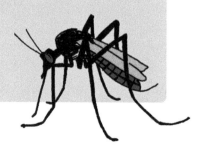

habitat and environmental control, personal protective measures, chemical control, and biological control. Many vector control measures can be effective against multiple vectors. The WHO refers to this as "integrated vector management," a cost-effective tool to protect populations from several diseases. Removing or modifying breeding grounds like stagnant water can help reduce vector populations. Personal protection includes using screens in doors and windows, using insect repellent, wearing long shirts and pants, and sleeping under insecticide-treated bed nets. Chemical vector control involves use of larvicides and insecticides, and spraying campaigns, ground and aerial. Biological control is a newer vector control method targeted at mosquito control. Scientists are designing and releasing genetically modified mosquitoes that do not survive to adulthood, and irradiated mosquitoes, which are sterilized male mosquitoes, for population control.

From Efficient Transmitter to Secret Weapon
Using Mice to Fight Lyme Disease in the US Northeast

White-footed mice are exceptionally efficient transmitters of Lyme disease, a zoonosis caused by the bacterium *Borrelia burgdorferi*. They can have up to one hundred ticks on their faces and ears and are able to infect roughly 95 percent of the ticks that feed on them.[29] Cases of Lyme disease are increasing exponentially. The geographic range of infected ticks has more than doubled and the US CDC reports more than 30,000 people infected with Lyme disease in the US each year, though recent studies estimate the number could be as high as 476,000.[30]

Scientists and tick-borne illness experts Rick Ostfeld and Felicia Keesing are trying to combat the increasing rates of disease by using the Tick Control System (TCS), fipronil-treated bait boxes that "weaponize" mice against Lyme.[31] Small mammals like mice are attracted to the TCS, a small dark box. When they enter it, their coats are brushed with a dose of fipronil, an insecticide that kills ticks but is safe for people, pets, and the environment.[32] The Tick Project research shows that TCS bait boxes reduced the number of ticks in observed yards by 50 percent, encouraging evidence for the effectiveness of neighborhood-based prevention measures to reduce Lyme and other tickborne diseases.[33]

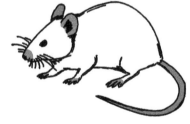

HYGIENE
Proper handwashing etiquette, limiting risky behaviors, and wearing appropriate gear while handling animals are key ways of preventing disease spread.

This can include wearing gloves, clothing, and boots used exclusively for animal area use. People should also avoid eating and drinking around animals to limit the possibility that germs from the animals enter their bodies.

Stop PDA (Poultry Displays of Affection)

Increase in Live-Poultry-Associated Salmonellosis (LPAS) Outbreaks in the US

For over a decade, the US CDC's salmonella outbreak investigations highlighted the increase in contact with backyard poultry as a source of human salmonella infections across the US and issued repeated guidance to avoid cuddling or kissing your feathered friends.

Backyard poultry, like chickens and ducks, can carry the *Salmonella* bacteria, which humans can ingest by touching their mouths after handling poultry or supplies and equipment used to care for them. Risky behaviors also include cuddling or kissing the birds and eating or drinking around them. A salmonella infection can cause diarrhea, fever, and stomach cramps, even hospitalization in severe cases, and in much rarer cases, death.

A 2016 study conducted by the US CDC looking at the increase in live-poultry-associated salmonellosis (LPAS) outbreaks from 1990 to 2014 found that 13 percent of case-patients reported kissing the birds and 49 percent reported cuddling.[34] Other high-risk practices included keeping poultry inside of the home; 46 percent of respondents said they kept the birds inside the house, of that group, 12 percent of case-patients kept poultry in the kitchen and 10 percent in their bedroom.

The solutions to avoiding an LPAS outbreak: always wash your hands thoroughly with soap and water after handling poultry, their eggs, or anything used in the area where they live and roam; keep them and any equipment and supplies used to care for them outside the house; and do not cuddle or kiss the birds.[35]

Chickens, Hedgehogs, Turtles, and Dragons

Salmonella outbreaks tied to live animals in the USA are not limited to chickens and ducks. In 2019, the US CDC conducted a multistate investigation of a *Salmonella typhimurium* outbreak that was linked to pet hedgehogs through epidemiologic and laboratory evidence. Between October 2018 and September 2019, fifty-four people across twenty-three states were identified with that particular outbreak strain of *Salmonella*.[36]

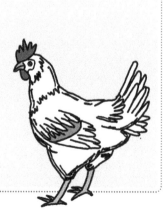

Pet turtles and bearded dragons are also recurring sources of salmonella outbreaks that the US CDC investigates each year.

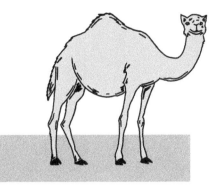

ROUTINE ANIMAL CARE

Animals can appear healthy and still carry diseases that can infect people. The individuals who interact frequently with animals, including pet owners, farmers, veterinarians, butchers, and hunters, should monitor the animals they interact with for signs of illness, report suspected disease, and seek veterinary care when appropriate.

MERS-CoV

Camels to Humans

Read about how MERS-CoV was discovered in the "Field Epidemiology Training Program in Action" case study in the Staffing and Training chapter.

Middle East respiratory syndrome coronavirus (MERS-CoV) is a zoonotic disease transmitted from infected dromedary camels to humans. Scientists found serological evidence that MERS-CoV had existed in camels for at least three decades before the first human infection was identified in 2012.[37]

Although dromedary camels are proven to be the primary reservoir for MERS-CoV, the specific mode of transmission for the disease between camels and humans has still not been identified. As a result, advised preventive measures address several potential routes, including practicing proper hand hygiene; avoiding touching eyes, nose, or mouth after contact with animals; wearing masks and protective clothing used only for contact with camels; and avoiding handling or consuming raw camel milk, urine, or meat.[38] Studies have shown that MERS-CoV is present in the raw milk of infected camels.[39]

Studies on risk factors for infection demonstrate a clear increased risk of MERS-CoV for people who have direct contact with dromedary camels, including camel-farm owners and workers, shepherds at camel barns, persons involved in camel racing, individuals who ingest raw camel milk, and veterinarians who care for camels.[40]

SANITIZING AND DECONTAMINATING ANIMAL INFRASTRUCTURE

Infrastructure used for animals—buildings, vehicles, equipment—need to be frequently cleaned to prevent and mitigate the spread of disease between animals and from animals to humans. This infrastructure exists in agricultural,

See the Disease Prevention and Mitigation chapter to learn about infrastructure sanitation and decontamination to avoid the spread of disease.

Learn more about mad cow disease in the case study on page 127.

Learn more about Nipah virus in the case study on page 31.

See the "Food Safety" section of the Disease Prevention and Mitigation chapter to learn more about preventing foodborne outbreaks.

research, food production, and educational facilities, as well as on smaller scales, like small farms or households. Proper sanitation can help reduce the risk of a disease transmission from an animal to a human during animal care and limit the chance that an infected animal becomes part of the food production, distribution, and consumption process.

Bacteria like *Salmonella* and *Escherichia coli* (*E. coli*) are common causes of disease resulting from interaction with or consumption of animals. Rarer are infections of bovine spongiform encephalopathy, also known as mad cow disease, and Nipah virus.

Maintaining clean animal spaces can also help avoid attracting animals like mice and rats, which can carry diseases like the plague, Hantavirus, and Lassa fever, and reduce breeding grounds for transmitters of vector-borne diseases like mosquitoes and ticks.

CASE STUDY

Biosecurity Response Zone in Australian Airports

to Prevent the Arrival of Foot and Mouth Disease

During the summer of 2022, the Australian Government launched a concerted effort to prevent the arrival of foot and mouth disease (FMD), a highly contagious disease affecting livestock like cows, sheep, and pigs.

FMD was spreading rapidly in Asian countries like Indonesia, and viral fragments of FMD had been found in meat products arriving from China. An FMD outbreak in Australia had the potential to decimate the livestock industry and experts estimated the economic cost of an FMD outbreak would be AU$80 billion.[41]

The government approved a AU$14 million biosecurity package to fund biosecurity measures to address the increased threat of FMD domestically in airports and mail centers, as well as fund international efforts like distributing FMD vaccines in outbreak hotspots like Bali.[42] The national strategy involved increasing surveillance, deploying biosecurity personnel and detector dogs in airports, providing traveler education, and establishing Biosecurity Response Zones in airports. Airport biosecurity measures included requiring all arriving and returning passengers from Indonesia to wipe their shoes on disinfecting mats, establishing strict passenger declaration, profiling all arriving and returning passengers from Indonesia, questioning passengers, and performing ongoing risk assessment.

At the time of writing, the biosecurity measures have been effective and Australia has not had a case of FMD.

Hantavirus Outbreak in Yosemite National Park

During the summer of 2012, a rare outbreak of hantavirus pulmonary syndrome (HPS) was traced to Yosemite National Park in the US state of California. HPS, the form of the virus that appears in the Americas, is characterized by fever, body aches, and in severe cases, fluid accumulation in the lungs.[43] Its primary reservoir is deer mice and it is generally contracted through inhalation of aerosolized mouse feces and urine.[44] Current estimates place the mortality rate between 30 and 50 percent.[45]

The first case of HPS from the 2012 Yosemite outbreak was reported to the California Department of Health (CDPH) in early July: an individual who had visited Yosemite National Park during June.[46] In mid-July, laboratory analysis of samples collected by the first case's doctor confirmed that the illness was hantavirus. A second case was reported and died shortly after.

Preliminary investigations by the CDPH revealed that both victims had recently travelled to Yosemite National Park and stayed in the Curry Village campsite, specifically the signature tent cabins. The ninety-one signature cabins were hard-sided with insulation and allowed food, unlike the other three hundred-odd canvas-sided cabins making up the majority of Curry Village, which do not allow food. The combination of food and insulated walls created ideal conditions for mice to live, and consequently for humans to be exposed to infected mice droppings.[47] In early August, the National Park Service (NPS) closed the signature tent cabins to carry out extensive sanitization efforts and implement vermin prevention measures by sealing off gaps in the walls.

The CDPH, US CDC, and NPS Office of Public Health initiated an investigation and announced the outbreak August 16. They sent out notices requesting potential cases, defined as anyone with flu-like symptoms between June 1 and October 31 who had visited Yosemite National Park within six weeks prior to symptom development, be tested for hantavirus.

Researchers identified at least ten people associated with the outbreak, including three deaths.[48] For each case, a control was recruited from their traveling companions who had not contracted the illness. Both case and control groups were interviewed for demographic information, travel history, illness history, and a description of various activities engaged in during their stay in Yosemite.[49] Of the ten hantavirus cases, nine had spent one or more nights in one of the signature tent cabins at the Curry Village campsite, suggesting a significant association between the Curry Village cabins and HPS infection. Environmental investigation revealed extensive mice infestation in the cabins, and live capture and testing of mice revealed that 14 percent of the mice trapped in the signature cabins carried hantavirus antibodies.

Despite rodent proofing attempts, the ninety-one signature tent cabins were permanently removed on August 28 to prevent further exposure and possible future outbreaks.[50]

Public Health Ally: The Possum

Opossums, or possums, are highly resistant and unlikely to develop or transmit Lyme disease and rabies. Not only are they rarely disease carriers for common zoonotic diseases like Lyme disease, but they also eat common disease vectors like ticks, mice, and rats![51] Their grooming habits help them quickly detect and eat nearly 96 percent of ticks on their bodies, helping reduce vector populations.[52]

Zoonotic Outbreak Response

For the most part, responding to a zoonotic outbreak will follow the same steps as a standard outbreak. In addition to those activities, there are several animal-outbreak specific response actions, including:

- designating infected zone(s) and animal population(s);
- implementing quarantine and movement restrictions on potentially contaminated animals, vehicles, and personnel (this could be international, cross-border, or subnational-level movement restrictions);
- humanely stamping out infected and exposed animal populations;
- safely disposing of carcasses and other potentially infected, hazardous materials; and
- disinfecting and cleaning infected premises.[53]

Unfortunate, but sometimes necessary, is the destruction and disposal of infected and exposed animals. In situations where treatment or vaccination is not available to prevent or contain a disease in an animal population, or a disease has the potential to spread rapidly to a human population and cause

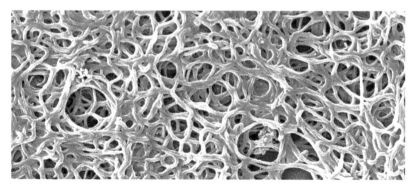

Borrelia burgdorferi, the bacteria that causes Lyme disease

severe disease or death, it may be necessary to destroy all infected and exposed animals.[54] This is referred to as culling or stamping out.

Once the disease is confirmed and the decision is made to cull an animal population, culling must be carried out rapidly and in accordance with relevant national culling policies and international animal welfare standards.[55] This typically involves ensuring that all personnel involved are trained in proper handling and disposal of hazardous waste, minimizing contact with the infected and exposed animals, and oversight by a designated authority such as a government veterinarian.

Often alternative outbreak prevention and control measures—vaccination (through baiting or campaign), livestock fencing, and improved biosecurity practices—are more cost-effective, have long-term positive impact on minimizing future disease spread, and are in line with a One Health approach.[56]

CASE STUDY

Implementing an Avian Influenza Prevention Zone (AIPZ)

to Stop the UK's Largest Bird Flu Outbreak

In 2022, the UK observed its largest outbreak to date of highly pathogenic avian influenza (HPAI) strain H5N1, also referred to as bird flu, in wild and domesticated flocks. Over a year-long period from October 2021 to September 2022 an estimated forty-eight million birds were culled across the UK and the EU.[57] To further control the spread of disease, in October 2022, UK chief veterinary officers declared an Avian Influenza Prevention Zone (AIPZ).[58] Establishment of an AIPZ meant that bird keepers across England, Scotland, Northern Ireland, and Wales were legally mandated to follow strict biosecurity measures, including restricting access to flocks to essential personnel only, keeping free-ranging birds within fenced areas, increasing cleaning and disinfection protocol for bird enclosures and vehicles, wearing and disinfecting clothing and footwear used exclusively for bird care, separating domestic ducks and geese from chickens, and preventing wild birds from sharing food and water sources with captive birds.

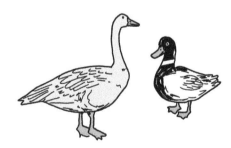

Only one person tested positive for H5N1 in the UK during this outbreak, a man in December 2021.[59] While no other human cases were detected in the UK during the 2022 to 2023 season, by following biosecurity protocols, the risk for further spread within flocks and thus the possibility of the virus mutating to a form where it can then infect people was lowered.[60]

When Culling Is Not the Answer

Culling may not always be effective, or be the right course of action for controlling a disease.

In 2009, a novel influenza A virus emerged—H1N1. Prior to the identification of a human case in the US in April 2009, the influenza A (H1N1) strain had not been detected in humans. The disease was initially referred to as swine flu, given genetic analyses that showed genetic similarity to influenza viruses in pigs. It spread rapidly around the world and by June 2009, when the WHO declared it a PHEIC, it had been laboratory confirmed in seventy-four countries.[61]

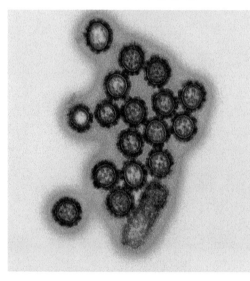

H1N1 influenza virus particles. Credit CDC PHIL, Copyright 2024, StatPearls Publishing LLC.

The UN FAO, WHO, and WOAH discouraged the use of the term "swine flu" to avoid confusion and create an unfounded fear of pigs. The FAO issued a formal statement stating there was no justification for culling, controlling movement, or quarantining pigs.[62] Without evidence suggesting that H1N1 could be contracted by eating pig products or interacting with pigs, culling was not an appropriate control measure.

However, despite no evidence that influenza A (H1N1) affected pigs or their meat, and against guidance from UN agencies, on April 28 the government of Egypt passed a bill ordering the culling of all pigs in the country.[63] The Egyptian pig population, roughly 300,000 animals, was slaughtered starting August 30. Health policies not backed by scientific evidence may misguidedly target minority populations on the basis of occupation, religion, and other elements of identity. Further, when policy decisions are made without scientific basis, it can erode confidence in public health decisions and acceptance of measures like culling during future health events.

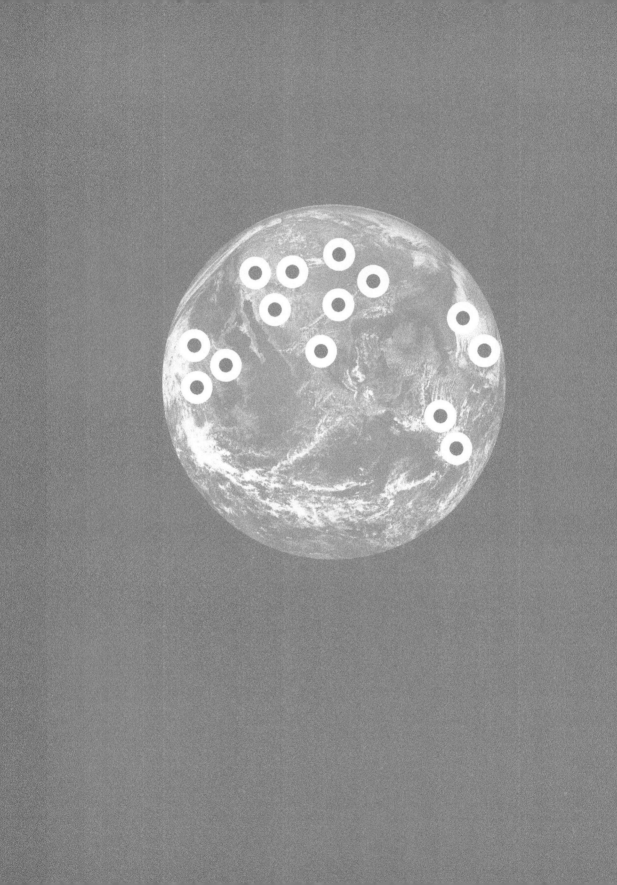

EMERGENCY OPERATIONS AND LOGISTICS
Mobilizing People, Supplies, and Equipment

Outbreak response operations, whether they deal with a small foodborne outbreak tied to a single restaurant or with a global pandemic, involve obtaining, transporting, cleaning, and disposing of a variety of supplies and equipment. A number of different professions are also involved in managing operations and preventing the spread of disease, and sometimes those personnel need to be moved to and from outbreak locations. Public health operations and logistics describe the acquisition and distribution of products and equipment needed for detecting and controlling infectious disease, and the movement and management of the personnel, supplies, and information gathered and used over the course of a disease event. In this chapter, we outline how countries map the resources available, manage complex procurement and movement of resources, and operationalize information using national emergency response plans to activate public health emergency operations centers (PHEOCs) to manage the outbreak response.

Mapping Resources for Outbreak Response

Officials map resources to get an accurate idea of what is available, how it is distributed, and what the capacity is. Here, *map* is used both spatially and organizationally. Resources can include the human workforce, vehicles, facilities, supplies, and equipment involved across the full spectrum of outbreak detection, investigation, and response.

Understanding in advance the amount and distribution of resources available helps officials create efficiencies for the mobilization of goods, personnel, and equipment during a response. Resource mapping allows countries to assess what is available to them, consider logistical aspects of ensuring these resources reach their intended targets, and identify gaps or redundancies in coverage, access to care, and response capabilities.[1] Mapping activities can be carried out by government personnel, research institutions, and public or private organizations. Geospatial software is often used to help assess key metrics in preparation for and in response to an outbreak, such as measuring the distance between facilities involved in outbreak management (clinics, hospitals, laboratories, isolation/quarantine facilities, etc.) or how much of the population is served by a given facility. Community resource mapping can be facilitated through partnerships between experts responsible for documentation and spatial analysis and community members familiar with the available resources.[2]

Mapping exercises can capture a wide array of data and information on the resources required for emergency response to a public health event. This can include mapping logistics infrastructure, like supply chains and stockpiles, transportation routes and vehicles, staffing levels and expertise, equipment, durable and consumable supplies, laboratory diagnostic and testing materials, financial resources, and locations, networks, and capabilities of facilities (health facilities, laboratories, POD locations, etc.). In addition to broad public health system mapping, governments may carry out sector-specific mapping for health care, laboratories, and security to get more nuanced images of the different fields that work together during a response.

Once resources are mapped, health officials can develop more accurate strategic response plans and allocate resources to strengthen gaps identified during the mapping process.

Transporting People and Things

Vehicles are necessary to safely transport responders, patients, biological samples, supplies, equipment, and waste to and from outbreak sites and designated care facilities during outbreaks. In order to transport people and things, you need vehicles. Around the world, a wide variety of transport vehicles are used—from boats and planes to motorcycles and cars. Health personnel identify vehicles dedicated to transportation of infectious and noninfectious persons, medical supplies, responders, drugs, and food prior to an outbreak. Identifying transportation resources early is 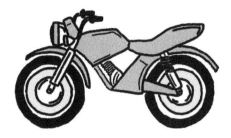 also vital for distributing personal protective equipment and other medical countermeasures often stockpiled at centralized facilities during an outbreak.[3]

Transport Health Care Personnel

To find, diagnose, and treat cases, response officials must ensure that health care personnel, including public health and medical responders, are able to reach their site of work. Conversely, if the location of an outbreak overlaps with an area of violent conflict, responders may need to be evacuated for their safety.

Public health staff may use commercial or public modes of transportation, or ground and air transport acquired specifically for outbreak response. The mode of transportation used will depend on what is accessible, safe, and effective in getting health staff to outbreak sites and/or care facilities. If public transportation is reduced or eliminated, this will impact essential workers' ability to reach sites of care. Officials must have plans and policies in place to provide alternative travel options for essential workers. This may involve making public transport available just for essential workers, and/or developing agreements with private carriers.

There are several scenarios during which health and humanitarian responders may need to be evacuated during an outbreak response: discovery that the outbreak is a novel pathogen or the result of an intentional release, political instability, natural disaster, and/or border closures. International organizations and countries should have mechanisms in place to help health workers find safety amid an infectious disease outbreak. Some countries and international organizations have developed their own medical evacuation

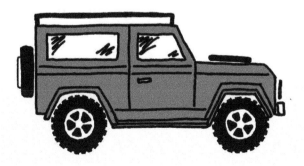

(medevac) capacity, while others may prefer to charter medevac flights from organizations dedicated to providing these services.

Under this framework, organizations must develop a clear set of eligibility criteria for evacuation and identify personnel who may be required to stay and maintain aid. If a patient is already infected, the medevac will be supervised by a clinical care team using ground or air ambulances, as appropriate. Clear procedures regarding medevac can increase feelings of safety and thus potentially increase the number of humanitarian workers willing to participate in a response.

When political instability transitions to violence that threatens the safety of health and humanitarian personnel and inhibits their ability to provide aid, countries and/or organizations may evacuate them. Under these circumstances, the parties responsible for evacuating responders must consider the risk both for potential exposure and to security when creating evacuation plans. Médecins Sans Frontiers was forced to make this decision when it evacuated its personnel from Northeast Syria in November 2019.

CASE STUDY

Public Transportation during the COVID-19 Pandemic

During the COVID-19 pandemic, public transportation services around the world adjusted their operating schedules to decrease population movement and increased IPC measures like cleaning to limit the spread of disease. Cities implemented a range of public transportation programs to ensure transport for essential workers and continuity of services by protecting transport workers. For example, in New York City, essential workers could access free rides from buses or cabs when the subways were closed between 1 and 5 a.m. for disinfection.[4] Buses in cities like Dar es Salaam, Abidjan, London, and Paris were outfitted with plastic shields and had passengers enter only from middle or rear doors to reduce infection risk for bus drivers. In Nyeri, Kenya, the Nyeri County Department of Health, supported by the WHO, hosted public health training sessions with minibus taxi owners and drivers, the primary means of transport in the area, to teach them about transmission risks for the passengers and drivers.[5]

Public transportation was also used to help offset the demand for ambulatory vehicles in nonemergency situations. The Seattle King County local government established a program to transport patients with presumed or confirmed positive COVID-19 infections to isolation/quarantine sites, medical facilities, homeless shelters, and assisted living facilities. By providing transportation services, they helped prevent further spread of disease from the suspected infected individual and did not utilize an emergency vehicle that might be needed for an urgent health matter.[6]

Transport Patients

During an outbreak, patients may need to be moved from their homes to a clinic site, or from clinical care to a specialized treatment unit. Patient transport should be executed in a way that ensures the safety of the patient and those transporting the patient. All those involved should use appropriate personal protective equipment to minimize secondary spread. The key elements of safe transfer involve clear communication between the transport vehicle and the receiving clinic; observation of general and disease-specific biosafety guidance for transporting infectious patients; pretransfer stabilization and preparation; choice of the appropriate mode of transfer; presence of trained personnel accompanying the patient; appropriate equipment and monitoring; and documentation and handover of the patient at the receiving facility.

Air medical transport (AMT) is a unique patient care setting.[7] Unlike ground medical transport, an aircraft usually does not stop or resupply during transport, the mission usually exceeds several hours, and a patient's condition can deteriorate, requiring additional interventions that could result in an increased risk of exposure for health care providers. Specific AMT standards have been developed for some diseases. Much work, for instance, was undertaken after the West Africa Ebola outbreak to develop viral hemorrhagic fever protocols for air transport.[8]

EMERGENCY RESPONSE VEHICLES

Emergency response vehicles, such as ambulances, are used for transporting patients infected by the outbreak disease while remaining available and operational for non-outbreak emergency health services. Emergency response vehicles require proper cleaning and sanitization of interior and high touch exterior surfaces, stocking with proper personal protective equipment and medications, and replacing air filters as needed (approximately every six months) to prevent disease transmission to health responders and potentially to noninfected individuals who ride in the ambulance after someone who is infected.[9] Ambulances must be staffed with paramedical staff trained to utilize the equipment to care for patients.[10] Currently, it is recommended that countries aim for a minimum of one ambulance per fifty thousand residents, though rural municipalities often need to have relatively higher ratios than urban populations.[11]

See the Disease Prevention and Mitigation chapter to learn about disinfection guidance during an outbreak.

TRANSPORT VEHICLES

To transport noncritical patients to quarantine, isolation, and/or care facilities, and health workers to and from their worksites, municipal vehicles, like buses and cars, can be adapted to prevent disease transmission, follow sanitation procedures, and inform the community regarding the availability of the resources.[12] These vehicles are not substitutes for emergency ambulances but can help ensure vulnerable populations can access medical resources while reducing disease transmission.

AIR TRANSPORTATION

Access to air transportation is particularly important for long distance transport and hard-to-reach locations, whether they are inaccessible due to conflict, geographical isolation, or natural disasters. Developing these assets increases a country's capacity to respond to an outbreak or disaster with equipment or to provide air ambulance services. International humanitarian programs and organizations as well as private sector entities may fill gaps in this capacity. First responders have utilized air ambulances (usually helicopters) and other aircraft adapted specifically to transport people for medical emergencies. These aircraft may need to be retrofitted with biocontainment units to prevent disease transmission during transportation.

Globally, two main organizations offer air support to vulnerable environments, the World Food Programme (WFP) and the European Union (EU). The WFP operates the United Nations Humanitarian Air Service (UNHAS), which currently serves more than four hundred regular destinations in 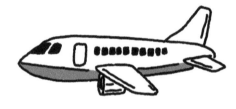 twenty-four countries, focusing on remote and under-resourced locations.[13] The EU operates the EU Humanitarian Aid Flight system, which serves sub-Saharan Africa to deliver passengers and cargo to crisis-affected areas.[14] While UNHAS and the EU Humanitarian Aid Flight systems both have their own aircraft, they also contract private companies to provide carrying services. Most NGOs, like MSF, operate using charter flights. The Humanitarian Air Services is another organization that provides airplane and helicopter transport to reach crises-affected areas in sub-Saharan Africa that lack reliable roads, ports, or commercial air strips, or are otherwise inaccessible.[15]

Governments may need to coordinate and negotiate with commercial airlines to keep flights open and available for moving outbreak personnel, patients, and goods and supplies.

Military Aircraft Reassigned for Emergency Public Health Response

Some nations may reassign military air transportation assets for use in an emergency. The UK's Royal Air Force and the French Air Force both reassigned military aircraft to transport patients during the COVID-19 pandemic.[16]

Infected Foreign Health Care Workers Medically Evacuated

during the 2014–2016 West Africa Ebola Outbreak

The 2003 severe acute respiratory syndrome (SARS) outbreak and subsequent avian flu outbreak brought global attention to the need for a safe mechanism for the transport of highly infectious patients to specified clinical facilities. The first single-patient isolator for aeromedical evacuation was developed in the 1970s for the UK's Royal Air Force (RAF). However, seeking a larger isolation unit, the US CDC, the US Department of Defense, and Phoenix Air, a private airline company, designed an airborne biological containment system (ABCS) that allowed medical personnel equipped with the appropriate PPE to be in the isolation unit with a highly infectious patient to provide care during transport.[17]

The ABCS accommodates one patient and is made up of a metal support system draped internally with a plastic liner that forms a tent-like isolation pod. The system is 1.57m × 1.8m × 3.65m. Within the metal frame there are two chambers. The smaller chamber at the unit's entrance is reserved for health care providers (one doctor and two nurses) to don and doff PPE. Behind this chamber is the larger patient isolation chamber. Inside are a stretcher, patient monitoring equipment, and a disposable toilet for the safe disposal of infectious wastes. A negative-pressure environment is maintained inside the unit to prevent air from leaking out, and the front and back sides of the unit each have an air filtration system that filters the air down to virus-sized particles. The entire unit is placed in a Gulfstream G-III aircraft. After each flight, the plastic liner and all equipment inside it is disinfected for twenty-four hours and then incinerated.[18]

Three ABCS units were finished in late 2011 and certified by the US Federal Aviation Administration (FAA).[19] The units were put in storage due to a lack of federal funds as well as the absence of a major infectious disease outbreak at the time.[20] The ABCS remained in storage until late July 2014, when the US State Department's Chief of Emergency Medicine called Phoenix Airlines to inquire if the containment units were suitable for the transportation of Ebola virus disease (EVD) patients. The US CDC and Phoenix Air medical personnel thoroughly assessed the ABCS and determined that it would protect against EVD in addition to the airborne diseases it was originally designed for.[21]

The 2014–2016 EVD outbreak in West Africa was the largest in history. Countries and nongovernmental organizations around the world sent health, humanitarian, and logistics experts to support the response. While caring for patients, a number of foreign response workers contracted EVD and were evacuated to their home countries for treatment.

On August 2, 2014, Phoenix Air retrieved the first American EVD patient from Liberia and flew him to Atlanta, Georgia, to be treated at Emory University Hospital.[22] Immediately after, the second American EVD patient was transported, also from Liberia to Atlanta. After the success of the first two flights, Phoenix Air transferred coordination responsibility to the US government, which was better equipped to mitigate challenges associated with customs officials and foreign airspace, and to determine treatment centers.[23]

While all patients were transported safely, Phoenix Air faced logistical difficulties. Staffing was initially a problem as many medical personnel employed by Phoenix Air also worked in other medical facilities. They were advised by their employers not to participate in the transportation of EVD patients as they would not be able return to work for twenty-one days after a flight, so Phoenix had to hire full-time medical staff. Other problems were not as easy to fix. Fear surrounding EVD meant that many foreign countries did not allow Phoenix Air flights to stop to refuel. In addition, Phoenix Air flights were only allowed to land at five airports in the US. Flights were complicated by these restrictions, sometimes requiring an extra stop.[24]

By the end of the outbreak, the ABCS had been used to successfully transport forty-one EVD patients back to the US and Europe for medical care during the outbreak.[25]

Containerized Biocontainment System (CBCS)

To increase capacity for infected-patient transport, the US State Department and US CDC partnered with MRIGlobal to design the containerized biocontainment system (CBCS), which can transport four highly infectious patients at a time, compared to ABCS's one. The CBCS features a patient treatment area, an anteroom where medical staff don and doff PPE and store medical and cleaning supplies, and a medical staff room where staff can rest without wearing PPE. With a steel inner wall and aluminum outer wall, it is sturdier than the ABCS.[26] The CBCS is flown in a B747–400 cargo aircraft.[27]

Air Transportation during COVID-19

The UN Humanitarian Air Service played a vital role during the COVID-19 response, transporting PPE, test kits, samples, and other medical supplies to hard-to-reach locations.[28] They also established a new Pacific Humanitarian Air Service dedicated to supporting supply chains among the Pacific Islands.[29] The EU Humanitarian Aid flight system set up the Humanitarian Air Bridge program to function on an ad-hoc basis as part of the global COVID-19 response.[30]

Maintaining Critical Transportation Infrastructure

During an outbreak, transportation can be both a vector of disease and a necessity for the secure movement of patients, health workers, and supplies. Health and transport officials should coordinate to develop an outbreak plan that addresses different transportation systems (e.g., transit, roads and highways, air travel) and assesses the systemic effects of changes to their operation.[31]

Once an outbreak is detected, health and transportation leaders should determine the existence and location of potential threats to the secure transportation of patients and supplies. With this in mind, the outbreak plan can guide the implementation of alternative transportation solutions such as clearing or maintaining necessary roads and infrastructure. Specific actions for this implementation may include coordinating regulatory waivers and exemptions, obtaining emergency funding to secure routes, and including pertinent engineering and contracting/procurement personnel and equipment. As with all restrictions and regulations implemented during an outbreak, transportation and health officials should work together to keep the public informed of any transportation-specific guidance.[32]

Procurement, Supply Chains, and Stockpiling

To respond to an outbreak, health personnel need supplies, equipment, and medicines. Those resources need to be procured, stored, and distributed according to need. The supplies required are outlined in national response plans and guidelines for laboratories and health facilities. Supplies may be standard, like basic personal protective equipment for responders and infected individuals, or specific to the disease and outbreak context, requiring, for example, a specific diagnostic assay to be identified, and a unique drug to treat the infection. To prepare for an outbreak, officials predict what materials will be needed and store them in stockpiles until they are used.

Logistics planning is important because resource stockpiles cannot be utilized if acquisition and distribution methods are not readily available.

Secure Supply Chains

Resilient national and global supply chains are critical to address increased need during public health emergency responses. During an outbreak, the supply chain must be effectively managed to ensure the availability, accessibility, and quality of necessary commodities. In general, supply chain systems for outbreak related materials include:

Demand: Definition of supply needs; identification of funding source; formulation, validation, and prioritization of supply request

Purchasing: Review of requests against availability; identification of suppliers; confirmation of order and funding source with requestor; commitment of supplies for distribution

Distribution: Shipment scheduling; transportation of supplies to distribution hubs; communication with recipient; receipt and processing of supplies for use[33]

When an outbreak is detected, the response team collaborates with suppliers (e.g., manufacturers, state or local stockpiles) to forecast and communicate the needed resource quantities and delivery timeframe. Timely communication and clear data on resource needs allow manufacturers to produce sufficient supplies to serve the target population.[34]

There are several difficulties to securing reliable supply chains, including state and local dispensing capacity, security, staffing, communication, transportation, and site selection.[35] Health and government officials and operations managers work with manufacturers, couriers, and security personnel to help maintain supply chains during a large-scale outbreak. Along the supply chain, any number of challenges can prevent necessary supplies and equipment from reaching their intended target. Closed factories due to worker shortages, broken cold chains damaging the integrity of products, limited transport options, and lost or stolen goods can all impede the overall response to an outbreak.

Project Last Mile

Coca-Cola Company leverages its distribution and system network to support transporting and storing medicines and vaccines across the African continent as part of "Project Last Mile."[36] This helps lower distribution costs, supports transportation route verification, ensures cold chain integrity, and identifies storage and distribution points.[37]

Procuring Resources and Equipment

Outbreak investigation and response involves an array of fields, each requiring different resources to perform their jobs, whether it is disinfecting buildings or conducting laboratory tests. Medical countermeasures (i.e., drugs and vaccines), sampling, diagnostics, laboratory testing materials, PPE, medical equipment, and decontamination agents and tools are among the consumable and durable resources procured in preparation for and in response to an outbreak. When an outbreak coincides with or triggers a humanitarian crisis, procurement also covers food aid, potable water, materials for temporary shelters, and general medical supplies.

Over the course of an outbreak, from early response through recovery, officials work to ensure that responders have the tools they need to stop the spread. When planning for an outbreak, governments and international agencies procure supplies and store them in stockpiles to be used in emergency situations. There are some generic supplies, like PPE, temporary cold chain support (e.g., coolers, dry ice), and nonspecific test reagents, like DNA/RNA extractives, that are commonly stocked and will be immediately available at the start of an outbreak. Other more specific supplies needed to address a particular pathogen in question, such as diagnostic testing kits and/or testing reagents or medicines, may need to be ordered, which takes valuable time.

See "Creating and Using Stockpiles" to learn more about stockpiles later in this chapter.

Basic inventory and purchasing management practices at laboratories and health facilities help ensure that supplies are available when needed, that high-quality supplies are obtained at fair cost, and that supplies are not lost due to improper storage or used beyond their expiration.[38] Of course, the particular nature of the outbreak—the offending pathogen and the drugs it is susceptible to, for instance—will dictate what supplies and how many of them will be needed.

Methods for procurement vary between countries and organizations, with some purchasing directly from manufacturers and others using national or regional procurement systems. Sometimes donors play a major role in the procurement of supplies and reagents, both during the preparedness phase and during outbreaks.

See the Governance chapter to learn about requesting aid.

Supplies used in outbreak detection and response are manufactured by both national and private companies, and it is possible that some or all of the necessary resources for an appropriate, safe response may not be produced or used in the region of the outbreak. If so, the response team will pursue purchasing arrangements with necessary vendors or request assistance from another country or international organization. In a large outbreak, pressures on supply chains may rise and bottleneck the availability of necessary sampling supplies.

Harvesting and manufacturing tends to be regionally or nationally focused (e.g., latex in Malaysia, surgical instruments in Pakistan, and generic drug production in India).[39] However, an overreliance on a small set of producers leaves supply chains vulnerable to bottlenecking if one part fails. Additionally, nationalization of manufacturing, border closures, and export restrictions can block countries without domestic manufacturing from obtaining important medical equipment during outbreaks. Transportation can also become a challenge when reductions in commercial air travel limit the amount of belly cargo space available for transport.[40] Countries and organizations address these challenges through advance planning, procurement, agreements with vendors or regional purchasing coalitions, and mutual-aid agreements. National regulatory agencies can issue more flexible emergency-use guidelines to adapt to shortages during emergencies or expand domestic manufacturing scope to try to reduce bottlenecking and transportation costs.[41]

Scaling Up Production of Supplies

In a large-scale outbreak, rapidly increasing the supply of consumable products, including PPE, syringes, diagnostics, medications, vaccines, and other medical items, may be necessary to maintain standards of care. Policymakers and international organizations should work with manufacturers to adopt new strategies that can stabilize supply chains during an outbreak response. For example, launching a vaccination campaign or developing novel countermeasures will likely require scale-up of existing manufacturing levels or initiation of research, development, and manufacturing for a new vaccine at a scale that can meet the need.

Countries may opt to work with manufacturers on these efforts directly, or to join forces with multilateral institutions working on global efforts toward countermeasure availability. Vendor partnerships are critical in accelerating the scale-up process. For example, vendors may be able to increase supply if notified of the type and quantity of items needed in a timely, clear manner. Medical countermeasure development and manufacturing is typically a function of biotechnology and pharmaceutical companies in the private sector, but it may be supported or even taken on directly by national governments.

The scale-up of medical countermeasure production will require a highly coordinated approach between governments and industry that considers a number of factors:

- Construction of the supply chain
- Design of the assembly process
- Establishment of testing and quality procedures
- Other safety, quality, and cost details[42]

CASE STUDY

The Defense Production Act

The Defense Production Act (DPA) was first passed in 1950, at the start of the Korean War. The purpose was to give the US president broad powers over the economy, including rationing consumer goods. It has continuously been reauthorized by Congress. The DPA allows the president to direct companies to prioritize orders from the federal government, increase domestic production of goods, and force coordination with other companies, all for national defense purposes.

The DPA was used during the COVID-19 pandemic, first to produce ventilators and masks for the federal government and prevent the hoarding of essential supplies. It was later used to assist with the production of vaccines and diagnostic tests. Between March 2020 and September 2021, the DPA was used to prioritize seventy-three contracts and orders, expand domestic production for N95 respirator masks by over fifty million per month, and enter into a public-private partnership to coordinate distribution of personal protective equipment.[43]

___

Managing Cold Chain

Lab reagents, medical countermeasures, and biological samples often require temperature-controlled environments throughout their production, storage, and distribution cycle. This may require separate temperatures, freezers, and other resources. Effective management of cold chain is critical to protecting individuals and communities by helping to ensure they have access to high-quality, necessary drugs and vaccines to stop an outbreak.

Cold chain is the system of transporting and storing samples and products within the optimum temperature to prevent degradation and maintain potency and integrity. It is made up of a network of cold rooms, freezers, refrigerators, and cold boxes that maintain the designated temperature throughout the manufacturing or sample collection process, through transportation, and finally to analysis or distribution. For vaccines, this temperature range is between 2 and 8°C (35–46°F), however there are instances where products need to be

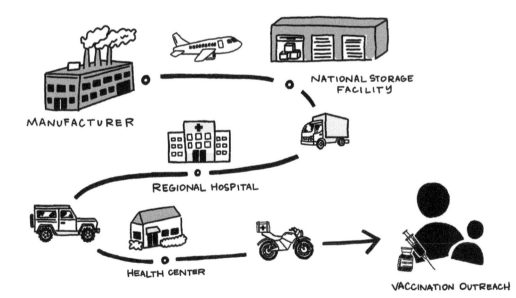

stored at ultra-cold temperatures. This range preserves the vaccine's potency, ensuring its function as a medical countermeasure.[44]

When an outbreak is detected, the response team should assess cold chain capacity applicable to the threat. This includes the identification of commodities that will need to be transported via cold chain, means for their storage, transportation required for them to reach their intended targets, and potential challenges to maintenance of cold chain.[45] Specific procedures and protocols are set in place along all steps in the supply chain to detect and deal with breaches in the cold chain.[46] Cold chain breaches occur when vaccines are managed or stored outside their recommended range of light or temperature.[47] These breaches may be detected by end-users via temperature indicator cards on external packaging. Should a breach be identified, the response team should be prepared to evaluate its impact on the vaccine's potency, communicate their findings with relevant personnel, and mobilize backup resources (e.g., revaccinate individuals who received compromised vaccines) as needed.

> From Ethiopia to Nepal, Afghanistan to Tanzania, health workers hike rough terrain to bring vaccines to remote communities.[48] These health trekkers are frequently women, navigating long distances with vaccine cooler boxes on their backs. They tackle arid deserts, steep hills, monsoons, and snow storms to provide lifesaving childhood vaccinations.
>
> Isolated hill communities are often far from formal vaccination sites and are not always accessible by road, making it difficult for people to travel round trip to receive immunizations. By bringing vaccines to the people and notifying community leaders ahead of time, immunization campaigns have been able to reach previously unreachable communities.

CASE STUDY

The 1925 Serum Run

In January of 1925, a diphtheria epidemic hit the town of Nome, a remote community just south of the Arctic Circle, in what was then considered the US territory of Alaska.

At the end of 1924, what were first thought to be unconnected tonsillitis cases were soon recognized as diphtheria, a serious bacterial infection affecting the respiratory system. Dr. Curtis Welch, the only doctor for Nome and the surrounding area, discovered that the diphtheria antitoxin in stock was expired and ineffective, and that the closest antitoxin was in Anchorage, more than a thousand miles away.

By the end of January, there were more than twenty cases and at least four children had died. In an emergency meeting, Dr. Welch and the town council implemented a quarantine in an effort to control the spread of disease. Dr. Welch sent a telegram to the US Public Health Service in Washington, DC, requesting one million units of diphtheria antitoxin, claiming that "an epidemic of diphtheria is almost inevitable here."[49] With Nome trapped between frozen sea and vast wilderness, transport of the antitoxin was not possible via sea or air, and so officials determined that sled dog relay would be the fastest way to get the antitoxin vials to Nome.

Over five and a half days, a relay of twenty mushers (sled drivers) and approximately 150 sled dogs made the dangerous 1,085 km (674 mile) journey across mountain ranges, frozen rivers, and blizzard conditions in temperatures as low as -65° Celsius (-85° Fahrenheit) with windchill to deliver the diphtheria antitoxin.

While Gunnar Kaasen and joint lead dogs Balto and Fox ran the roughly fifty-three-mile final leg into Nome, it was Leonhard Seppala and lead dog Togo who covered more than ninety-one miles over the most hazardous and technical section of the route.

Sensational coverage of the journey via newspaper and radio catalyzed inoculation campaigns around the country. The present day Iditarod Trail Sled Dog Race commemorates many aspects of the Serum Run.

CASE STUDY

Measles Outbreak Resulting from Vaccine Failure

in the Federated States of Micronesia

For twenty years, the Federated States of Micronesia (FSM) had no reported cases of measles, but in 2014, 393 cases occurred between February and August in three of the four states, Pohnpei, Kosrae, and Chuuk.[50]

Cases were initially diagnosed as dengue fever or chikungunya, allowing measles to spread undetected. Febrile rash illness was not part of the measles case definition in FSM as it had not been seen on the islands for decades. Eventually patient samples were tested and proved positive for measles-specific antibodies. The FSM Department of Health and Social Affairs and the Department of Health Services, supported by the WHO, UNICEF, and US CDC, continued testing samples and conducting active case finding and contact tracing. In response to the outbreak, officials launched a renewed measles vaccination campaign across all four states targeting children aged six months to adults aged fifty-seven years without documentation of two doses of measles-containing vaccine (MCV), which ended the outbreak.

Over the course of the outbreak, two-thirds of cases were adults, of whom 71 percent had received at least one dose of MCV prior to the outbreak, and many with at least two doses of MCV. Children less than twelve months old accounted for 65 percent of the unvaccinated cases, making them ineligible for measles vaccination. The low incidence of child cases suggested that the robust child vaccination programs were successful and dispelled the hypothesis that recent cold chain practices were inadequate. Measles is typically a disease that affects children and given that the bulk of the cases were vaccinated adults, investigators suspected that vaccine failure was the cause of the rapid spread of disease.[51] Upon further investigation, researchers proposed that the larger number of adult cases and suspected diminished vaccine effectiveness could be attributed to historical cold chain failures, such as improper vaccine storage and handling that damaged the potency of the vaccines used decades prior.[52] The environment of FSM poses distinct challenges to vaccine storage, such as high ambient temperatures, power outages, and difficulty with inter-island shipping.

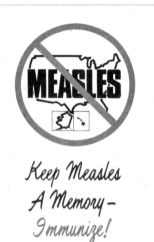

Courtesy of NLM.

The cost of the outbreak is approximated at $4,000,000, nearly $10,000 per case.[53] This estimate includes medical and containment expenses, as well as the indirect cost of productivity lost for infected persons. The outbreak illuminated challenges with cold chain management in resource-limited settings, as well as the need for more thermostable vaccines.

Go to the Treating Patients chapter to learn about how health facilities respond to surge capacity.

CASE STUDY

Dippin' Dots Cold Chain Mobilized for COVID-19 Vaccine

The Pfizer-BioNTech vaccine developed to protect people against COVID-19 needs to be stored at -94° Fahrenheit (-70° Celsius). What also requires transportation and storage at extremely low temperatures? Dippin' Dots, the "Ice Cream of the Future"—ice cream beads developed by microbiologists. It can only maintain its frozen beaded form when stored at -49°F (-45°C), compared to traditional ice cream which needs 0°F (-17.7°C).[54] Many of the locations that planned on distributing COVID-19 vaccine doses, such as pharmacies, clinics, and emergency PODs, did not have the facilities to store the vaccine at the appropriate temperature. Health experts looked at Dippin' Dots' logistics and cold chain, which utilized freezers operating at -122° Fahrenheit (-85.5°C) and are thus capable of maintaining the integrity of the vaccine.[55] The ice cream company reported receiving requests for the lease or purchase of these special freezers for COVID-19 vaccine storage.[56]

Creating and Using Stockpiles

Outbreaks and other public health emergencies can create demands that challenge or exceed the available resources of an affected area. This may cause health facilities to resort to crisis standards of care, potentially hindering the ability to provide adequate care. To prepare for potential surge needs, manage the initial spike in demand at the start of an outbreak, mitigate bottlenecks in supply availability, and avoid purchasing at surge prices, health officials and organizations create stockpiles. Stockpiles may be managed by individual health facilities, groups of health care centers (e.g., a centralized facility for joint stockpile use), national governments, or international organizations. Outbreak stockpiles typically contain critical resources such as medicines, vaccines, personal protective equipment, and medical supplies and devices that can be readily distributed during health crises.

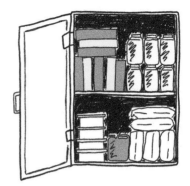

When a stockpile is prepared, officials outline criteria for its release, implement communication plans related to usage, and provide guidance on replenishing stockpiles after an outbreak is over.[57] Overall logistics planning is important because resource stockpiles cannot be utilized if acquisition and distribution methods are not readily available. Stockpile resources may be distributed to outbreak sites when local public health resources cannot meet demand, following a clear, evidence-based decision-making process. Deployment is often triggered by emergency use declarations to protect public health and safety. Governments may designate state agencies to determine criteria for deployment of national stockpiles through evaluation standards of health emergency situations. Countries and international organizations, such as the WHO, also may select dedicated groups to understand laws and policies related to preparedness plans and disease response. Epidemiological data, laboratory information, the availability of stocks in affected areas, and requests received are taken into consideration during the development of stockpile deployment standards.

CASE STUDY

Deployment of the US Strategic National Stockpile

during the H1N1 Influenza Pandemic

In mid-April 2009, the US CDC reported two confirmed cases of a new strain of influenza A (H1N1) in California. Cases had also been identified in Texas, Kansas, and New York. Experts were particularly concerned due to the irregular timing of the influenza outbreak outside of regular flu seasons, as well as the virulence and observed high mortality in young, healthy patients. By April 26, 2009, there were a total of twenty-one cases in the United States. That same day, the US government declared a nationwide public health emergency.

In response to the growing outbreak, the US CDC released 25 percent of its influenza supplies from the Strategic National Stockpile (SNS), including antiviral drugs and PPE (e.g., masks and respirators, gowns, gloves, and face shields), and distributed them across states based on state populations.[58] SNS personnel worked with state and local health department staff to identify supply needs and infrastructure capability to receive resources. Once the materials left federal control, states were responsible for their maintenance, storage, security, and deployment.

By June 11, 2009, the WHO had declared the first human influenza pandemic in more than four decades. From April 2009 to April 2010, the US CDC estimated that there were as many as eighty-nine million US cases, disproportionately children. Of these, there were as many as 403,000 hospitalizations and 18,300 deaths.

The deployment of the SNS in response to the H1N1 influenza outbreak was considered an overall success, delivering useful supplies to states in an appropriate time frame. While the virus was less virulent than predicted during planning scenarios, the resources deployed from the SNS were still well-received and illuminated areas of improvement for its use in future epidemics, highlighting, for example, the need for improving integration of operations of the SNS with the day-to-day medical supply chain, and for clarifying points of confusion for state and local partners who were not clear on certain aspects of the supply chain.[59] There were also issues with materials expected by states versus those delivered and unclear or even nonexistent long-term storage guidelines.[60]

More targeted use of the SNS could be facilitated by improved predictive methods that ensure the appropriate disbursement of resources.[61]

CASE STUDY

Smallpox Vaccine Stockpile Used for Mpox Outbreak

While smallpox was eradicated in the late twentieth century and no longer is part of routine immunization schedules, many countries keep limited stockpiles of smallpox vaccine in case of a biological terror event.[62]

In early 2022, cases of mpox, a virus closely linked to smallpox and rarely seen outside of the African continent, began spreading exponentially around the world. In response to the rapidly growing outbreak, several countries mobilized portions of their vaccine stockpiles against smallpox as a preventive measure to curb the spread of mpox. Health authorities in Britain, Japan, Canada, and the US approved the use of stockpiled smallpox vaccine to prevent mpox.[63] A two-dose shot, given twenty-eight days apart, developed by Bavarian Nordic and named differently around the world—Imvanex (UK and Europe), Jynneos (US), and Imvamune (Canada)—was used to control the outbreak. It was estimated to be 85 percent effective in preventing mpox.[64]

Emergency Response and Operations

Ensuring Power Is Available

In addition to acquiring necessary supplies, vehicles, and staff, public health response operations require power. Power and fuel are critical resources for maintaining public health facility operations, constant communication capabilities, data information systems, transportation abilities, integrity of biological samples, and safe storage of temperature-vulnerable supplies. Clinics, hospitals, laboratories, and emergency operations centers all rely on power and/or the necessary fuel to ensure they can remain running during a health threat. Power outages and fuel shortages have the potential to threaten an effective response, furthering the spread of disease. Emergency generators, fuel, and lighting allow key public health facilities to remain operational in supporting the community's emergency response. Vehicles moving responders, patients, and supplies to, from, and between these facilities also need to be provided with fuel.

Public Health Emergency Operations Center (PHEOC)

A public health emergency operations center (PHEOC) is a central location for coordinating operational information and resources to support incident management during a major public health emergency.[65] At a PHEOC, staff and scientific experts can monitor outbreak and response activities, manage

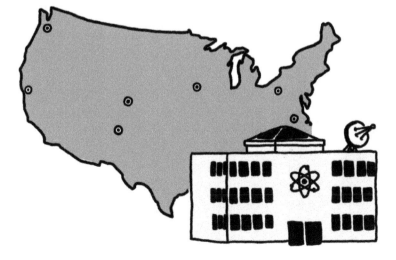

supplies and equipment before delivery to incident sites, facilitate communication among stakeholders, and make decisions about the response.[66]

PHEOCs may be permanent facilities that have ongoing baseline operations or be facilities that are set up in response to a disease outbreak.[67] Others may be stood up and activated only when needed. Regardless of whether an PHEOC is set up in a dedicated space or located in a repurposed facility, it must be physically and environmentally secure, with the appropriate general and emergency energy sources, communication networks, work spaces, sanitary facilities, security measures (control systems, barriers, secure areas, surveillance devices, etc.), and when relevant, food, water, and rest areas.

Some jurisdictions have protocols in place that specify when a PHEOC should be activated; others use an action committee or other authority to determine when to activate it.[68] Common activation triggers for PHEOCs include:

- Requests for assistance from overwhelmed subnational jurisdictions or countries
- Need for significant external partner coordination
- High level of expected political or media interest
- Need to coordinate risk communication messages with diverse partners
- Need for significant internal coordination across multiple agency programs
- Presence of a new disease agent or known agent exhibiting new characteristics
- Activation of other PHEOCs by external response partners[69]

See "Coordinating Response Efforts across Sectors" later in this chapter for more information on multisectoral coordination.

Incident command systems (ICS) or alternative frameworks may be used to manage staff, resources, and information at a PHEOC. They help provide a clear command structure, shared terminology, and standard protocols for effectively managing a public health emergency, evaluating its impact on the population and preparing for recovery.[70] Common PHEOC staff sections include command, operations, planning, logistics, finance, and administration. Liaisons from other organizations and/or agencies are useful to ensure collaboration and coordination.

Another common part of PHEOCs is an emergency response plan (ERP), which clearly lays out the operational roles, responsibilities, and resources attributed to the different entities involved in the response.

Given the important role PHEOCs play as central locations for coordinating operational information to support decision-making and management of public health emergencies, they must have the capacity to collate and share data and information among public health staff and stakeholders. This means having available and reliable information and communications technology, software, hardware, systems, and trained personnel that allow PHEOCs to collect, analyze, interpret, visualize, and disseminate information. Properly built data processing sharing platforms allow PHEOCs to receive information, process and analyze it, and share it back out to other actors in a timely fashion. These systems can be purchased or custom built. Backup systems, redundancy, and security requirements are also critical for ensuring that PHEOCs' information and data management systems remain functional even if initial systems glitch or fail.

Eventually when an outbreak ends, stabilizes, or is no longer a major threat, PHEOCs are no longer needed to manage the threat and are deactivated.[71] To make this decision, health authorities and other relevant leadership must assess certain factors:

- Incident status
- Nature and magnitude of the incident
- Hazards and safety concerns
- Priorities and resource requirements
- Activation level and staffing

Each country's public health emergency response plan should contain guidance for deactivation, including who can authorize deactivation, how to reduce staff levels, how to ensure critical activities remain supported, and what forms, reports, and other assessments will be required prior to deactivation.[72]

CASE STUDY

The Role of Public Health Emergency Operation Centers

in the Eradication of Polio in Nigeria

In 2012, Nigeria was one of three countries still struggling with uninterrupted wild poliovirus (WPV) transmission internally and had also been identified as the origin of imported WPV to twenty-five previously polio-free countries.[73] The continued spread of the disease was attributed to inadequate immunization, civil unrest and mistrust, and poor coordination between government and partner organizations.[74] As confirmed new cases continued to rise, it became increasingly clear that more intensive action was needed.

In March 2012, the Nigerian government established a presidential task force to guide the country's efforts to eradicate polio through improved immunization (supplemental and routine) campaigns and surveillance. Nigeria's Ministry of Health established public health emergency operations centers (PHEOCs) to implement initiatives in areas of highest priority, improve coordination, and closely monitor progress. Programmatic efforts were coordinated

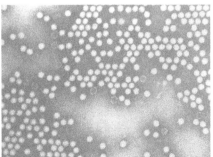

Poliovirus. Credit: CDC PHIL

with national and international organizations like the National Primary Health Care Development Agency, WHO, UNICEF, US CDC, the Bill and Melinda Gates Foundation, McKinsey and Company, and Rotary International.

A national PHEOC was established in the capital, Abuja, in October 2012, and subnational PHEOCs for each state were established between 2013 and 2014. The national PHEOC set the country's National Polio Eradication Emergency Plan (NPEEP) at the start of each year, outlining priorities, strategies, objectives, and milestones. An Expert Review Committee made up of representatives from the WHO, US CDC, UNICEF, and other partner organizations recommended activities for implementation. PHEOC members in the field determined which activities to prioritize and implement with the support of government and partners.

The success of NPEEP rested on clear collaboration between the national and state PHEOCs, allowing health officials and workers to make dynamic, evidence-based decisions using real-time field data at the state level while staying in line with the country's national agenda.[75] The state PHEOCs, in conjunction with the national PHEOC and other key stakeholders, used epidemiological data and community input and information to identify particularly vulnerable populations and to inform the design and implementation of tailored initiatives. For example, several states, including Borno and Yobe, faced security complications. Their polio emergency plans were adjusted accordingly to adapt to the higher risk. Kano and other states in northern Nigeria struggled with misinformation about the oral polio vaccine, such as it being a sterilization tool from Western powers, and general mistrust of the Nigerian government. In response, state PHEOCs launched trust-building activities implemented by key local field staff.[76] The eleven states at greatest risk of being polio strongholds were able to maintain autonomy while continuing to collaborate with the national PHEOC through decentralized coordination and resource distribution activities.

Implementation rates of the NPEEP increased in 2013 and 2014, resulting in significant declines in the number of children paralyzed by polio. One assessment of the PHEOCs' efficacy noted that more than 90 percent of planned activities with agreed milestones were achieved; at least 80 percent of the wards achieved more than 80 percent coverage with polio supplemental immunization; and more than 80 percent of the local government areas reached at least 80 percent coverage. Moreover, there was a 90 percent reduction in wild poliovirus cases from 122 in 2012 to 6 in 2014. In 2015, transmission was deemed "interrupted."[77] The PHEOC model's effectiveness in Nigeria's eradication of polio stemmed from clear leadership and a chain of command, the establishment of a joint agenda, and strong relationships built on collaboration, coordination, communication, and trust at both national and local levels.

The last polio case in Nigeria was detected in 2016. In June 2020, the Africa Regional Certification Commission for polio eradication certified Nigeria as WPV-free, and two months later in August 2020, certified the entire WHO Africa Region as WPV-free.[78]

Coordinating Response Efforts across Sectors

Public health events are not addressed solely by the health sector. Given the complex nature of diseases, a multidisciplinary response coordinated across sectors is necessary for effective outbreak preparedness, response, and recovery. Countries, ministries, relevant sectors, and stakeholders must jointly work to both create and implement health security measures. Health, laboratory, animal, environment, finance, foreign policy, transportation, commercial, agriculture, security and law enforcement, research, and private sectors all serve various purposes during an emergency public health response, and by coordinating efforts, they can lead a more efficient response. Personnel from public and private sectors should work to strengthen existing partnerships and build new ones to facilitate potential agreements in an outbreak context.

Office for the Coordination of Humanitarian Affairs

UN Office for the Coordination of Humanitarian Affairs (OCHA) supports response efforts across sectors. During the COVID-19 pandemic, OCHA boosted the UN systemwide response by creating an Inter-Agency Standing Committee to coordinate humanitarian agencies and NGOs.[79] Furthermore, OCHA released the COVID-19 Global Humanitarian Response Plan (GHRP) to further target intersectoral response coordination, and the plan included partnerships with a range of agencies such as FAO, IOM, UNDP, UNHCR, UNICEF, WFP, WHO, NGOs, the rest of the UN system and the Red Cross and Red Crescent Movement.[80] Under the same UN umbrella, the United Nations Country Team (UNCT) exists in 132 countries and targets interagency coordination and decision-making at a country level.[81]

For more information, see the "International Health Regulations" section in the Governance chapter, and the Risk chapter.

During humanitarian emergencies, WHO is the designated lead for health in coordination meetings among different partners, called the Humanitarian Cluster System. The cluster system is designed to ensure all of the stakeholders involved in a response are organized, connect to the partner governments, and are—ideally—coordinated in their actions.

The UN's Inter-Agency Standing Committee (IASC) has specific protocols for the control of infectious disease events, first adopted in 2016 and later revised.[82] The protocol is triggered by the WHO risk assessment process linked to the IHR. Activation of the protocol then leads to defined coordination activities: deployment of supplies and logistics, establishment of coordination hubs, deployment of surge capacity, and creation of response reporting. It addresses funding, ongoing rapid assessments, and coordinated humanitarian response efforts throughout an outbreak.

Global Outbreak Alert and Response Network

The Global Outbreak Alert and Response Network (GOARN) is a partnership of agencies established by the WHO to identify, confirm, and respond to global public health emergencies.[83] GOARN includes more than 270 technical institutions and networks (and their members) that span medical and surveillance initiatives, regional technical networks, networks of laboratories, UN organizations (such as UNICEF, UNHCR), the International Federation of Red Cross and Red Crescent Societies (IFRC), international humanitarian nongovernmental organizations (such as Médecins Sans Frontières and International Rescue Committee), and national public health institutions.

Operational Communication

Reliable and consistent operational communication during an outbreak is critical for effective planning and response. Regular communication between government officials and response partners is required to ensure the coordination of technical and operational support and timely, accurate sharing of information. Before an outbreak even happens, public health officials develop an operational communication strategy. Officials leading the response identify the agencies, organizations, and partners that need to be engaged in operational communication during an outbreak, identify key communication contacts, and define their roles. While the specific strategy, the groups involved, and the resources available will depend on the outbreak, most operational communication strategies present frameworks for sharing information between response organizers, covering:

- Processes for clearance and approval of information, materials, etc.
- Means of sharing information (email, call, text, in-person or teleconference meetings, web-based information sharing systems)
- Timing for sharing information
- Types of operational communications reports to develop during and after the outbreak
- Training programs for operational communications personnel[84]

Go to the Money chapter to learn about how countries and organizations manage the financial impacts of outbreaks.

Operational communications guidance considers which information channels government officials and partners have access to, prefer, and are appropriate for the messages' content, and the timing and frequency of messaging appropriate for the magnitude, scope, and nature of the threat. Maintaining partner channels relies on the establishment of a "trust triangle" between communicators, technical staff, and policymakers. To maintain that trust, the mechanisms used for communication should be accessible, timely, and accurate, and foster collaboration.

After an outbreak, operational communications reports can identify successes, failures, challenges, and strengths of the response. Operational reports may broadly cover the full response, or focus on one or more fields of operation, including supply chain management, resource procurement, distribution processes, and the capacity of health departments to meet surge needs. This information can guide the establishment of best practices, inform future emergency response plans, and provide critical insight into the events of the outbreak and its response.[85]

Go to the Community Engagement and Humanitarian Response chapter to read more about enhancing community resilience following an outbreak.

Recovery

In the aftermath of disease outbreaks, even well-resourced communities can experience severe disruptions to regular services, supply chains, available resources, and financial systems.[86] Thorough planning for disease outbreak recovery helps reduce social, economic, and health impacts, and ensures an organized and effective response and recovery.[87] Recovery processes offer a unique opportunity to plan for and reduce future public health risks.

Health officials begin the recovery planning process by creating a collaborative, interdisciplinary, community-based planning team to assess the impact of the outbreak on the public health system and on communities.[88] Using epidemiological research and analysis, they determine and prioritize short- and long-term recovery efforts.[89] Ultimately, the ideal recovery plan balances the competing interests of constituents to build long-term community health and resilience.[90]

Recovery plans capture both the social and economic aspects of a response, addressing how a government plans to revitalize and return the economy to pre-outbreak conditions, rebuild and strengthen social service delivery capacity, and provide support to the most vulnerable community members, including care (economic or otherwise) for individuals incapacitated by long term effects of infection as well as the bereaved families of those who died during the outbreak. Public health personnel use situation monitoring and assessment to quantify the effectiveness of recovery measures and help update protocols, guidelines, and public health priorities.[91] Once recovery plans are updated or new information regarding the outbreak arises, health officials must keep the public and relevant stakeholders informed. It is also important to establish systems for monitoring and treatment of individuals with long term health problems resulting from the outbreak. For example, more than 75 percent of Ebola survivors suffer from significant long-term complications, including headaches, joint pain, and vision problems.[92] Following the Zika outbreak, a registry was created to monitor the long term effects of babies born with at least one Zika-related birth defect.[93] Similarly, in July 2023, US Health and Human Services announced the creation of the Long COVID Research and Practice office to support the somewhere between 7.7 and 23 million Americans who developed Long COVID.[94]

Document Lessons Learned during Recovery

After-action reviews (AARs) document lessons learned from the public health crisis. They are retrospective, qualitative assessments of actions taken from preparedness for a public health event through to recovery. AARs evaluate organizational capacity gaps, challenges, and best practices by looking at emergency operations plans, information sharing methods, how coordination with local, state, and other relevant stakeholders was carried out, staff and resource management, logistics and supply chains, infection prevention measures, laboratory and testing capabilities, case management protocols, medical countermeasure use, and administrative and financial management.[95]

The WHO suggests AARs focus on four central questions: (1) what was supposed to happen, (2) what actually happened, (3) why was there a difference, (4) and what can be learned from this.[96] These questions should help stakeholders understand the root cause of the problems to identify where health officials can improve their emergency response.[97] For public health preparedness, identifying, documenting, and sharing lessons learned can strengthen institutional capacities to better prepare for and prevent mistakes, as well as minimize moral and financial harm in future public health crises.[98] Ultimately, AARs help ensure critical thinking about infectious disease outbreaks, build consensus on critical issues, promote cross-sectoral learning, and strengthen capacities for preparedness and response.[99]

What Does It Mean to Return to Normal?

WRAPPING UP

Learning from the Past to Prepare for the Future

During a public health emergency, normal operations may cease because medical and public health professionals are focused on outbreak response; businesses may close to stop the spread of disease or for lack of staff due to infection; elective medical procedures and routine check-ups may be cancelled; and lockdowns, curfews, and other physical distancing limitations may affect professional and educational environments, as well as public transportation access and events of all sizes.

Disease outbreaks, whether a small cluster or a global pandemic, impact people differently.

A "return to normal" should be guided by evidence and the epidemiological reality of the situation, and maybe even an acceptance that our concepts of normality can change—the impact of disease certainly has that ability. Health systems must resume addressing nonemergent patients, especially those whose conditions may have been exacerbated by reduced access to care during the outbreak.[1] Workplaces, schools, and other public environments must eventually lift restrictions. Government officials must resume addressing regular concerns for their constituents, as well as any additional issues resulting from the outbreak, such as unemployment, housing insecurity, and the financial consequences of illness and death.

Our hope—as public health professionals—is that people learn from the outbreak, and become better acquainted with basic preventive practices to stop the next one.

CASE STUDY AND FACTS INDEX

GLOSSARY

A

AFTER-ACTION REVIEW (AAR): A qualitative review of the actions taken during a public health event response, project, or intervention, used to identify and document best practices and challenges encountered during the response to the event or the implementation of the project

AGENT: Any infectious microorganism, including bacteria, viruses, fungi, and parasites, capable of causing disease

ANTIMICROBIAL RESISTANCE (AMR): When bacteria, viruses, fungi, and parasites no longer respond to medicines as a result of a mutation. This makes treating infections harder and increases the risk of disease spread, severe illness, and death

ASYMPTOMATIC: When an infected human or animal does not show symptoms associated with a disease they are infected with (also see **carrier**)

ATTRIBUTION ASSESSMENT: The task of determining who was responsible for a deliberate event

B

BIODEFENSE: Defensive measures taken to prevent, detect, respond to, and recover from harm or damage caused by intentional use of a biological agent

BIOLOGICAL AND TOXINS WEAPONS CONVENTION (BWC): An international treaty adopted in 1972 prohibiting the development, production, proliferation, and retention of biological or toxin weapons

BIOSAFETY: The practices, equipment, and infrastructure implemented to safely contain and prevent unintentional exposure to pathogens and toxins, or their accidental release

BIOSAFETY LEVELS: The biosafety measures taken to safely contain increasingly dangerous hazardous biological materials or agents

BIOSECURITY: The set of processes used to protect and control biological materials as well as information and research related to these materials, to prevent their unauthorized access, loss, theft, misuse, diversion, or intentional release

C

CARRIER: An infected person or animal that can transmit an infectious agent to others but does not exhibit symptoms of the disease (also see **asymptomatic**)

CASE: A person or animal who has the particular disease that meets the case definitions for surveillance and outbreak investigation purposes. The definition of a case for surveillance and outbreak investigation purpose is not necessarily the same as the ordinary clinical definition

CASE DEFINITION: A set of diagnostic criteria that must be fulfilled for an individual to be regarded as a case of a particular disease for surveillance and outbreak investigation purposes. Case definitions can be based on clinical criteria, laboratory criteria, or a combination of the two, and incorporates specific information on time and place of exposure, as well as characteristics about the person

CLADE: Organisms that originate from a common ancestor. In virology, it describes clusters of similar viruses based on genetic sequences. For COVID, SARS-CoV-2 is a clade within the larger family of Coronaviruses (including SARS and MERS). These are the "branches" in the phylogenic tree

COLD CHAIN: A system of storing and transporting medical countermeasures at recommended temperatures from the point of manufacture to the point of use

COMMUNICABLE DISEASE: An illness caused by an infectious agent or its toxins that occurs through direct or indirect transmission from an infected individual, animal, vector, or the environment to another susceptible host. Often simply defined as a disease transmitted from person to person

COMMUNITY ASSESSMENT FOR PUBLIC HEALTH EMERGENCY RESPONSE (CASPER): A method used in disaster epidemiology to rapidly collect health information in a representative manner

COMMUNITY-BASED SURVEILLANCE (CBS): The starting point for event notification at the community level, generally done by a community worker; it can be active (looking for cases) or passive (reporting cases). It may be particularly useful during an outbreak and where syndromic case definitions can be used

CONTACT: An individual who has been in close proximity to another individual who is, or is suspected of being, infected with an infectious disease agent

CONTACT TRACING: The set of processes involved in identifying, interviewing, and monitoring contacts of cases to determine if they have been infected

CONTAMINATION: The presence of an infectious or toxic agent or matter on the body surface of a human or animal, in or on a product prepared for consumption or on other inanimate objects, including conveyances that may constitute a public health risk

D

DECONTAMINATION: Procedures used to control or kill infectious agents on living or inanimate surfaces

DISEASE: An illness or medical condition caused by a specific agent and manifesting through the presentation of distinctive signs or symptoms

DOCUMENTED PROCEDURES: Agreed and approved strategies for operation, standard operating procedures, roles and responsibilities, agreements, terms of reference, chains of command, and reporting mechanisms, among others

E

EARLY WARNING SYSTEM (EWAR): A specific procedure in disease surveillance to detect any abnormal occurrence, or departure from the usual or normally observed frequency of phenomena (such as one case of Ebola fever), as early as possible. An early warning system is only useful if it is linked to mechanisms for early response

EMERGING INFECTIOUS DISEASE (EID): An infectious disease that has not been seen before or is novel in its epidemiologic range (geographic or host) or transmission mode

ENDEMIC: A disease that occurs regularly and is limited to a geographic area or population

EPIDEMIC: An occurrence of disease in a population that is greater than would otherwise be expected at a particular time and place; the number of cases indicating the presence of an epidemic varies according to the agent, size and type of population exposed, previous experience or lack of exposure to the disease, and time and place of occurrence (used in the same way as **outbreak**)

EPIDEMIOLOGY: The scientific field that studies the patterns of health and illness and health determinants at the population level

ETHYLENEDIAMINETETRAACETIC ACID (EDTA): An anticoagulant used for most procedures related to blood; the purple tubes used when blood is drawn contain EDTA.

ETIOLOGY: The cause(s) or origin(s) of a disease

EVENT: A manifestation of disease or an occurrence that creates a potential for disease

EVENT-BASED SURVEILLANCE (EBS): The organized and rapid capture of information about events that are a potential risk to public health. This information can be rumors and other ad hoc reports transmitted through formal channels (e.g., established routine reporting systems) and informal channels (e.g., the media, health workers, and reports from nongovernmental organizations), including events related to the occurrence of disease in humans and events related to potential human exposure

EXPOSURE: Any factor that may be associated with the infection or disease

F

FIELD EPIDEMIOLOGY (SHOE LEATHER EPIDEMIOLOGY): A type of epidemiology in which experts work on response to urgent public health events in order to collect pertinent information and guide interventions to mitigate the impacts of the event. The term "shoe leather epidemiologist" refers to people who go out in the community and personally investigate disease

FIELD EPIDEMIOLOGY TRAINING PROGRAM (FETP): A training program designed to build capacity in conducting timely outbreak detection, public health response, and public health surveillance

FOMITE: Object or material that can carry and/or spread disease and infectious agents

G

GLOBAL HEALTH SECURITY: The existence of strong and resilient public health systems that can prepare for; prevent, detect, and respond to; and recover from acute public health emergencies with the potential for international spread, irrespective of biologic origin or geographic location

H

HAZARD: The inherent capability of an agent or situation to have an adverse effect; a factor or exposure that may adversely affect health

HEALTH CARE WORKER: An individual working in the provision of health services, whether or not professionally trained, and whether or not subject to public regulation; includes a variety of professions, such as clinicians, therapists, social workers, pharmacists, and other technicians

HEALTH EVENT: Any event relating to the health of an individual, such as the occurrence of a case of a specific disease or syndrome, the administration of a vaccine, or an admission to hospital

HEALTH MEASURE: A procedure applied to prevent the spread of disease or contamination; not inclusive of law enforcement or security measures

HEALTH SECURITY: Multisectoral efforts geared toward minimizing the impact of acute public health emergencies on populations, economies, and political stability

HEALTH THREAT: A risk to public health in the context of national or global security

I

INCIDENCE: The number of new cases of disease during a specific period of time in a specific population

INCIDENT COMMAND SYSTEM: The standardized approach or hierarchy for the command, control, and coordination of emergency response personnel often across multiple agencies and organizations

INCUBATION PERIOD: The time interval between exposure to a biological agent and the first appearance of disease symptoms

INDEX CASE: The first confirmed case of an outbreak

INDICATOR-BASED SURVEILLANCE (IBS):
The routine reporting of cases of disease, including from notifiable diseases surveillance, sentinel surveillance, or laboratory-based surveillance. This routine reporting is commonly health care facility–based with reporting done on a weekly or monthly basis

INFECTION: The entry and development or multiplication of an infectious agent in the body of humans and animals that may constitute a public health risk

INFECTION PREVENTION AND CONTROL (IPC): Measures used to prevent, control, and contain the spread of infectious disease, based on how the agent is transmitted

INTERNATIONAL HEALTH REGULATIONS (IHR): An international, legally binding treaty requiring all member states of the WHO to uphold specific practices and procedures to detect, report, and respond to potential public health emergencies of international concern

ISOLATION: Separation and restriction of movement of people or animals that are believed to have a communicable disease

J

JOINT EXTERNAL EVALUATION TOOL (JEE):
A voluntary, collaborative, multisectoral process as part of the IHR Monitoring and Evaluation Framework to assess country capacities to prevent, detect, and rapidly respond to public health risks whether occurring naturally or due to deliberate or accidental events; the JEE helps countries identify the most critical gaps within their public health systems in order to prioritize opportunities for enhanced preparedness and response

L

LITERATURE REVIEW: a comprehensive review of previous research on a given topic

M

MEDICAL COUNTERMEASURES (MCM):
Regulated products and equipment (e.g., drugs, vaccines, diagnostic tests, ventilators) that both prevent the harmful effects of a biological agent and mitigate consequences for those who become ill

MORBIDITY: Having a disease or symptom of disease

MORTALITY: Death

MULTISECTORAL: A holistic approach involving the efforts of multiple organizations, institutes, and agencies. It encourages interdisciplinary participation, collaboration, and coordination of people of concern and resources from these key organizations for promoting health security, to achieve a specific goal

N

NOTIFIABLE DISEASE: A disease that must be reported to appropriate authorities, as mandated by either law or regulation

NOTIFICATION: The processes by which cases or outbreaks are brought to the knowledge of the health authorities

O

ONE HEALTH: Term used to refer to using a multisectoral approach to achieve optimal health outcomes recognizing the interconnection between people, animals, plants, and their shared environment

OUTBREAK: An epidemic limited to localized increase in the incidence of a disease, such as in a village, town, or closed institution

P

PANDEMIC: Spread of a disease across a wide geographic area and affecting multiple populations, often at a global scale. Some official definitions require spread to two or more WHO regions, as well as serious severity of disease

PATHOGEN: See agent

PERSONAL PROTECTIVE EQUIPMENT (PPE): Specialized clothing and equipment designed to create a barrier and protect against health and safety hazards; equipment may include masks, respiratory protective devices, protective clothing, and other forms of protection

PHYSICAL DISTANCING: An infection control strategy that includes methods taken to restrict when and where people can gather with the intent of stopping or slowing the spread of communicable diseases

POINT OF ENTRY (POE): A passage for international entry or exit of travelers, baggage, cargo, containers, conveyances, goods, and postal parcels, and the agencies and areas providing services to them upon entry or exit. Also designated as an international entry point by nations under the IHR

POSITIVE PREDICTIVE VALUE: The proportion of individuals with a positive test result that actually have the disease

PREPAREDNESS: The actions and policies associated with preventing, protecting against, responding to, and recovering from an event

PREVALENCE: The number of instances of illness or of persons ill, in a specified population, without any distinction between new and old cases

PUBLIC HEALTH: There are multiple definitions of public health, but at its simplest, it is the science of protecting and improving health of populations and their communities

PUBLIC HEALTH EMERGENCY: An acute event capable of causing large-scale morbidity and mortality, either immediately or over time; these events have the ability to overwhelm normal public health capabilities

PUBLIC HEALTH EMERGENCY OF INTERNATIONAL CONCERN (PHEIC): An extraordinary event (as defined in the IHR) that constitutes both a public health risk to other states through the international spread of disease and that may require a coordinated, international response. PHEICs are declared by the Director General of the WHO through processes defined by the IHR

PUBLIC HEALTH EMERGENCY OPERATIONS CENTER (PHEOC): A central facility responsible for carrying out the principles of emergency preparedness and management or disaster management functions at a strategic level during a public health emergency

PUBLIC HEALTH LITERACY: The ability of individuals to obtain, understand, and use information necessary to make public health decisions

PUBLIC HEALTH RISK: The likelihood of an event that may adversely affect the health of human populations, with an emphasis on whether it may spread internationally or present a serious and direct danger

Q

QUALITATIVE DATA: Information that is measured by types instead of numbers

QUANTITATIVE DATA: Data that can be counted, including numeric variables

QUARANTINE: The separation and restriction of movement of people or animals that may have been exposed to an infectious agent

R

RAPID RESPONSE TEAM: A group of trained individuals that is ready to respond quickly to an event. The composition and terms of reference are determined by the concerned country or organization

READINESS: The ability to quickly and appropriately respond when required to any emergency

RESERVOIR: The principal source in which an infectious agent normally lives, the presence of which may constitute a public health risk

RISK COMMUNICATION: A range of communication capacities required through the preparedness, response, and recovery phases of a serious public health event to encourage informed decision making, positive behavior change, and the maintenance of trust

S

SENSITIVITY: The ability of a test to identify an individual with disease as positive

SPECIFICITY: The ability of a test to identify an individual who does not have a disease as negative

STRATEGIC STOCKPILE: A stockpile of drugs, vaccines, and medical equipment that can be rapidly deployed in response to a public health emergency

SURGE CAPACITY: The ability of a health care system (such as clinical care facilities and laboratories) to accommodate a sharp increase in demand beyond normal services during a public health emergency

SURVEILLANCE: The systematic ongoing collection, collation, and analysis of data for public health purposes, and the timely dissemination of public health information for assessment and public health response

SYMPTOMS: Effects of infection apparent to an infected individual

T

TECHNICAL EXPERTISE/GUIDANCE: Guidance published or provided by a recognized authority, including governments, international organizations, or professional experts

TRANSMISSION: An agent leaving its reservoir or host and infecting a susceptible host; also, how an agent is spread from one entity to another

V

VACCINE: Induces immunity in humans and animals against a pathogenic agent

VERIFICATION: The provision of information by a State Party to WHO confirming the status of an event within the territory or territories of that State Party

VIRULENCE: The ability of an infectious agent to cause disease and death

W

WORLD HEALTH ORGANIZATION: The directing and coordinating authority for human health within the UN system. It is responsible for providing leadership on public health matters, setting research agendas, articulating evidence-based policy options, and providing technical support to countries

WORLD ORGANISATION FOR ANIMAL HEALTH (WOAH, FORMERLY OIE): An international organization that directs and coordinates activities associated with animal health. It is responsible for informing governments of the occurrence and prevention of animal disease, setting research agendas, and harmonizing trade regulations for animals and animal products

Z

ZOONOSIS/ZOONOTIC DISEASE: A disease that is transmitted from animals to humans

NOTES

Book epigraph. Katherine F. Smith, Michael Goldberg, Samantha Rosenthal, Lynn Carlson, Jane Chen, Cici Chen, and Sohini Ramachandran, "Global Rise in Human Infectious Disease Outbreaks," *Journal of the Royal Society Interface* 11, no. 101 (December 2014): 20140950. https://doi.org/10.1098/rsif.2014.0950.

INTRODUCTION

1. Georgetown Outbreak Activity Library (GOAL), outbreaklibrary.org; "Outbreak Activity Library: An Online, User-Friendly Compilation of Activities Essential for Effective Outbreak Response," Research brief 2020-05, Georgetown University Center for Global Health Science and Security, 2020, https://georgetown.app.box.com/s/p64gdearegdw9rdtnn004408ole7g7nv.

CHAPTER 1

1. Sonja A. Rasmussen, and Richard A. Goodman, "The CDC Field Epidemiology Manual," Centers for Disease Control and Prevention, last modified December 2018, https://www.cdc.gov/eis/field-epi-manual/index.html.
2. Julia M. Baker, Markus Buchfellner, William Britt, Veronica Sanchez, Jennifer L. Potter, L. Amanda Ingram, Henry Shiau, et al., "Acute Hepatitis and Adenovirus Infection among Children—Alabama, October 2021–February 2022," *Morbidity and Mortality Weekly Report* 71, no. 18 (May 2022): 638-40, http://dx.doi.org/10.15585/mmwr.mm7118e1.
3. Anita K Kambhampati, "Trends in Acute Hepatitis of Unspecified Etiology and Adenovirus Stool Testing Results in Children—United States, 2017–2022," *Morbidity and Mortality Weekly Report* 71 (June 2022): 797-802, http://dx.doi.org/10.15585/mmwr.mm7124e1.
4. "Multi-Country — Acute, Severe Hepatitis of Unknown Origin in Children," World Health Organization, last modified April 23, 2022, https://www.who.int/emergencies/disease-outbreak-news/item/2022-DON376.
5. "Red Book Online Outbreaks: Hepatitis Cases Possibly Associated with Adenoviral Infection," American Academy of Pediatrics, last modified December 7, 2023, https://publications.aap.org/redbook/resources/20171.
6. Nelson, Amy, Lauren N. Bradley, and FOCUS Workgroup, "Laboratory Diagnosis: An Overview," *FOCUS on Field Epidemiology* 4, no. 3 (2007), https://nciph.sph.unc.edu/focus/vol4/issue3/4-3LabOverview_issue.pdf.
7. "Lesson 1: Introduction to Epidemiology," Centers for Disease Control and Prevention, last modified May 18, 2012, https://www.cdc.gov/csels/dsepd/ss1978/lesson1/section5.html.
8. "Background: Constructing a Case Definition," European Centre for Disease Prevention and Control, last modified January 1, 2012, https://www.ecdc.europa.eu/sites/default/files/media/en/healthtopics/food_and_waterborne_disease/toolkit/Documents/tool-03-3-case-definitions-background.pdf.
9. Neil Gupta, "Introduction to Outbreak Investigations of Healthcare—Associated Infections," Pan American Health Organization (Online Webinar), February 13, 2018, https://www.paho.org/en/documents/introduction-outbreak-investigations-healthcare-associated-infections-february-2018.

10. "Outbreak Case Definitions," Centers for Disease Control and Prevention, accessed December 6, 2023, https://www.cdc.gov/urdo/downloads/CaseDefinitions.pdf.

11. Robert E Fontaine, "The CDC Field Epidemiology Manual: Describing Epidemiologic Data," Centers for Disease Control and Prevention, last modified December 13, 2018, https://www.cdc.gov/eis/field-epi-manual/chapters/Describing-Epi-Data.html.

12. "Chapter 1. What is Epidemiology?" *BMJ*, accessed December 6, 2023, https://www.bmj.com/about-bmj/resources-readers/publications/epidemiology-uninitiated/1-what-epidemiology.

13. "Case Definitions," Outbreak Toolkit, National Collaborating Centre for Infectious Diseases Canada, accessed December 6, 2023, https://outbreaktools.ca/background/case-definitions.

14. "Community-Based Surveillance: Guiding Principles," International Federation of Red Cross and Red Crescent Societies, March 2017, https://www.ifrc.org/sites/default/files/CommunityBasedSurveillance_Global-LR.pdf.

15. Wayne W. LaMorte, "Step 3: Establish a Case Definition; Identify Cases," Outbreak Investigations, Boston University School of Public Health, last modified May 3, 2016, https://sphweb.bumc.bu.edu/otlt/mph-modules/ph/outbreak/Outbreak4.html.

16. "Outbreak Investigation Steps. Step 2: Define and Find Cases," Centers for Disease Control and Prevention, last modified June 20, 2018, https://www.cdc.gov/foodsafety/outbreaks/steps/defining-cases.html.

17. "Lesson 6: Investigating an Outbreak," Centers for Disease Control and Prevention, last modified September 15, 2016, https://www.cdc.gov/csels/dsepd/ss1978/lesson6/section2.html.

18. "Initial Case-Patient Interviewing," Centers for Disease Control and Prevention, last modified April 12, 2019, https://www.cdc.gov/foodcore/practice/case-patient-interviewing.html.

19. "Contact Tracing in the Context of COVID-19: Interim Guidance," World Health Organization, last modified February 1, 2021, https://apps.who.int/iris/handle/10665/339128.

20. "Bioterrorism Response Planning: Public Health Response Activities," Centers for Disease Control and Prevention, last modified July 24, 2017, https://www.cdc.gov/smallpox/bioterrorism-response-planning/public-health/epidemiological-investigation.html.

21. "Infection Prevention and Control: Contact Tracing," World Health Organization, last modified May 9, 2017, https://www.who.int/news-room/questions-and-answers/item/contact-tracing.

22. Vincent Wong, Daniel Cooney, and Yaneer Bar-Yam, "Beyond Contact Tracing: Community-Based Early Detection for Ebola Response," *PLoS Currents* 8 (May 2016), doi: 10.1371/currents.outbreaks.322427f4c3cc2b9c1a5b3395e7d20894.

23. Olushayo Oluseun Olu, Margaret Lamunu, Miriam Nanyunja, Foday Dafae, Thomas Samba, Noah Sempiira, Fredson Kuti-George, et al., "Contact Tracing during an Outbreak of Ebola Virus Disease in the Western Area Districts of Sierra Leone: Lessons for Future Ebola Outbreak Response," *Frontiers in Public Health*, no. 4 (June 2016): 130, https://doi.org/10.3389/fpubh.2016.00130.

24. World Health Organization, Disease Surveillance and Response Programme Area, Disease Prevention and Control Cluster. *Contact Tracing during an Outbreak of Ebola Virus Disease* (Brazzaville: World Health Organization Regional Office for Africa, 2014), https://apps.who.int/iris/bitstream/handle/10665/159040/9789290232575.pdf.

25. Krista C. Swanson, Chiara Altare, Chea Sanford Wesseh, Tolbert Nyenswah, Tashrik Ahmed, Nir Eyal, Esther L. Hamblion, Justin Lessler, David H. Peters, and Mathias Altmann, "Contact Tracing Performance during the Ebola Epidemic in Liberia,

2014–2015," *PLoS Neglected Tropical Diseases* 12, no. 9 (September 2018): e0006762, https://doi.org/10.1371/journal.pntd.0006762.

26. Saurabh RamBihariLal Shrivastava, Prateek Saurabh Shrivastava, and Jegadeesh Ramasamy, "Utility of Contact Tracing in Reducing the Magnitude of Ebola Disease," *Germs* 4, no. 4 (December 2014): 97, https://doi.org/10.11599/germs.2014.1063.

27. Mikiko Senga, Alpha Koi, Lina Moses, Nadia Wauquier, Philippe Barboza, Maria Dolores Fernandez-Garcia, Etsub Engedashet, et al., "Contact Tracing Performance during the Ebola Virus Disease Outbreak in Kenema District, Sierra Leone," *Philosophical Transactions of the Royal Society B: Biological Sciences* 372, no. 1721 (April 2017), https://doi.org/10.1098/rstb.2016.0300.

28. Cordelia E. Coltart, M. Benjamin Lindsey, Isaac Ghinai, Anne M. Johnson, and David L. Heymann, "The Ebola Outbreak, 2013–2016: Old Lessons for New Epidemics." *Philosophical Transactions of the Royal Society B: Biological Sciences* 372, no. 1721 (April 2017): https://doi.org/10.1098/rstb.2016.0297; Wong, Cooney, and Bar-Yam, "Beyond Contact Tracing."

29. Gerardo Chowell and Hiroshi Nishiura, "Transmission Dynamics and Control of Ebola Virus Disease (EVD): A Review." *BMC Medicine* 12, no. 1 (October 2014): 1–17. https://doi.org/10.1186/s12916-014-0196-0; Olu et al., "Contact Tracing during an Outbreak"; Shrivastava et al., "Utility of Contact Tracing," 97.

30. Jilian A Sacks, Elizabeth Zehe, Cindil Redick, Alhoussaine Bah, Kai Cowger, Mamady Camara, Aboubacar Diallo, Abdel Nasser Iro Gigo, Ranu S. Dhillon, and Anne Liu, "Introduction of Mobile Health Tools to Support Ebola Surveillance and Contact Tracing in Guinea," *Global Health: Science and Practice* 3, no. 4 (2015): 646–59, http://dx.doi.org/10.9745/GHSP-D-15-00207.

31. Clarence Roy-Macaulay, "Sierra Leone Makes Hiding Ebola Patients Illegal," Associated Press, last modified July 14, 2016, https://www.aol.com/article/2014/08/23/sierra-leone-makes-hiding-ebola-patients-illegal/20951542.

32. Sacks et al., "Introduction of Mobile Health Tools."

33. Olu et al., "Contact Tracing during an Outbreak."

34. Ayesha Rascoe, "What's Driving the Rise in STIs?" National Public Radio, September 25, 2022, podcast, audio. https://www.npr.org/2022/09/25/1124974244/whats-driving-the-rise-in-stis.; "Reported STDs Reach All-Time High for 6th Consecutive Year," Centers for Disease Control and Prevention, last modified April 13, 2021, https://www.cdc.gov/media/releases/2021/p0413-stds.html.

35. Tomas Folke and Anatole Sebastian Menon-Johansson, "An Evaluation of Digital Partner Notification Tool Engagement and Impact for Patients Diagnosed with Gonorrhea and Syphilis," *Sexually Transmitted Diseases* 49, no. 12 (December 2022): 815–21, https://doi.org/10.1097/OLQ.0000000000001707.

36. Kristin N. Harper, Molly K. Zuckerman, Megan L. Harper, John D. Kingston, and George J. Armelagos, "The Origin and Antiquity of Syphilis Revisited: An Appraisal of Old World Pre-Columbian Evidence for Treponemal Infection," *American Journal of Physical Anthropology* 146, no. S53 (November 2011): 99–133, https://doi.org/10.1002/ajpa.21613.

37. Maria A. Spyrou, Guido A. Lyazzat Musralina, Gnecchi Ruscone, Arthur Kocher, Pier-Giorgio Borbone, Valeri I. Khartanovich, Alexandra Buzhilova Leyla Djansugurova, Kirsten Bos, Denise Kuhnert, Wolfgang Haak, Philip Slavin, and Johannes Krause, "The Source of the Black Death in Fourteenth-Century Central Eurasia," *Nature* 606, no. 7915 (June 2022): 718–24, https://doi.org/10.1038/s41586-022-04800-3.

38. Michelle Torok, "Case Finding and Line Listing: A Guide for Investigators," *FOCUS on Field Epidemiology* 1, no. 4, accessed December 8, 2023, https://nciph.sph.unc.edu/focus/vol1/issue4/1-4CaseFinding_issue.pdf.

39. "Line List Template," Centers for Disease Control and Prevention, last modified January 2008, https://www.cdc.gov/urdo/downloads/linelisttemplate.pdf.; "Line Lists," Outbreak Toolkit, National Collaborating Centre for Infectious Disease Canada, accessed December 8, 2023, https://outbreaktools.ca/background/line-lists.

40. Wayne W. LaMorte, "Descriptive Epidemiology," Boston University School of Public Health, last modified May 5, 2017, https://sphweb.bumc.bu.edu/otlt/MPH-Modules/EP/EP713_DescriptiveEpi.

41. "Quick-Learn Lesson: Using an Epi Curve to Determine Mode of Spread," Centers for Disease Control and Prevention, accessed December 9, 2023, https://www.cdc.gov/training/QuickLearns/epimode.

42. Tom Koch, "Knowing Its Place: Mapping As Medical Investigation," *Lancet* 379, no. 9819 (March 2012): 887–88, https://doi.org/10.1016/S0140-6736(12)60383-3.

43. "John Snow's Map 1 (1854)," UCLA, Fielding School of Public Health, accessed December 9, 2023, https://www.ph.ucla.edu/epi/snow/snowmap1_1854_lge.htm.

44. "Epidemiological Research Methods: Epidemiologic Hypotheses, Designs, and Populations," Penn State Eberly College of Science, accessed December 9, 2023, https://online.stat.psu.edu/stat507/lesson/1/1.4-0.

45. Michelle Torok, "Hypothesis Generation during Outbreaks," FOCUS on Field Epidemiology 1, no. 4, accessed December 12, 2023, https://nciph.sph.unc.edu/focus/vol1/issue6/1-6Hypothesis_issue.pdf.

46. "Section 10: Chain of Infection," Centers for Disease Control and Prevention, last modified May 18, 2012, https://archive.cdc.gov/www_cdc_gov/csels/dsepd/ss1978/lesson1/section10.html.

47. Paul L Delamater, Erica J. Street, Timothy F. Leslie, Y. Tony Yang, and Kathryn H. Jacobsen, "Complexity of the Basic Reproduction Number (R_0)," *Emerging Infectious Diseases* 25, no. 1 (January 2019): 1–4, https://doi.org/10.3201/eid2501.171901.

48. Seoyun Choe, Hee-Sung Kim, and Sunmi Lee, "Exploration of Superspreading Events in 2015 MERS-CoV Outbreak in Korea by Branching Process Models," *International Journal of Environmental Research and Public Health* 17, no. 17 (August 2020): 6137, https://doi.org/10.3390/ijerph17176137.

49. Filio Marineli, Gregory Tsoucalas, Marianna Karamanou, and George Androutsos, "Mary Mallon (1869–1938) and the History of Typhoid Fever," *Annals of Gastroenterology* 26, no. 2 (2013): 132–34, https://www.ncbi.nlm.nih.gov/pmc/articles/PMC3959940.

50. Lorraine K. Alexander, Brettania Lopes, Kristen Ricchetti-Masterson, and Karin B. Yeatts, "Cohort Studies," *ERIC Notebook*, 2nd ed., no. 6 (2014–2015): 1–4, https://sph.unc.edu/wp-content/uploads/sites/112/2015/07/nciph_ERIC6.pdf.

51. Communicable Diseases Network Australia, *Guidelines for the Public Health Management of Gastroenteritis Outbreaks Due to Norovirus or Suspected Viral Agents in Australia* (Canberra: Australian Government Department of Health and Ageing, 2010): chap. 7, https://www.health.gov.au/sites/default/files/documents/2020/03/norovirus-and-suspected-viral-gastroenteritis-cdna-national-guidelines-for-public-health-units-guidelines.pdf.

52. Meike Ressing, Maria Blettner, and Stefanie J. Klug, "Data Analysis of Epidemiological Studies: Part 11 of a Series on Evaluation of Scientific Publications." Deutsches Ärzteblatt International 107, no. 11 (March2010): 187–92, https://doi.org/10.3238/arztebl.2010.0187. https://doi.org/10.3238/arztebl.2010.0187.

53. Meredith Anderson, Amy Nelson, and FOCUS Workgroup, "Data Analysis: Simple Statistical Tests," *FOCUS on Field Epidemiology* 3, no. 6, https://nciph.sph.unc.edu/focus/vol3/issue6/3-6DataTests_issue.pdf.

54. Vladimir Trkulja and Pero Hrabač, "The Role of t Test in Beer Brewing," *Croatian Medical Journal* 61, no. 1 (February 2020): 69–72, doi:10.3325/cmj.2020.61.69.

55. Lorraine K. Alexander, Brettania Lopes, Kristen Ricchetti-Masterson, and Karin B. Yeatts, "Common Statistical Tests and Applications in Epidemiological Literature," *ERIC Notebook*, 2nd ed., no 2 (2014–2015), https://sph.unc.edu/wp-content/uploads/sites/112/2015/07/nciph_ERIC2.pdf.

56. "Outbreak Investigations," Boston University School of Public Health, accessed December 9, 2023, https://sphweb.bumc.bu.edu/otlt/mph-modules/ph/outbreak/outbreak_print.html.

57. Michael E. King, Diana M. Bensyl, Richard A. Goodman, and Sonja A. Rasmussen, "Conducting a Field Investigation," CDC Field Epidemiology Manual. Centers for Disease Control and Prevention, last modified 2018, https://www.cdc.gov/eis/field-epi-manual/chapters/Field-Investigation.html.

58. Barbara L Herwaldt, Marta-Louise Ackers, and Cyclospora Working Group, "An Outbreak in 1996 of Cyclosporiasis Associated with Imported Raspberries," *New England Journal of Medicine* 336, no. 22 (May 1997): 1548–56, doi: 10.1056/NEJM199705293362202.

59. Linda Calvin, Luis Flores, and William E. Foster, "Case Study: Guatemalan Raspberries and Cyclospora." No. 569-2016-39036. Food Safety in Food Security and Food Trade 10, no. 7 (September 2003), https://www.researchgate.net/publication/5055676_Case_study_Guatemalan_raspberries_and_cyclospora.

60. Calvin, Flores, and Foster, "Case Study."

61. "What Is Anthrax?" Centers for Disease Control and Prevention, last modified February 15, 2022, https://www.cdc.gov/anthrax/basics/index.html.

62. Susan Scutti, "Russian Officials Blame Thawed Reindeer Carcass in Anthrax Outbreak," CNN, July 28, 2016, https://www.cnn.com/2016/07/28/health/anthrax-thawed-reindeer-siberia.

63. Elisa Stella, Lorenzo Mari, Jacopo Gabrieli, Carlo Barbante, and Enrico Bertuzzo, "Permafrost Dynamics and the Risk of Anthrax Transmission: A Modelling Study," *Scientific Reports* 10, no. 1 (October 2020): 1–12, https://doi.org/10.1038/s41598-020-72440-6.; Elena A. Liskova, Irina Y. Egorova, Yuri O. Selyaninov, Irina V. Razheva, Nadezhda A. Gladkova, Nadezhda N. Toropova, Olga I. Zakharova, et al.,"Reindeer Anthrax in the Russian Arctic, 2016: Climatic Determinants of the Outbreak and Vaccination Effectiveness," *Frontiers in Veterinary Science* 8 (June 2021), https://doi.org/10.3389/fvets.2021.668420.

64. "Child, 12, Died from Anthrax, as Nine Cases Confirmed of the Deadly Disease," *Siberian Times*, August 1, 2016, http://siberiantimes.com/other/others/news/n0693-eight-people-have-contracted-anthrax-amid-reports-that-one-has-died.

65. "UPDATED First Anthrax Outbreak since 1941: 9 Hospitalised, with Two Feared to Have Disease," *Siberian Times*, July 26, 2016, http://siberiantimes.com/other/others/news/n0686-first-anthrax-outbreak-since-1941-9-hospitalised-with-two-feared-to-have-disease.

66. Michaeleen Doucleff, "Anthrax Outbreak in Russia Thought to Be Result of Thawing Permafrost," National Public Radio, August 3, 2016, https://www.npr.org/sections/goatsandsoda/2016/08/03/488400947/anthrax-outbreak-in-russia-thought-to-be-result-of-thawing-permafrost.

67. "Siberia Anthrax Outbreak: 12yo Boy Killed, 8 Infected As Disease Returns After 75 Years," RT August 1, 2016, https://www.rt.com/news/354139-anthrax-siberia-boy-dead.

68. "Child, 12, Died from Anthrax."

69. Stephanie Pappas, "'Zombie' Anthrax Goes on a Killing Spree in Siberia—How?" *Scientific American*, August 3, 2016, https://www.scientificamerican.com/article/zombie-anthrax-goes-on-a-killing-spree-in-siberia-how.

70. "40 Now Hospitalised after Anthrax Outbreak in Yamal, More Than Half Are Children," *Siberian Times*, July 30, 2016, http://siberiantimes.com/other/others/news/n0691-40-now-hospitalised-after-anthrax-outbreak-in-yamal-more-than-half-are-children.

71. Ekaterina Ezhova, Dmitry Orlov, Elli Suhonen, Dmitry Kaverin, Alexander Mahura, Victor Gennadinik, Ilmo Kukkonen, et al., "Climatic Factors Influencing the Anthrax Outbreak of 2016 in Siberia, Russia," *EcoHealth* 18, no. 2 (August 2021): 217–28, https://doi.org/10.1007/s10393-021-01549-5; A. Yu Popova, Yu V. Demina, E. B. Ezhlova, A. N. Kulichenko, A. G. Ryazanova, V. V. Maleev, A. A. Ploskireva, et al., "Outbreak of Anthrax in the Yamalo-Nenets Autonomous District in 2016, Epidemiological Peculiarities," *Problems of Particularly Dangerous Infections* 4 (2016): 42–46, https://doi.org/10.21055/0370-1069-2016-4-42-46.

72. Olga Gertcyk, "Yamal Trims Back Reindeer Cull to 100,000 as Herders Fear Future of Nomadic Lifestyle," *Siberian Times*, October 7, 2016, http://siberiantimes.com/other/others/features/f0260-yamal-trims-back-reindeer-cull-to-100000-as-herders-fear-future-of-nomadic-lifestyle.

73. "20 People Now Infected by Zombie Anthrax Outbreak in Siberia, Say Officials," *Siberian Times*, August 2, 2016, http://siberiantimes.com/other/others/news/n0694-20-people-now-infected-by-zombie-anthrax-outbreak-in-siberia-say-officials.

74. "20 People Now Infected by Zombie Anthrax Outbreak in Siberia."

75. "Five Week Delay' in Issuing Warning of Anthrax Outbreak, Claims Senior Veterinary Regulator," *Siberian Times*, August 3, 2016, http://siberiantimes.com/other/others/news/n0696-five-week-delay-in-issuing-warning-of-anthrax-outbreak-claims-senior-veterinary-regulator.

76. "Two More Outbreaks of Anthrax Hit Northern Siberia Due to Thawing Permafrost," *Siberian Times*, August 31, 2016, http://siberiantimes.com/other/others/features/f0253-deadly-anthrax-infection-spread-250-kilometres-in-15-days-due-to-mosquitoes.

77. Olga Gertcyk, "Huge Cull of 250,000 Reindeer by Christmas in Yamalo-Nenets after Anthrax Outbreak," *Siberian Times*, September 19, 2016, http://siberiantimes.com/other/others/news/n0738-huge-cull-of-250000-reindeer-by-christmas-in-yamelo-nenets-after-anthrax-outbreak.

78. Gertcyk, "Huge Cull.".

79. Elle Hunt, "Nightmare before Christmas: Siberia Plans to Cull 250,000 Reindeer Amid Anthrax Fears," *Guardian*, September 29, 2016, https://www.theguardian.com/world/2016/sep/30/nightmare-before-christmas-siberia-plans-to-cull-250000-reindeer-amid-anthrax-fears.

80. Anna Nemtsova, "The Nenets Herders, Last Nomads of the North," Russia Beyond, June 29, 2011, https://www.rbth.com/articles/2011/06/29/the_nenets_herders_last_nomads_of_the_north_13098.html.

81. "Beware of Action that Would Put Age-Old Tundra Nomadism at Risk in Yamal, Says Expert." *Siberian Times*, September 23, 2016, http://siberiantimes.com/other/others/features/f0257-beware-of-action-that-would-put-age-old-tundra-nomadism-at-risk-in-yamal-says-expert.

82. Olga Gertcyk, "Huge Cull."

83. "New Rudolphs for Christmas—All 2,349 Reindeer Killed in Anthrax Outbreak Are Replaced." *Siberian Times*, December 23, 2016, http://siberiantimes.com/other/others/news/n0833-new-rudolphs-for-christmas-all-2349-reindeer-killed-in-anthrax-outbreak-are-replaced.

84. "New Rudolphs for Christmas."

85. Rebecca Katz and Burton Singer, "Can an Attribution Assessment Be Made for Yellow Rain? Systematic Reanalysis in a Chemical-and-Biological-Weapons Use

Investigation," *Politics and the Life Sciences* 26, no. 1 (March 2007): 24–42, https://doi.org/10.2990/26_1_24.

86. Arunmozhi Balajee, Stephanie J. Salyer, Blanche Greene-Cramer, Mahmoud Sadek, and Anthony W. Mounts, "The Practice of Event-Based Surveillance: Concept and Methods," *Global Security: Health, Science and Policy* 6, no. 1 (January 2021), https://doi.org/10.1080/23779497.2020.1848444.

87. "Global Health Protection and Security: Event Based Surveillance," Centers for Disease Control and Prevention, last modified April 18, 2023, https://www.cdc.gov/globalhealth/healthprotection/gddopscenter/how.html.

88. "Event-Based Surveillance Curriculum," Center for Global Health Science and Security, accessed December 10, 2023, https://ghss.georgetown.edu/ebs.

89. World Health Organization Emergency Programme, Booklet 1: "Introduction," *Technical Guidelines for Integrated Disease Surveillance and Response in the African Region*, 3rd ed. (Atlanta, GA: Centers for Disease Control and Prevention Center for Global Health; Brazzaville: World Health Organization Regional Office for Africa, 2019), https://apps.who.int/iris/bitstream/handle/10665/325015/WHO-AF-WHE-CPI-05.2019-eng.pdf.

90. CDC, "Global Health Protection and Security: Event Based Surveillance."

91. World Health Organization Emergency Programme, introduction to *Technical Guidelines for Integrated Disease Surveillance*.

92. World Health Organization Western Pacific Region, *A Guide to Establishing Event-Based Surveillance* (Geneva: World Health Organization, 2008), https://www.who.int/publications/i/item/9789290613213.

93. World Health Organization, *Early Detection, Assessment and Response to Acute Public Health Events: Implementation of Early Warning and Response with a Focus on Event-Based Surveillance*, interim version (Lyon: World Health Organization, 2014), https://iris.who.int/bitstream/handle/10665/112667/WHO_HSE_GCR_LYO_2014.4_eng.pdf.

94. Tammy L. Stuart Chester, Marsha Taylor, Jat Sandhu, Sara Forsting, Andrea Ellis, Rob Stirling, and Eleni Galanis, "Use of a Web Forum and an Online Questionnaire in the Detection and Investigation of an Outbreak," *Online Journal of Public Health Informatics* 3, no. 1 (June 2011), https://doi.org/10.5210/ojphi.v3i1.3506.

95. Tammy L. Stuart Chester, J. Sandhu, R. Stirling, J. Corder, A. Ellis, P. Misa, S. Goh, B. Wong, P. Martiquet, L. Hoang, and E. Galanis, "Campylobacteriosis Outbreak Associated with Ingestion of Mud during a Mountain Bike Race," *Epidemiology and Infection* 138, no. 12 (December 2010), https://doi.org/10.1017/S095026881000049X.

96. Juliette Morgan, Shari L. Bornstein, Adam M. Karpati, Michael Bruce, Carole A. Bolin, Constance C. Austin, Christopher W. Woods, et al., "Outbreak of Leptospirosis Among Triathlon Participants and Community Residents in Springfield, Illinois, 1998," *Clinical Infectious Diseases* 34, no. 12 (June 2002): 1593–99, https://doi.org/10.1086/340615; Stefan Brockmann, Isolde Piechotowski, Oswinde Bock-Hensley, Christian Winter, Rainer Oehme, Stefan Zimmermann, Katrin Hartelt, et al., "Outbreak of Leptospirosis Among Triathlon Participants in Germany, 2006," *BMC Infectious Diseases* 10, no. 91 (April 2010): 1-5, https://doi.org/10.1186/1471-2334-10-91; F. Pagès, S. Larrieu, J. Simoes, P. Lenabat, B. Kurtkowiak, Vanina Guernier, Gildas Le Minter, et al., "Investigation of a Leptospirosis Outbreak in Triathlon Participants, Réunion Island, 2013," *Epidemiology and Infection* 144, no. 3 (July 2015): 661-669, https://doi.org/10.1017/S0950268815001740.

97. Fern Greenwell and Shannon Salentine, "Module 10: Public Health Surveillance System," Health Information System Strengthening: Standards and Best Practices for Data Sources, MEASURE Evaluation, 2018, https://www.measureevaluation.org/resources/hisdatasourcesguide/module-10-public-health-surveillance-system.

98. CDC, "Global Health Protection and Security: Event Based Surveillance."

99. World Health Organization, *Early Detection, Assessment and Response*; World Health Organization Emergency Programme, "Booklet 1: Introduction."

100. World Health Organization, *Early Detection, Assessment and Response*.

101. Fern and Salentine, "Module 10: Public Health Surveillance System."

102. World Health Organization, *Early Detection, Assessment and Response*.

103. Anna Kuehne, Patrick Keating, Jonathan Polonsky, Christopher Haskew, Karl Schenkel, Olivier Le Polain De Waroux, and Ruwan Ratnayake, "Event-Based Surveillance at Health Facility and Community Level in Low-Income and Middle-Income Countries: A Systematic Review," *BMJ Global Health* 4, no. 6 (2019): e001878, http://dx.doi.org/10.1136/bmjgh-2019-001878.

104. A. M. Naser, M. J. Hossain, H. M. S. Sazzad, N. Homaira, E. S. Gurley, G. Podder, S. Afroj, et al., "Integrated Cluster-and Case-Based Surveillance for Detecting Stage III Zoonotic Pathogens: An Example of Nipah Virus Surveillance in Bangladesh," *Epidemiology and Infection* 143, no. 9 (2015): 1922–30, https://doi.org/10.1017/S0950268814002635.

105. "2009 H1N1 Influenza Surveillance Systems," Behavioral Health System Baltimore, last modified 2011, https://baltimorecity.md.networkofcare.org/mh/model-practice-detail.aspx?pid=5502; E. O. Kara, A. J. Elliot, H. Bagnall, D. G. F. Foord, R. Pnaiser, H. Osman, G. E. Smith, and Babatunde Olowokure, "Absenteeism in Schools during the 2009 Influenza a (H1N1) pandemic: A Useful Tool for Early Detection of Influenza Activity in the Community?" *Epidemiology and Infection* 140, no. 7 (2012): 1328–36, https://doi.org/10.1017/S0950268811002093; Asami Sasaki, Anne Gatewood Hoen, Al Ozonoff, Hiroshi Suzuki, Naohito Tanabe, Nao Seki, Reiko Saito, and John S. Brownstein, "Evidence-Based Tool for Triggering School Closures during Influenza Outbreaks, Japan," *Emerging Infectious Diseases* 15, no. 11 (November 2009): 1841–43, https://doi.org/10.3201/eid1511.090798.

106. Jonathan L. Temte, Shari Barlow, Maureen Goss, Emily Temte, Amber Schemmel, Cristalyne Bell, Erik Reisdorf, et al., "Cause-Specific Student Absenteeism Monitoring in K-12 Schools for Detection of Increased Influenza Activity in the Surrounding Community—Dane County, Wisconsin, 2014–2020," *PLOS One* 17, no. 4 (April 2022): e0267111, https://doi.org/10.1371/journal.pone.0267111.

107. World Health Organization, *Coordinated Public Health Surveillance between Points of Entry and National Health Surveillance Systems: Advising Principles* (Lyon: World Health Organization 2014), https://apps.who.int/iris/bitstream/handle/10665/144805/WHO_HSE_GCR_LYO_2014.12_eng.pdf.

108. WHO, *Coordinated Public Health Surveillance*.

109. "Ebola Virus Disease POE Preparedness at Screening Points – Kanungu District (1-31 January 2020)." Flow Monitoring, Global Data Institute Displacement Tracking Matrix, accessed December 11, 2023, https://migration.iom.int/node/7769.

110. WHO, *Early Detection, Assessment and Response*.

111. WHO, *Early Detection, Assessment and Response*.

112. James W. Buehler, Richard S. Hopkins, J. Marc Overhage, Daniel M. Sosin, and Van Tong, "Framework for Evaluating Public Health Surveillance Systems for Early Detection of Outbreaks: Recommendations from the CDC Working Group," *MMWR Recommendations and Reports*, Centers for Disease Control and Prevention, last modified May 7, 2004, https://www.cdc.gov/mmwr/preview/mmwrhtml/rr5305a1.htm.; Epidemiological Surveillance Strengthening Team of the WHO Lyon Office for National Epidemic Preparedness and Response. *Communicable Disease Surveillance and Response Systems: Guide to Monitoring and Evaluating* (Lyon: World Health Organization, 2006), https://iris.who.int/bitstream/handle/10665/69331/WHO_CDS_EPR_LYO_2006_2_eng.pdf; World Health Organization Department of Communicable Disease Surveillance and Response, *Protocol*

for the Assessment of National Communicable Disease Surveillance and Response Systems: Guidelines for Assessment Teams (Lyon: World Health Organization, 2001), https://iris.who.int/bitstream/handle/10665/66787/WHO_CDS_CSR_ISR_2001.2_text_annexes1-11.pdf.

113. WHO, *Early Detection, Assessment and Response.*

114. Epidemiological Surveillance Strengthening Team, *Communicable Disease Surveillance.*

115. Eric Yirenkyi Adjei, Keziah Laurencia Malm, Kofi Nyarko Mensah, Samuel Oko Sackey, Donne Ameme, Ernest Kenu, Marijanatu Abdulai, Richael Mills, Edwin Afari, "Evaluation of Cholera Surveillance System in Osu Klottey District, Accra, Ghana (2011-2013)," *Pan African Medical Journal* 28 (2017), DOI: 10.11604/pamj.2017.28.224.10737.

CHAPTER 2

1. "Flu & Ebola Map," Health Map, accessed December 12, 2023, https://healthmap.org/en.

2. G. Namara, "Strengthening Epidemic Intelligence in Africa: Activities of the WHO Hub for Pandemic and Epidemic Intelligence," Webinar for GET Consortia, August 31, 2022.

3. European Centre for Disease Prevention and Control, *Operational Tool on Rapid Risk Assessment Methodology* (Stockholm: ECDC, 2019), https://www.ecdc.europa.eu/sites/default/files/documents/operational-tool-rapid-risk-assessment-methodolgy-ecdc-2019.pdf.

4. D. L. Heymann, *Control of Communicable Diseases Manual* (Washington, DC: American Public Health Association, 2022), https://www.apha.org/Publications/Published-Books/CCDM.

5. Michaeleen Doucleff, "He Discovered the Origin of the Monkeypox Outbreak — and Tried to Warn the World," *National Public Radio*, July 29, 2022, https://www.npr.org/sections/goatsandsoda/2022/07/28/1114183886/a-doctor-in-nigeria-tried-to-warn-the-world-that-monkeypox-had-become-a-global-t?.

6. Chikwe Ihekweazu, Adesola Yinka-Ogunleye, Swaib Lule, and Abubakar Ibrahim, "Importance of Epidemiological Research of Monkeypox: Is Incidence Increasing?" *Expert Review of Anti-infective Therapy* 18, no. 5 (March 2020): 389–92, https://doi.org/10.1080/14787210.2020.1735361.

7. "Human Health Risk Assessment," United States Environmental Protection Agency, last modified December 6, 2023, https://www.epa.gov/risk/human-health-risk-assessment#tab-1.

8. "Risk Assessment," Pan American Health Organization, accessed December 12, 2023, https://www.paho.org/en/detection-verification-and-risk-assessment-dva/risk-assessment.

9. "Operational Tool on Rapid Risk Assessment Methodology," European Centre for Disease Prevention and Control, last modified March, 19, 2019, https://www.ecdc.europa.eu/en/publications-data/operational-tool-rapid-risk-assessment-methodology-ecdc-2019.

10. United Nations Conference on Environment and Development, Rio Declaration on Environment and Development (Rio de Janeiro: United Nations, 1992), Principle 15, https://culturalrights.net/descargas/drets_culturals411.pdf.

11. "Risk Assessment of Infectious Disease Threats," European Centre for Disease Prevention and Control, accessed December 12, 2023, https://www.ecdc.europa.eu/en/publications-and-data/risk-assessment.

12. Centers for Disease Control and Prevention, National Center for Environmental Health Environmental Hazards and Health Effects Health Studies Branch,

Community Assessment for Public Health Emergency Response (CASPER) Toolkit (Atlanta: CDC, 2012), https://www.cdc.gov/disasters/surveillance/pdf/casper_toolkit_version_2_0_508_compliant.pdf.

13. Long Beach Department of Health and Human Services, *Long Beach Zika Community Assessment for Public Health Emergency Response (CASPER)* (Long Beach, CA: City of Long Beach: Long Beach Department of Health and Human Services, 2017), https://www.longbeach.gov/globalassets/health/media-library/documents/diseases-and-condition/information-on/zika/lb-zika-casper-final-report.

CHAPTER 3

1. World Health Organization, *Laboratory Biosafety Manual*, 4th ed. (Geneva: World Health Organization, 2020), https://iris.who.int/bitstream/handle/10665/337956/9789240011311-eng.pdf.

2. N. Wurtz, A. Papa, M. Hukic, A. Di Caro, I. Leparc-Goffart, Eric Leroy, M. P. Landini, et al., "Survey of Laboratory-Acquired Infections Around the World in Biosafety Level 3 and 4 Laboratories," *European Journal of Clinical Microbiology and Infectious Diseases* 35, no. 8 (May 2016): 1247–58, https://doi.org/10.1007/s10096-016-2657-1.

3. West Nile Virus: Centers for Disease Control and Prevention, "Laboratory-Acquired West Nile Virus Infections--United States, 2002," *Morbidity and Mortality Weekly Report* 51, no. 50 (December 2002): 1133–35, https://www.cdc.gov/mmwr/preview/mmwrhtml/mm5150a2.htm; SARS: Kathryn Senio, "Recent Singapore SARS Case a Laboratory Accident," *Lancet Infectious Diseases* 3, no. 11 (November 2003): 679, https://doi.org/10.1016/S1473-3099(03)00815-6; Plague: Carlos Sadovi, "U. of C. Researcher Dies after Exposure to Plague Bacteria," *Chicago Tribune*, September 19, 2009, https://www.chicagotribune.com/news/ct-bn-xpm-2009-09-19-28504883-story.html; Dengue: Sumudu Britton, Andrew F. van den Hurk, Russell J. Simmons, Alyssa T. Pyke, Judith A. Northill, James McCarthy, and Joe McCormack, "Laboratory-Acquired Dengue Virus Infection — A Case Report," *PLoS Neglected Tropical Diseases* 5, no. 11 (2011): e1324, https://doi.org/10.1371/journal.pntd.0001324; Changhwan Lee, Eun Jung Jang, Donghyok Kwon, Heun Choi, Jung Wan Park, and Geun-Ryang Bae, "Laboratory-Acquired Dengue Virus Infection by Needlestick Injury: A Case Report, South Korea, 2014," *Annals of Occupational and Environmental Medicine* 28, no. 1 (2016): 1–8, https://doi.org/10.1186/s40557-016-0104-5; Meningitis: Lieff Beryl Benderly, "Suit Brought for Wrongful Death of Lab Worker," *Science*, May 10, 2013, https://www.science.org/content/article/suit-brought-wrongful-death-lab-worker; Zika: Michael Nedelman, "Researcher Infected with Zika Virus during Laboratory Accident in Pittsburgh," ABC News, June 9, 2016, https://abcnews.go.com/Health/researcher-infected-zika-virus-laboratory-accident-pittsburgh/story?id=39736836; Creutzfeldt-Jakob Disease: Jean-Philippe Brandel, M. Bustuchina Vlaicu, Audrey Culeux, Maxime Belondrade, Daisy Bougard, Katarina Grznarova, Angeline Denouel, et al., "Variant Creutzfeldt-Jakob Disease Diagnosed 7.5 Years after Occupational Exposure," *New England Journal of Medicine* 383, no. 1 (2020): 83–85, doi: 10.1056/NEJMc2000687.

4. Georgios Pappas, "The Lanzhou Brucella Leak: The Largest Laboratory Accident in the History of Infectious Diseases?" *Clinical Infectious Diseases* 75, no 10 (November2022); 1347, https://doi.org/10.1093/cid/ciac463.

5. Reuters, "Explainer: How Thousands in China Got Infected by Brucellosis in One Single Outbreak," Reuters, November 6, 2020, https://www.reuters.com/article/us-health-brucellosis-china-explainer/explainer-how-thousands-in-china-got-infected-by-brucellosis-in-one-single-outbreak-idUSKBN27M0JM.

6. Reuters, "Over 6,000 people in China's Lanzhou Test Positive for Brucellosis - State Media," Reuters, November 5, 2020, https://www.reuters.com/article/us-health-

brucellosis-china/over-6000-people-in-chinas-lanzhou-test-positive-for-brucellosis-state-media-idUSKBN27L1LA.

7. "Tularemia Fact Sheet," Federation of American Scientists, accessed December 13, 2023, https://programs.fas.org/bio/factsheets/tularemia.html.

8. William A. Agger, "Tularemia, Lawn Mowers, and Rabbits' Nests," *Journal of Clinical Microbiology* 43, no. 8 (August 2005): 4304–5, https://doi.org/10.1128/JCM.43.8.4304-4305.2005.; David L Belding and Beulah Merrill, "Tularemia in Imported Rabbits in Massachusetts," *New England Journal of Medicine* 224, no. 26 (1941): 1085–87, https://www.nejm.org/doi/pdf/10.1056/NEJM194106262242602.

9. Katherine A. Feldman, Donna Stiles-Enos, Kathleen Julian, Bela T. Matyas, Sam R. Telford III, May C. Chu, Lyle R. Petersen, and Edward B. Hayes, "Tularemia on Martha's Vineyard: Seroprevalence and Occupational Risk," *Emerging Infectious Diseases* 9, no. 3 (March 2003): 350–54, https://doi.org/10.3201/eid0903.020462.

10. Katherine A. Feldman, Russell E. Enscore, Sarah L. Lathrop, Bela T. Matyas, Michael McGuill, Martin E. Schriefer, Donna Stiles-Enos, David T. Dennis, Lyle R. Petersen, and Edward B. Hayes, "An Outbreak of Primary Pneumonic Tularemia on Martha's Vineyard," *New England Journal of Medicine* 345, no. 22 (2001): 1601–6, doi: 10.1056/NEJMoa011374.

11. "Disease Commodity Packages," World Health Organization, accessed December 13, 2023, https://www.who.int/emergencies/disease-commodity-packages.

12. Kazunobu Kojima, Lisa Stevens, and Rica Zinsky, *Guidance on Regulations for the Transport of Infectious Substances 2021–2022* (Geneva: World Health Organization, 2021), https://iris.who.int/bitstream/handle/10665/339825/9789240019720-eng.pdf.

13. Zahid Naeem, "Zika - Global Concern," *International Journal of Health Sciences* 10, no. 3 (July 2016): 5–7, https://www.ncbi.nlm.nih.gov/pmc/articles/PMC5003575.

14. Maria Cheng, Raphael Satter, and Joshua Goodman, "Few Zika Samples Being Shared by Brazil," AP News, February 4, 2016, https://apnews.com/article/2db2a3581d2a42a08f5b031419cb09ed.

15. Nurith Aizenman, "Scientists Say It's Time to End 'Parachute Research,'" National Public Radio, April 2, 2016, https://www.npr.org/sections/goatsandsoda/2016/04/02/472686809/scientists-say-its-time-to-end-parachute-research.

16. Roosecelis Brasil Martines, "Notes from the Field: Evidence of Zika Virus Infection in Brain and Placental Tissues from Two Congenitally Infected Newborns and Two Fetal Losses—Brazil, 2015," *Morbidity and Mortality Weekly Report* 65 (February 2016): 159–60, https://doi.org/10.15585/mmwr.mm6506e1.

17. OIE Ad Hoc Group on Biosafety and Biosecurity in Veterinary Laboratories, *Manual of Diagnostic Tests and Vaccines for Terrestrial Animals*, 7th ed. (Paris: World Organisation for Animal Health, 2018), chap. 1.1.2, https://www.woah.org/fileadmin/Home/eng/Health_standards/tahm/1.01.02_COLLECTION_DIAG_SPECIMENS.pdf.

18. OIE Ad Hoc Group on Biosafety and Biosecurity, *Manual of Diagnostic Tests.*

19. OIE Ad Hoc Group on Biosafety and Biosecurity, *Manual of Diagnostic Tests.*

20. Laura Annaratone, Giuseppe De Palma, Giuseppina Bonizzi, Anna Sapino, Gerardo Botti, Enrico Berrino, Chiara Mannelli, et al., "Basic Principles of Biobanking: From Biological Samples to Precision Medicine for Patients," *Virchows Archiv* 479, no. 2 (July 2021): 233–46, https://doi.org/10.1007/s00428-021-03151-0.

21. "Smallpox," American Museum of Natural History, accessed December 13, 2023, https://www.amnh.org/explore/science-topics/disease-eradication/countdown-to-zero/smallpox.

22. "Smallpox," Disease & Conditions, National Institute of Allergy and Infectious Diseases, accessed December 13, 2023, https://www.niaid.nih.gov/diseases-conditions/smallpox.

23. Brandy Dennis and Lena H. Sun, "FDA Found More Than Smallpox Vials in Storage Room," *Washington Post*, July 16, 2014, https://www.washingtonpost.com/national/health-science/fda-found-more-than-smallpox-vials-in-storage-room/2014/07/16/850d4b12-0d22-11e4-8341-b8072b1e7348_story.html.

24. Jocelyn Kaiser, "Six Vials of Smallpox Discovered in U.S. Lab," *Science*, July 8, 2014, https://www.science.org/content/article/six-vials-smallpox-discovered-us-lab.

25. Alexandra Flemming, "The Origins of Vaccination," *Nature*, September 28, 2020, https://www.nature.com/articles/d42859-020-00006-7.

26. Antti Vasala, Vesa P. Hytönen, and Olli H. Laitinen, "Modern Tools for Rapid Diagnostics of Antimicrobial Resistance," *Frontiers in Cellular and Infection Microbiology* 10 (July 2020): 308, https://doi.org/10.3389/fcimb.2020.00308.

27. "IRR," International Reagent Resource, accessed December 13, 2023, https://www.internationalreagentresource.org/About/IRR.aspx.

28. R. G. Van der Merwe, P. D. Van Helden, R. M. Warren, S. L. Sampson, and N. C. Gey van Pittius, "Phage-Based Detection of Bacterial Pathogens," *Analyst* 139, no. 11 (2014): 2617–26, https://doi.org/10.1039/C4AN00208C; A. J. Sabat, A. Budimir, D. Nashev, R. Sá-Leão, J. M. Van Dijl, F. Laurent, H. Grundmann, A. W. Friedrich, and ESCMID Study Group of Epidemiological Markers, "Overview of Molecular Typing Methods for Outbreak Detection and Epidemiological Surveillance," *Eurosurveillance* 18, no. 4 (2013): 20380, https://doi.org/10.2807/ese.18.04.20380-en; Ricardo Franco-Duarte, Lucia Černáková, Snehal Kadam, Karishma S. Kaushik, Bahare Salehi, Antonio Bevilacqua, Maria Rosaria Corbo, et al., "Advances in Chemical and Biological Methods to Identify Microorganisms—from Past to Present," *Microorganisms* 7, no. 5 (May 2019): 130, https://doi.org/10.3390/microorganisms7050130.

29. Maria T. Vazquez-Pertejo, "Introduction to Laboratory Diagnosis of Infectious Disease," Merck Manual, September 2022, https://www.merckmanuals.com/professional/infectious-diseases/laboratory-diagnosis-of-infectious-disease/introduction-to-laboratory-diagnosis-of-infectious-disease.

30. Van der Merwe et al., "Phage-Based Detection of Bacterial Pathogens."

31. World Health Organization, "Managing Epidemics: Key Facts about Major Deadly Diseases," World Health Organization, accessed December 13, 2018, https://apps.who.int/iris/handle/10665/272442.

32. "Rapid Data Sharing and Genomics Vital to China Virus Response," Yale School of Public Health, last modified January 23, 2020, https://ysph.yale.edu/news-article/rapid-data-sharing-and-genomics-vital-to-china-virus-response; Oana Stroe, "Pathogen Data Sharing – Key to Pandemic Preparedness," *EMBL-EBI*. March 24, 2022, https://www.ebi.ac.uk/about/news/perspectives/pathogen-data-sharing-principles.

33. Christopher JL Murray, Kevin Shunji Ikuta, Fablina Sharara, Lucien Swetschinski, Gisela Robles Aguilar, Authia Gray, Chieh Han, et al., "Global Burden of Bacterial Antimicrobial Resistance in 2019: A Systematic Analysis," *Lancet* 399, no. 10325 (2022): 629–55, https://doi.org/10.1016/S0140-6736(21)02724-0.

34. "Influenza Antiviral Drug Resistance," Influenza (Flu), Centers for Disease Control and Prevention, last modified September 9, 2021, https://www.cdc.gov/flu/treatment/antiviralresistance.htm.

35. Deenan Pillay and Maria Zambon, "Antiviral Drug Resistance," *BMJ* 317, no. 7159 (1998): 660–62, https://doi.org/10.1136/bmj.317.7159.660.

36. "Whole Genome Sequencing," PulseNet, Centers for Disease Control and Prevention, last modified August 15, 2022, https://www.cdc.gov/pulsenet/pathogens/wgs.html.

CHAPTER 4

1. "Rocky Mountain Spotted Fever," Health, Johns Hopkins Medicine, accessed December 13, 2023, https://www.hopkinsmedicine.org/health/conditions-and-diseases/rocky-mountain-spotted-fever.

2. Naomi A. Drexler, Marc S. Traeger, Jennifer H. McQuiston, Velda Williams, Charlene Hamilton, and Joanna J. Regan, "Medical and Indirect Costs Associated with a Rocky Mountain Spotted Fever Epidemic in Arizona, 2002–2011," *American Journal of Tropical Medicine and Hygiene* 93, no. 3 (2015): 549–51, https://doi.org/10.4269/ajtmh.15-0104.

3. "Prevention and Early Treatment of RMSF in Arizona May Save Millions by Preventing Premature Death and Disability," Centers for Disease Control and Prevention, last modified June 19, 2015, https://archive.cdc.gov/#/details?url=https://www.cdc.gov/media/releases/2015/p0619-RMSF.html

4. "One Health Office Fact Sheet," One Health, Centers for Disease Control and Prevention, last modified February 3, 2020, https://www.cdc.gov/onehealth/who-we-are/one-health-office-fact-sheet.html.

5. "Alpha-Gal Syndrome," Ticks, Centers for Disease Control and Prevention, last modified March 28, 2022, https://www.cdc.gov/ticks/alpha-gal/index.html.

6. José Guerra, Pratikshya Acharya, and Céline Barnadas, "Community-Based Surveillance: A Scoping Review," *PLoS One* 14, no. 4 (April2019): e0215278, https://doi: 10.1371/journal.pone.0215278.

7. M. S. Lado, Mackoy, B. Steve, and J. Rumunu, "Evaluation of Community-Based Surveillance for Guinea Worm, South Sudan, 2006," *South Sudan Medical Journal* 5, no. 3 (2012): 72–74, https://www.ajol.info/index.php/ssmj/article/view/132494.

8. Alain Metuge, Lundi-Anne Omam, Elizabeth Jarman, and Esther Omam Njomo, "Humanitarian Led Community-Based Surveillance: Case Study in Ekondo-Titi, Cameroon," *Conflict and Health* 15, no. 1 (March 2021): 1–12, https://doi.org/10.1186/s13031-021-00354-9.

9. A. Kongelf, T. Tingberg, A. L. McClelland, M. C. Jean, and B. D. Dalzie, "Community-Based Cholera Surveillance by Volunteers with Mobile Phones: A Case Study from Western Area, Haiti," *International Journal of Infectious Diseases* 53 (December 2016): 115–16, https://doi.org/10.1016/j.ijid.2016.11.289.

10. Elburg Van Boetzelaer, Samiur Chowdhury, Berhe Etsay, Abu Faruque, Annick Lenglet, Anna Kuehne, Isidro Carrion-Martin, et al., "Evaluation of Community Based Surveillance in the Rohingya Refugee Camps in Cox's Bazar, Bangladesh, 2019," *PLoS One* 15, no. 12 (December 2020): e0244214, https://doi.org/10.1371/journal.pone.0244214.

11. PAHO and WHO Regional Office for the Americas, "COVID-19 Risk Communication and Community Engagement (RCCE)," Pan American Health Organization, accessed December 13, 2023, https://www.paho.org/en/documents/covid-19-risk-communication-and-community-engagement-rcce.

12. "Centering Communities in Pandemic Preparedness and Response," Independent Panel for Pandemic Preparedness and Response, May 2021, https://theindependentpanel.org/wp-content/uploads/2021/05/Background-paper-10-community-involvement.pdf.

13. Douglas S. Lloyd, "Circular Letter #12-32," State Department of Health, State of Connecticut, August 3, 1976, https://portal.ct.gov/-/media/Departments-and-Agencies/DPH/dph/infectious_diseases/lyme/1976circularletterpdf.pdf.

14. Edward D Harris Jr, "Lyme Disease — Success for Academia and the Community," *New England Journal of Medicine* 308, no. 13 (March 1983): 773-775, doi: 10.1056/NEJM198303313081309.

15. "A Brief History of Lyme Disease in Connecticut," Connecticut State Department of Public Health, last modified July 1, 2019, https://portal.ct.gov/DPH/Epidemiology-and-Emerging-Infections/A-Brief-History-of-Lyme-Disease-in-Connecticut.

16. FEMA, *Effective Coordination of Recovery Resources for State, Tribal, Territorial and Local Incidents* (Washington, DC: FEMA, 2015), https://www.fema.gov/sites/default/files/2020-07/fema_effective-coordination-recovery-resources-guide_020515.pdf.

17. Karl Blanchet, Sara L. Nam, Ben Ramalingam, and Francisco Pozo-Martin, "Governance and Capacity to Manage Resilience of Health Systems: Towards a New Conceptual Framework," *International Journal of Health Policy and Management* 6, no. 8 (2017): 431–35, https://doi.org/10.15171/ijhpm.2017.36.

18. Marie Paule Kieny and Delanyo Dovlo, "Beyond Ebola: A New Agenda for Resilient Health Systems," *Lancet* 385, no. 9963 (January 2015): 91-92, https://doi.org/10.1016/S0140-6736(14)62479-X.

19. Allison Boyd, J. Barry Hokanson, Laurie A. Johnson, James C. Schwab, and Kenneth C. Topping, *Planning for Post-Disaster Recovery: Next Generation* (Washington, DC: American Planning Association, 2014), https://www.fema.gov/sites/default/files/2020-06/apa_planning-for-post-disaster-recovery-next-generation_03-04-2015.pdf.

20. Blanchet et al., "Governance and Capacity."

21. Paul H. Wise and Michele Barry, "Civil War and the Global Threat of Pandemics," *Daedalus* 146, no. 4 (2017): 71–84, https://doi.org/10.1162/DAED_a_00460.

22. Darryl Stellmach, Isabel Beshar, Juliet Bedford, Philipp Du Cros, and Beverley Stringer, "Anthropology in Public Health Emergencies: What is Anthropology Good for?" *BMJ Global Health* 3, no. 2 (2018): e000534, http://dx.doi.org/10.1136/bmjgh-2017-000534.

23. Christos Lynteris and Branwyn Poleykett, "The Anthropology of Epidemic Control: Technologies and Materialities," *Medical Anthropology* 37, no. 6 (November 2018): 433–41, https://doi.org/10.1080/01459740.2018.1484740.

24. "Kuru," National Institute of Neurological Disorders and Stroke, last modified November 28, 2023, https://www.ninds.nih.gov/health-information/disorders/kuru.

25. Michael P Alpers, "The Epidemiology of Kuru: Monitoring the Epidemic from Its Peak to Its End," *Philosophical Transactions of the Royal Society B: Biological Sciences* 363, no. 1510 (November 2008): 3707–13, https://doi.org/10.1098/rstb.2008.0071.

26. June Goodfield, "Cannibalism and Kuru," *Nature* 387, no. 6636 (June 1997): 841–41, https://doi.org/10.1038/43043.

27. Alpers, "The Epidemiology of Kuru."

28. Goodfield, "Cannibalism and Kuru."

29. Zartash Zafar, "Kuru: Background, Pathophysiology, Epidemiology," *Medscape*, last modified March 15, 2019, https://emedicine.medscape.com/article/220043-overview.

30. John Collinge, Jerome Whitfield, Edward McKintosh, John Beck, Simon Mead, Dafydd J. Thomas, and Michael P. Alpers, "Kuru in the Twenty-First Century — An Acquired Human Prion Disease with Very Long Incubation Perods," *Lancet* 367, no. 9528 (June 2006): 2068–74, https://doi.org/10.1016/S0140-6736(06)68930-7.

31. International Committee of the Red Cross, *Acquiring and Analysing Data in Support of Evidence-Based Decisions: A Guide for Humanitarian Work* (Geneva: International Committee of the Red Cross, 2020), https://www.icrc.org/en/publication/acquiring-and-analysing-data-support-evidence-based-decisions-guide-humanitarian-work.

32. Maximo Torero, "How to Stop a Looming Food Crisis." *Foreign Policy*, April 14, 2020, https://foreignpolicy.com/2020/04/14/how-to-stop-food-crisis-coronavirus-economy-trade; World Food Programme, *Responding to the Development Emergency Caused by COVID-19: WFP's Medium-Term Programme Framework* (Rome: World Food Programme, 2020), https://www.wfp.org/publications/responding-development-emergency-caused-covid-19-wfps-medium-term-programming.

33. "Coronavirus Food Shortage: Crisis within a Crisis," Vision of Humanity, accessed December 13, 2023, https://www.visionofhumanity.org/crisis-within-a-crisis-food-insecurity-and-the-pandemic.

34. "COVID-19: The Role of the Water Convention and the Protocol on Water and Health," UNECE Environmental Policy: Water, United Nations Economic Commission for Europe, last modified November 22, 2021, https://unece.org/environment-policy/water/covid-19-role-water-convention-and-protocol-water-and-health.

35. "Yemen Cholera Killing One Person Nearly Every Hour," Oxfam International, last modified June 7, 2017, https://www.oxfam.org/en/press-releases/yemen-cholera-killing-one-person-nearly-every-hour.

36. "Epidemic and Pandemic-Prone Diseases," World Health Organization Eastern Mediterranean Region, accessed December 13, 2023, https://www.emro.who.int/pandemic-epidemic-diseases/outbreaks/index.html.

37. "Cholera – Vibrio Cholerae Infection General Information," Centers for Disease Control and Prevention, last modified August 7, 2023, https://www.cdc.gov/cholera/general/index.html.

38. "Yemen," UN News, accessed December 13, 2023,https://news.un.org/en/focus/yemen.

39. Frederik Federspiel and Mohammad Ali, "The Cholera Outbreak in Yemen: Lessons Learned and Way Forward," *BMC Public Health* 18, no. 1 (December 2018): 1–8, https://doi.org/10.1186/s12889-018-6227-6.

40. Lydia Lindsay, "Disease Management of Cholera in Yemen among People Displaced by Conflict," *OJIN: The Online Journal of Issues in Nursing* 26, no. 3 (July 2021), https://doi.org/10.3912/OJIN.Vol26No03PPT29.

41. Anton Camacho, Malika Bouhenia, Reema Alyusfi, Abdulhakeem Alkohlani, Munna Abdulla Mohammed Naji, Xavier de Radiguès, Abdinasir M. Abubakar, et al., "Cholera Epidemic in Yemen, 2016–18: An Analysis of Surveillance Data," *Lancet Global Health* 6, no. 6 (2018): e680–e690, https://doi.org/10.1016/S2214-109X(18)30230-4; Kate Lyons, "Yemen's Cholera Outbreak Now the Worst in History as Millionth Case Looms," *Guardian*, October 12, 2017, https://www.theguardian.com/global-development/2017/oct/12/yemen-cholera-outbreak-worst-in-history-1-million-cases-by-end-of-year; Humanitarian Country Team, *2018 Humanitarian Needs Overview – Yemen* (New York: UN Office for the Coordination of Humanitarian Affairs, December 2017), https://reliefweb.int/sites/reliefweb.int/files/resources/yemen_humanitarian_needs_overview_hno_2018_20171204_0.pdf.

42. Stephen Snyder, "Thousands in Yemen Get Sick in an Entirely Preventable Cholera Outbreak," *The World*, May 15, 2017, https://theworld.org/stories/2017-05-15/thousands-yemen-get-sick-entirely-preventable-cholera-outbreak.

43. Gregory Härtl, "Cholera Count Reaches 500,000 in Yemen," *World Health Organization*, August 14, 2017, https://www.who.int/en/news-room/detail/14-08-2017-cholera-count-reaches-500-000-in-yemen.

44. Snyder, "Thousands in Yemen."

45. "Evaluation of the UNICEF Level 3 Response to the Cholera Epidemic in Yemen: Crisis within a Crisis: Executive Summary," United Nations Digital Library, accessed December 13, 2023, https://digitallibrary.un.org/record/1637498?ln=en; "Coping with Risks in Yemen while Providing Hope," World Bank, January 15, 2019, https://www.worldbank.org/en/news/feature/2019/01/15/coping-with-risks-in-yemen-while-providing-hope.

46. "Coping with Risks in Yemen."

47. WASH Cluster, Yemen Acute Watery Diarrhea and Cholera Outbreak Standard Operating Procedures, March 2018, http://Yemen Acute Watery Diarrhea and Cholera Outbreak Standard Operating Procedures; Mohammed Al-Ghorbani, and Sabrin Al-Aghbari, "Rapid Response Teams Reach Yemen's Most Remote Areas to Help Eliminate Cholera," UNICEF last modified January 31, 2019, https://www.unicef.org/yemen/stories/ rapid-response-teams-reach-yemens-most-remote-areas-help-eliminate-cholera.

48. Johns Hopkins Center for Humanitarian Health, *Brief Report Cholera in Yemen: A Case Study of Epidemic Preparedness and Response* (Baltimore, MD: Johns Hopkins Center for Humanitarian Health, USAID, 2018), http://hopkinshumanitarianhealth. org/assets/documents/CHOLERA_YEMEN_BRIEF_Low_Res_Dec_4_2018.pdf; UNICEF Yemen, "Cholera Rapid Response Teams Strengthen Communities' Role in Outbreak Prevention and Response," UNICEF, November 22, 2018, https://www. unicef.org/yemen/stories/cholera-rapid-response-teams-strengthen-communities- role-outbreak-prevention-and-response.

49. Yemen WASH Cluster, *Yemen Acute Watery Diarrhea and Cholera Outbreak Standard Operating Procedures* (New York: Global WASH Cluster, March 2018), https:// drive.google.com/file/d/1pfnBOiRON7wvcb5NPNdcLsP9ZwZYqpbT/view; Yemen Humanitarian Situation Reports from 2018 to 2023 are available through the UNICEF website, at https://www.unicef.org/appeals/yemen/situation-reports; Johns Hopkins Center for Humanitarian Health, *Brief Report Cholera in Yemen*; United Nations CERF, *Resident/Humanitarian Coordinator – Report on the Use of Cerf Funds Yemen Rapid Response Disruption of Basic Services* (Geneva: United Nations, 2018), https://cerf.un.org/sites/default/files/resources/18-RR-YEM-28632- NR01_Yemen_RCHC.Report.pdf.

50. UNICEF Yemen, "Cholera Rapid Response Teams."

51. United Nations Digital Library, "Evaluation of the UNICEF."

52. "Emergency Shelter Standard," UN Refugee Agency, accessed December 13, 2023, https://emergency.unhcr.org/entry/36774/emergency-shelter-standard.

53. Angel N. Desai, John W. Ramatowski, Nina Marano, Lawrence C. Madoff, and Britta Lassmann, "Infectious Disease Outbreaks among Forcibly Displaced Persons: An Analysis of ProMED Reports 1996–2016," *Conflict and Health* 14, no. 1 (2020): 1–10, https://doi.org/10.1186/s13031-020-00295-9.

54. World Health Organization, Western Pacific Region, *Repurposing Facilities for Quarantine or Isolation and Management of Mild COVID-19 Cases* (Geneva: World Health Organization, 2022), https://iris.who.int/bitstream/handle/10665/332273/ WPR-DSE-2020-006-eng.pdf; Mark Johanson, "Today's Hotel Is Tomorrow's Coronavirus Hospital," CNN, March 25, 2020, https://www.cnn.com/travel/article/ hotels-turned-hospitals-coronavirus/index.html.

55. Anya Grahn, "Tuberculosis Sanitariums: Reminders of the White Plague," National Trust for Historic Preservation, August 6, 2015, https://savingplaces.org/stories/ tuberculosis-sanitariums-reminders-of-the-white-plaque.

56. Chiara Altare, Vincent Kahi, Moise Ngwa, Amelia Goldsmith, Heiko Hering, Ann Burton, and Paul Spiegel, "Infectious Disease Epidemics in Refugee Camps: A Retrospective Analysis of UNHCR Data (2009–2017)," *Journal of Global Health Reports* 3 (September 2019): e2019064, https://doi.org/10.29392/joghr.3.e2019064.

CHAPTER 5

1. Samuel L Groseclose, and David L. Buckeridge, "Public Health Surveillance Systems: Recent Advances in their Use and Evaluation," *Annual Review of Public Health* 38 (March 2017): 57–79, https://doi.org/10.1146/annurev-publhealth-031816-044348.

2. P. Gregg Greenough and Erica L. Nelson, "Beyond Mapping: A Case for Geospatial Analytics in Humanitarian Health," *Conflict and Health* 13, no. 1 (November 2019): 1–14, https://doi.org/10.1186/s13031-019-0234-9.

3. Antoine Kaboré, Sharon McDonnell, and Bradley A. Perkins, "Technical Guidelines for Integrated Disease Surveillance and Response in the African Region," (Atlanta: Centers for Disease Control, World Health Organization, 2001), https://stacks.cdc.gov/view/cdc/12082.

CHAPTER 6

1. World Health Organization, *WHO Guidelines for Investigation of Human Cases of Avian Influenza A (H5N1)*, Rev. (Geneva: World Health Organization, 2007), https://iris.who.int/bitstream/handle/10665/69416/WHO_CDS_EPR_GIP_2006_4r1.pdf.

2. Sarah Kliff and Margot Sanger-Katz, "Bottleneck for U.S. Coronavirus Response: The Fax Machine," *New York Times*, July 13, 2020, https://www.nytimes.com/2020/07/13/upshot/coronavirus-response-fax-machines.html.

3. World Health Organization, *International Health Regulations*, 3rd ed. (Geneva: World Health Organization, 2005), https://iris.who.int/bitstream/handle/10665/246107/9789241580496-eng.pdf.

4. "National Outbreak Reporting System (NORS)," Centers for Disease Control and Prevention, accessed December 14, 2023, https://www.cdc.gov/nors/index.html.

5. "Public Health Emergency Declaration," Administration for Strategic Preparedness and Response, U.S. Department of Health and Human Services, accessed December 14, 2023, https://www.phe.gov/Preparedness/legal/Pages/phedeclaration.aspx.

6. "A Guide to the Disaster Declaration Process and Federal Disaster Assistance," FEMA, accessed December 14, 2023, https://www.fema.gov/pdf/rrr/dec_proc.pdf.

7. "Emergency Declarations and Authorities Fact Sheet." Association of State and Territorial Health Officials (ASTHO), accessed December 14, 2023, https://www.astho.org/globalassets/pdf/legal-preparedness/04-emerg-dec-authorities.pdf.

8. "Covid-19 Timeline." David J. Sencer CDC Museum, in association with the Smithsonian Institution, Centers for Disease Control and Prevention, last modified March 15, 2023, https://www.cdc.gov/museum/timeline/covid19.html.

9. Jessie Yeung, Joshua Berlinger, Adam Renton, Meg Wagner, Meg Wagner, Mike Hayes, and Veronica Rocha, "March 13 Coronavirus News," CNN, March 13, 2020. https://edition.cnn.com/world/live-news/coronavirus-outbreak-03-13-20-intl-hnk/h_77fa590398cb13df77c6cea892954db0.

10. "COVID-19 Emergency Declaration," HQ-20-017-FactSheet, 3 C.F.R., FEMA, March 14, 2020, https://www.fema.gov/press-release/20210318/covid-19-emergency-declaration.

11. World Organisation for Animal Health, *Immediate Notification and Follow-Up Reports of a Disease, an Infection or Any Other Significant Epidemiological Event* (Paris: World Organisation for Animal Health, 2011), https://www.woah.org/fileadmin/Home/eng/Animal_Health_in_the_World/docs/pdf/OIE_Guidelines_Terra_2011.pdf.

12. World Health Organization, *International Health Regulations*, Article 5 (Geneva: World Health Organization, 2005), https://iris.who.int/bitstream/handle/10665/43883/9789241580410_eng.pdf.

13. World Health Organization, *International Health Regulations*, Articles 6-8, 10.

14. Government of Canada, and National Collaborating Centre for Infectious Disease, "Declaring the Outbreak Over," Outbreak Toolkit, accessed December 15, 2023, https://outbreaktools.ca/case-study-overview/module-4-concluding-the-investigation-2/declaring-outbreak-over.

15. World Health Organization, "WHO Recommended Criteria for Declaring the End of the Ebola Virus Disease Outbreak," last modified March 4, 2020,

https://www.who.int/publications/m/item/who-recommended-criteria-for-declaring-the-end-of-the-ebola-virus-disease-outbreak.

16. "Step 7: Decide an Outbreak Is Over," Foodborne Outbreaks, Centers for Disease Control and Prevention, last modified December 13, 2022, https://www.cdc.gov/foodsafety/outbreaks/steps/decision.html.

17. Australian Government, *Guidelines for the Public Health Management*, chap 7, section 7.5.

CHAPTER 7

1. Randall N. Hyer and Vincent T. Covello, *Effective Media Communication during Public Health Emergencies: A WHO Field Guide* (Geneva: World Health Organization,2005), https://iris.who.int/bitstream/handle/10665/43477/WHO_CDS_2005.31a_eng.pdf.

2. Interagency Standing Committee, "IASC Guidelines on Mental Health and Psychosocial Support in Emergency Settings," June 1, 2007, https://interagencystandingcommittee.org/iasc-task-force-mental-health-and-psychosocial-support-emergency-settings/iasc-guidelines-mental-health-and-psychosocial-support-emergency-settings-2007.

3. Breakthrough ACTION, *Establishing and Maintaining a Hotline: A Technical Brief* (United States: USAID, 2021), https://covid19communicationnetwork.org/wp-content/uploads/2020/04/EstablishingHotlineBrief_ENGLISH.pdf.

4. "Hotline in a Box," Guide and Tools, Community Engagement, British Red Cross, accessed December 14, 2023, https://communityengagementhub.org/guides-and-tools/hotline-in-a-box.

5. Adele Daleke Lisi Aluma, Sam Koulmini, Souley Kalilou, Obianuju Igweonu, Amadou Felix Kouassi, Mohamed Alimou Traore, Benoit Ntezayabo, et al., "Use of Call Centers in Polio Eradication Efforts in Island Settlement in Chad," *Journal of Immunological Sciences* 2 (2021): 1113, https://doi.org/10.29245/2578-3009/2021/S2.1113.

6. "The Polio Endgame Strategy 2019–2023: Eradication, Integration, Containment and Certification," Polio Endgame Strategy, Global Polio Eradication Initiative, accessed December 14, 2023, https://polioeradication.org/who-we-are/polio-endgame-strategy-2019-2023.

7. Aluma et al., "Use of Call Centers."

8. Aluma et al., "Use of Call Centers," 88.

9. Aluma et al., "Use of Call Centers," 88.

10. "Certification," Global Polio Eradication Initiative, accessed December 14, 2023, https://polioeradication.org/polio-today/preparing-for-a-polio-free-world/certification.

11. Katherine J. Igoe, "Developing Public Health Communication Strategies—and Combating Misinformation—During Covid-19," Harvard School of Public Health, accessed December 14, 2023, https://www.hsph.harvard.edu/ecpe/public-health-communication-strategies-covid-19.

12. Carolyn M. Greene, Jennita Reefhuis, Christina Tan, Anthony E. Fiore, Susan Goldstein, Michael J. Beach, Stephen C. Redd, et al., "Epidemiologic Investigations of Bioterrorism-Related Anthrax, New Jersey, 2001," *Emerging Infectious Diseases* 8, no. 10 (October 2002): 1048-1055, https://doi.org/10.3201/eid0810.020329.

13. Caron Chess, and Lee Clarke, "Facilitation of Risk Communication During the Anthrax Attacks of 2001: The Organizational Backstory," *American Journal of Public Health* 97, no. 9 (October 2007): 1578–83, https://doi.org/10.2105/AJPH.2006.099267.

14. Larry M. Bush and Maria T. Perez, "The Anthrax Attacks 10 Years Later," *Annals of Internal Medicine* 156, no. 1 (January 2012): 41–44, https://doi.org/10.7326/0003-4819-

155-12-201112200-00373; Edward A. Belongia, Burney Kieke, Ruth Lynfield, Jeffrey P. Davis, and Richard E. Besser, "Demand for Prophylaxis after Bioterrorism-Related Anthrax Cases, 2001," *Emerging Infectious Diseases* 11, no. 1 (January 2005): 42, https://doi.org/10.3201/eid1101.040272.

15. World Health Organization Department of Communications, *Evidence Syntheses to Support the Guideline on Emergency Risk Communication* (Detroit: World Health Organization, 2016), https://cdn.who.int/media/docs/default-source/meeting-reports/systematic-review-question-10.pdf.

16. World Health Organization, *Communicating Risk in Public Health Emergencies: A WHO Guideline for Emergency Risk Communication (ERC) Policy and Practice* (Geneva: World Health Organization, 2017), https://iris.who.int/bitstream/handle/10665/259807/9789241550208-eng.pdf.

17. Institute of Medicine (US) Committee on Assuring the Health of the Public in the Twenty-First Century, "Media," in *The Future of the Public's Health in the Twenty-First Century* (Washington DC: National Academies Press, 2002), https://www.ncbi.nlm.nih.gov/books/NBK221224.

18. Institute of Medicine (US) Committee, *The Future of the Public's Health*.

19. "CDC Media Statement: Measles Cases in the U.S. Are Highest Since Measles Was Eliminated in 2000," Centers for Disease Control and Prevention, April 25, 2019, https://archive.cdc.gov/#/details?url=https://www.cdc.gov/media/releases/2019/s0424-highest-measles-cases-since-elimination.html.

20. Jessica Bursztynsky, "Jewish Nurses Debunk Anti-Vaxxer Misinformation as Measles Spreads in NYC Ultra-Orthodox Community," *CNBC*, April 21, 2019, https://www.cnbc.com/2019/04/18/jewish-nurses-debunk-anti-vaxxer-misinformation-as-measles-spreads.html; Gwynne Hogan and WNYC Staff, "How Orthodox Jewish Nurses Are Fighting 'Anti-Vaccination Propaganda' Targeting Their Community," *Gothamist*, March 26, 2019, https://gothamist.com/news/how-orthodox-jewish-nurses-are-fighting-anti-vaccination-propaganda-targeting-their-community.

21. Betsy McKay and Melanie Grayce West, "What Can Stop the Measles Outbreak? Officials Lean on an Unlikely Band of Locals," *Wall Street Journal*, May 5, 2019, https://www.wsj.com/articles/what-can-finally-stop-the-measles-outbreak-officials-lean-on-an-unlikely-band-of-locals-11557077101.

22. Amanda Schaffer, "Amid a Measles Outbreak, an Ultra-Orthodox Nurse Fights Vaccination Fears in Her Community," *New Yorker*, January 25, 2019, https://www.newyorker.com/news/as-told-to/amid-a-measles-outbreak-an-ultra-orthodox-nurse-fights-vaccination-fears-in-her-community.

23. Devona Overton, Selena Ramkeesoon, Kevin Kirkpatrick, and Esther Pak, "Lessons from COVID-19 on Executing Communications and Engagement at the Community Level During a Health Crisis," National Academies Sciences, Engineering, and Medicine, December 7, 2021, https://www.nationalacademies.org/news/2021/12/lessons-from-covid-19-on-executing-communications-and-engagement-at-the-community-level-during-a-health-crisis.

24. Rohit Valecha, Srikrishna Krishnarao Srinivasan, Tejaswi Volety, K. Hazel Kwon, Manish Agrawal, and H. Raghav Rao, "Fake News Sharing: An Investigation of Threat and Coping Cues in the Context of the Zika Virus," *Digital Threats: Research and Practice* 2, no. 2 (April 2021): 1–16, https://doi.org/10.1145/3410025.

25. Jan-Willem Van Prooijen, and Eric Van Dijk, "When Consequence Size Predicts Belief in Conspiracy Theories: The Moderating Role of Perspective Taking," *Journal of Experimental Social Psychology* 55 (2014): 63–73, https://doi.org/10.1016/j.jesp.2014.06.006.

26. Anand Venkatraman, Dhruvika Mukhija, Nilay Kumar, and Sajan Jiv Singh Nagpal, "Zika Virus Misinformation on the Internet," *Travel Medicine and Infectious Disease* 14, no. 4 (2016): 421–22, https://doi.org/10.1016/j.tmaid.2016.05.018; Michele Miller, Tanvi Banerjee, Roopteja Muppalla, William Romine, and Amit Sheth, "What Are People Tweeting about Zika? An Exploratory Study Concerning Its Symptoms, Treatment, Transmission, and Prevention." *JMIR Public Health and Surveillance* 3, no. 2 (2017): e7157, https://doi.org/10.2196/publichealth.7157.

27. Mark Dredze, David A. Broniatowski, and Karen M. Hilyard, "Zika Vaccine Misconceptions: A Social Media Analysis," *Vaccine* 34, no. 30 (June 2016): 3441, https://doi.org/10.1016/j.vaccine.2016.05.008.

28. Silvia Sommariva, Cheryl Vamos, Alexios Mantzarlis, Lillie Uyên-Loan Dào, and Dinorah Martinez Tyson, "Spreading the (Fake) News: Exploring Health Messages on Social Media and the Implications for Health Professionals Using a Case Study," *American Journal of Health Education* 49, no. 4 (2018): 246–55, https://doi.org/10.1080/19325037.2018.1473178.

29. Michael J. Wood, "Propagating and Debunking Conspiracy Theories on Twitter During the 2015–2016 Zika Virus Outbreak," *Cyberpsychology, Behavior, and Social Networking* 21, no. 8 (August 2018): 485–90, https://doi.org/10.1089/cyber.2017.0669.

30. Jovan Byford, *Conspiracy Theories: A Critical Introduction* (New York City: Springer, 2011), 91; Wood, "Propagating and Debunking."

31. John M. Carey, Victoria Chi, D. J. Flynn, Brendan Nyhan, and Thomas Zeitzoff, "The Effects of Corrective Information about Disease Epidemics and Outbreaks: Evidence from Zika and Yellow Fever in Brazil," *Science Advances* 6, no. 5 (January 2020), https://doi.org/10.1126/sciadv.aaw7449.

32. "Zika February 12–16, 2016 Survey (Week 1): Appendix," Annenberg Public Policy Center, accessed December 14, 2023, https://cdn.annenbergpublicpolicycenter.org/wp-content/uploads/ZikaWeek1Appendix.pdf.

33. Casey A. Klofstad, Joseph E. Uscinski, Jennifer M. Connolly, and Jonathan P. West, "What Drives People to Believe in Zika Conspiracy Theories?" *Palgrave Communications* 5, no. 1 (April 2019): 1–8, https://doi.org/10.1057/s41599-019-0243-8

34. Carey et al., "Effects of Corrective Information."

35. Center for Countering Digital Hate, *The Disinformation Dozen: Why Platforms Must Act on Twelve Leading Online Anti-Vaxxers* (Washington, DC: CCDH, 2021), https://counterhate.com/research/the-disinformation-dozen.

CHAPTER 8

1. J. Sylvester Squire, K. Hann, O. Denisiuk, M. Kamara, D. Tamang, and R. Zachariah, "The Ebola Outbreak and Staffing in Public Health Facilities in Rural Sierra Leone: Who is Left to Do the Job?" *Public Health Action* 7, no. 1 (June 2017): S47–S54, doi:10.5588/pha.16.0089; Federal Healthcare Resilience Taskforce, *Federal Healthcare Resilience Taskforce Alternate Care Site Toolkit*, 3rd ed. (Washington, DC: US Department of Health and Human Services, 2020), https://files.asprtracie.hhs.gov/documents/acs-toolkit-ed1-20200330-1022.pdf.

2. Kyle Mattice, "Ensuring Healthcare Staffing Preparedness for the Next Epidemic," *Becker's Hospital Review*, May 22, 2015, https://www.beckershospitalreview.com/hr/ensuring-healthcare-staffing-preparedness-for-the-next-epidemic.html.

3. Centers for Disease Control and Prevention, *Public Health Emergency Preparedness and Response Capabilities: National Standards for State, Local, Tribal, and Territorial Public Health* (Atlanta: US Department of Health and Human Services, 2019) https://www.cdc.gov/cpr/readiness/00_docs/CDC_PreparednesResponseCapabilities_

October2018_Final_508.pdf; Homeland Security Council, *National Strategy for Pandemic Influenza Implementation Plan* (Washington, DC: Homeland Security Council, 2006), https://www.cdc.gov/flu/pandemic-resources/pdf/pandemic-influenza-implementation.pdf.

4. Occupational Safety and Health Administration, *Pandemic Influenza Preparedness and Response Guidance for Healthcare Workers and Healthcare Employers*, OSHA 3328-05R (Washington, DC: US Department of Labor, 2009), https://www.osha.gov/sites/default/files/publications/OSHA_pandemic_health.pdf.

5. World Health Organization, *Occupational Safety and Health in Public Health Emergencies: A Manual for Protecting Health Workers and Responders* (Geneva: World Health Organization and International Labour Organization, 2018), https://iris.who.int/bitstream/handle/10665/275385/9789241514347-eng.pdf.

6. Jennifer Garvin, "Dentists, Dental Students among Providers Now Authorized to Administer COVID-19 Vaccine Nationwide," *American Dental Association News*, March 12, 2021, https://www.ada.org/publications/ada-news/2021/march/dentists-dental-students-among-providers-now-authorized-to-administer-covid-19-vaccine-nationwide.

7. World Health Organization, *Hospital Preparedness Checklist for Pandemic Influenza: Focus on Pandemic (H1N1) 2009*, No. EUR/08/5085079 (Copenhagen: WHO Regional Office for Europe, 2009), https://iris.who.int/bitstream/handle/10665/350605/WHO-EURO-2009-4543-44306-62586-eng.pdf.

8. "Health Workforce Estimator (HWFE)," Europe, World Health Organization, accessed December 15, 2023, https://www.who.int/europe/tools-and-toolkits/strengthening-the-health-system-response-to-covid-19/Surge-planning-tools/health-workforce-estimator-(hwfe).

9. Rupa Narra, Jeremy Sobel, Catherine Piper, Deborah Gould, Nahid Bhadelia, Mary Dott, Anthony Fiore, and William A. Fischer, "CDC Safety Training Course for Ebola Virus Disease Healthcare Workers," *Emerging Infectious Diseases* 23, suppl. 1 (December 2017): S217, https://doi.org/10.3201/eid2313.170549.

10. Mackenzie Moore and Kate Toole, *Contact Tracing during the COVID-19 Pandemic: A Systematic Comparison of Global Practices and Influencing Factors* (Washington, DC: Georgetown Center for Global Health Science and Security, 2021), https://georgetown.app.box.com/s/4f891fctc5gv04hfav1esm9bqvpxc7np.

11. "FETP - Field Epidemiology Training Program - Disease Detectives in Action," Centers for Disease Control and Prevention, last modified July 19, 2017, https://archive.cdc.gov/#/details?url=https://www.cdc.gov/globalhealth/infographics/uncategorized/fetp.htm.

12. A. McKenzie André, Augusto Lopez, Samantha Perkins, Stephanie Lambert, Lesley Chace, Nestor Noudeke, Aissatou Fall, and Biagio Pedalino, "Frontline Field Epidemiology Training Programs as a Strategy to Improve Disease Surveillance and Response," *Emerging Infectious Diseases* 23, suppl 1 (2017): S166, https://dx.doi.org/10.3201/eid2313.170803; "Training Programs," TEPHINET, Task Force for Global Health, https://www.tephinet.org/training-programs.

13. Ali M. Zaki, Sander Van Boheemen, Theo M. Bestebroer, Albert D. M. E. Osterhaus, and Ron A. M. Fouchier, "Isolation of a Novel Coronavirus from a Man with Pneumonia in Saudi Arabia," *New England Journal of Medicine* 367, no. 19 (November 2012): 1814–20, doi: 10.1056/NEJMoa1211721; Ali M. Zaki, Sander Van Boheemen, Theo M. Bestebroer, Albert D. M. E Osterhaus, and Ron A. M. Fouchier, "Isolation of a Novel Coronavirus from a Man with Pneumonia in Saudi Arabia," *New England Journal of Medicine* 367, no. 19 (2012): 1814–20, doi: 10.1056/NEJMoa1211721.

14. European Centre for Disease Prevention and Control, "Communicable Disease Threats Report, 29 April–5 May 2012, Week 18," European Centre for Disease Prevention and Control, May 4, 2012, https://www.ecdc.europa.eu/en/

publications-data/communicable-disease-threats-report-29-april-5-may-2012-week-18.

15. Mohannad Al Nsour, Ibrahim Iblan, and Mohammed Rasoul Tarawneh, "Jordan Field Epidemiology Training Program: Critical Role in National and Regional Capacity Building," *JMIR Medical Education* 4, no. 1 (2018): e9516, doi: 10.2196/mededu.9516.

16. Mohammad Mousa al-Abdallat, Daniel C. Payne, Sultan Alqasrawi, Brian Rha, Rania A. Tohme, Glen R. Abedi, Mohannad al Nsour, et al., "Hospital-Associated Outbreak of Middle East Respiratory Syndrome Coronavirus: A Serologic, Epidemiologic, and Clinical Description," *Clinical Infectious Diseases* 59, no. 9 (November 2014): 1225–33, https://doi.org/10.1093/cid/ciu359; Daniel C. Payne, Ibrahim Iblan, Sultan Alqasrawi, Mohannad al Nsour, Brian Rha, Rania A. Tohme, Glen R. Abedi, et al., "Stillbirth during Infection with Middle East Respiratory Syndrome Coronavirus," *Journal of Infectious Diseases* 209, no. 12 (June 2014): 1870–72, https://doi.org/10.1093/infdis/jiu068.

17. "Rapid Response Team Training," World Health Organization, accessed December 15, 2023, https://extranet.who.int/sph/rapid-response-team-training.

18. "Tanzania Launches Training for National Rapid Response Teams with Focus on Ebola," World Health Organization United Republic of Tanzania, July 17, 2018, https://www.afro.who.int/news/tanzania-launches-training-national-rapid-response-teams-focus-ebola.

CHAPTER 9

1. "No Such Thing as the Handshake Police," episode 357, May 14, 2021, in *No Such Thing as a Fish*, produced by Quite Interesting, podcast, audio, https://audioboom.com/posts/7864627-no-such-thing-as-the-handshake-police.

2. Ella al-Shamahi, *The Handshake: A Gripping History* (London: Profile Books, 2021).

3. "WASH in Health Care Facilities," Water Sanitation and Health, World Health Organization, accessed December 16, 2023, https://www.who.int/teams/environment-climate-change-and-health/water-sanitation-and-health-(wash)/health-care-facilities/wash-in-health-care-facilities.

4. Anita Patel, Maryann M. D'Alessandro, Karen J. Ireland, W. Greg Burel, Elaine B. Wencil, and Sonja A. Rasmussen, "Personal Protective Equipment Supply Chain: Lessons Learned from Recent Public Health Emergency Responses," *Health Security* 15, no. 3 (June 2017): 244–52, https://doi.org/10.1089/hs.2016.0129.

5. World Health Organization. *Health Worker Ebola Infections in Guinea, Liberia and Sierra Leone: A Preliminary Report 21 May 2015* (Geneva: World Health Organization, 2015), https://iris.who.int/bitstream/handle/10665/171823/WHO_EVD_SDS_REPORT_2015.1_eng.pdf.

6. William A. Fischer, II, Noreen A. Hynes, and Trish M. Perl. "Protecting Health Care Workers from Ebola: Personal Protective Equipment Is Critical But is Not Enough." *Annals of Internal Medicine* 161, no. 10 (December 2014): 753–54, https://doi.org/10.7326/M14-1953.

7. Fischer, Hynes, and Perl, "Protecting Health Care Workers."

8. "Steps to Put on Personal Protective Equipment (PPE) Including Gown," World Health Organization, accessed December 16, 2023, https://apps.who.int/iris/bitstream/handle/10665/150115/WHO_HIS_SDS_2015.1_eng.pdf.

9. Margaret Glancey, Patience Osei, William Alexander Patterson, Matthew Petney, Laura Scavo, Chandrakant Ruparelia, Soumyadipta Acharya, and Youseph Yazdi, "Design Improvements for Personal Protective Equipment Used in Ebola and Other

Epidemic Outbreaks," *Global Health: Science and Practice* 5, no. 2 (June 2017): 325–28, https://doi.org/10.9745/GHSP-D-17-00152.

10. Narra et al., "CDC Safety Training Course for Ebola."

11. Fischer, Hynes, and Perl, "Protecting Health Care Workers."

12. "Guidance on Community Physical Distancing during COVID-19 Pandemic," Fact Sheets and Brochures, Africa CDC, May 12, 2020. https://africacdc.org/download/guidance-on-community-social-distancing-during-covid-19-outbreak.

13. European Centre for Disease Prevention and Control. *Considerations Relating to Social Distancing Measures in Response to COVID-19 – Second Update* (Stockholm: European Centre for Disease Prevention and Control, 2020), https://www.ecdc.europa.eu/sites/default/files/documents/covid-19-social-distancing-measuresg-guide-second-update.pdf.

14. World Health Organization. *Overview of Public Health and Social Measures in the Context of COVID-19* (Geneva: World Health Organization, 2020). https://iris.who.int/bitstream/handle/10665/332115/WHO-2019-nCoV-PHSM_Overview-2020.1-eng.pdf.

15. Per Nilsen, Ida Seing, Carin Ericsson, Ove Andersen, Nina Thórný Stefánsdóttir, Tine Tjørnhøj-Thomsen, Thomas Kallemose, and Jeanette Wassar Kirk, "Implementing Social Distancing Policy Measures in the Battle against the Coronavirus: Protocol of a Comparative Study of Denmark and Sweden," *Implementation Science Communications* 1, no. 1 (September 2020): 1–10, https://doi.org/10.1186/s43058-020-00065-x.

16. Philip A. Mackowiak and Paul S. Sehdev, "The Origin of Quarantine." *Clinical Infectious Diseases* 35, no. 9 (November 2002): 1071–72, https://doi.org/10.1086/344062.

17. Zlata Blazina Tomic and Vesna Blazina, *Expelling the Plague: The Health Office and the Implementation of Quarantine in Dubrovnik* (Montreal: McGill University Press, 2015) 1377–533, https://www.mqup.ca/expelling-the-plague-products-9780773545397.php.

18. Rob Schmitz, "How a Medieval City Dealing with the Black Death Invented Quarantine," All Things Considered (podcast), National Public Radio, July 6, 2021, https://www.npr.org/2021/07/06/1012490871/how-a-medieval-city-dealing-with-the-black-death-invented-quarantine.

19. Alex Chase-Levenson, introduction to *The Yellow Flag Quarantine and the British Mediterranean World, 1780–1860* (Cambridge: Cambridge University Press, 2020).

20. World Health Organization, *WHO MERS-CoV Global Summary and Risk Assessment* (Geneva: World Health Organization, 2016), https://www.who.int/publications/m/item/who-mers-cov-global-summary-and-risk-assessment---5-december-2016.

21. Jung Wan Park, Keon Joo Lee, Kang Hyoung Lee, Sang Hyup Lee, Jung Rae Cho, Jin Won Mo, Soo Young Choi, et al., "Hospital Outbreaks of Middle East Respiratory Syndrome, Daejeon, South Korea, 2015," *Emerging Infectious Diseases* 23, no. 6 (2017): 898, https://doi.org/10.3201/eid2306.160120.

22. Madison Park, "South Korea Grapples to Contain MERS as 1,369 in Quarantine," CNN, June 4, 2015, https://www.cnn.com/2015/06/03/world/south-korea-mers/index.html.

23. Ju-min Park, "Quarantine Area: Korean Patients Tested by MERS Lockdown," Reuters, June 17, 2015. https://www.reuters.com/article/us-health-mers-southkorea-hospitals/quarantine-area-korean-patients-tested-by-mers-lockdown-idUSKB-N0OX2P320150618.

24. Choe Sang-Hun, "After MERS, South Korea Authorizes Prison for Quarantine Scofflaws," *New York Times*, June 26, 2015, https://www.nytimes.com/2015/06/27/world/asia/after-mers-south-korea-authorizes-prison-for-quarantine-scofflaws.html.

25. "South Korea to Track Mobile Phones to Enforce MERS Virus Quarantine Rules," *Guardian*, June 7, 2015, https://www.theguardian.com/world/2015/jun/07/mers-virus-outbreak-south-korea-reports-fifth-death-as-cases-rise-to-64.

26. Park et al., "Hospital Outbreaks."

27. "Overview, History, and How the Safety Process Works," Vaccine Safety, Centers for Disease Control and Prevention, September 9, 2020, https://www.cdc.gov/vaccine-safety/ensuringsafety/history/index.html.

28. "Tuberculosis," Global Health Centers for Disease Control and Prevention, last modified April 6, 2020, https://www.cdc.gov/globalhealth/newsroom/topics/tb/index.html.

29. Eliud Wandwalo, "Why Drug-Resistant Tuberculosis Poses a Major Risk to Global Health Security," Global Fund, November 19, 2020, https://www.theglobalfund.org/en/opinion/2020/2020-11-19-why-drug-resistant-tuberculosis-poses-a-major-risk-to-global-health-security.

30. James Millard, Cesar Ugarte-Gil, and David A. J. Moore, "Multidrug Resistant Tuberculosis," *BMJ* 350 (February 2015), https://doi.org/10.1136/bmj.h882.

31. "Multidrug Resistant Tuberculosis." Science Direct, accessed December 16, 2023, https://www.sciencedirect.com/topics/medicine-and-dentistry/multidrug-resistant-tuberculosis.

32. "Ensuring the Safety of Vaccines in the United States," FDA, July 2011, https://www.fda.gov/files/vaccines,%20blood%20&%20biologics/published/Ensuring-the-Safety-of-Vaccines-in-the-United-States.pdf.

33. Jeffrey C. Kwong, Julie Foisy, Sherman Quan, Christine Heidebrecht, Faron Kolbe, Julie A. Bettinger, David L. Buckeridge, et al., "Why Collect Individual-Level Vaccination Data?," *CMAJ* 182, no 3 (February 2010): 273–75, https://doi.org/10.1503/cmaj.091515.

34. Michael M. McNeil, Julianne Gee, Eric S. Weintraub, Edward A. Belongia, Grace M. Lee, Jason M. Glanz, James D. Nordin, et al., "The Vaccine Safety Datalink: Successes and Challenges Monitoring Vaccine Safety," *Vaccine* 32, no. 42 (September 2014): 5390–98, https://doi.org/10.1016/j.vaccine.2014.07.073.

35. Christopher Nelson, Edward W. Chan, Anita Chandra, Paul Sorensen, Henry H. Willis, Katherine Comanor, Hayoung Park, Karen A. Ricci, Leah B. Caldarone, Molly Shea, John A. Zambrano, and Lydia Hansell, *Recommended Infrastructure Standards for Mass Antibiotic Dispensing* (Santa Monica, CA: RAND Health Center for Domestic and International Health Security, 2008), https://www.rand.org/content/dam/rand/pubs/technical_reports/2008/RAND_TR553.pdf.

36. "Closed POD Evaluation, Planning and Selection Checklist," Mecklenburg County, accessed December 18, 2023, https://mecknc.widencollective.com/portals/w1i8lfyi/ClosedPointofDispensing(POD)Toolkit; Capitol Region Council of Governments, *Points of Dispensing (POD) Template Plan* (Hartford, CT: Capitol Region Council of Governments, 2017), https://crcog.org/wp-content/uploads/2017/12/POD-Template-Plan.pdf; Centers for Disease Control and Prevention, "Point of Dispensing (POD) Standards," Coordinating Office for Terrorism Preparedness and Emergency Response, last modified April 2008, https://www.cdc.gov/cpr/documents/coopagreement-archive/fy2008/dispensingstandards.pdf.

37. "Infection Prevention and Control," World Health Organization, accessed December 16, 2023, https://www.who.int/teams/integrated-health-services/infection-prevention-control.

38. Humanitarian Standards Partnership, *The Sphere Handbook: Humanitarian Charter and Minimum Standards in Humanitarian Response* (Geneva: Sphere Association, 2018), https://handbook.spherestandards.org/en/sphere/#ch002; Benedetta Allegranzi, "The Core Components of Infection Prevention and Control Programs: From Guidelines to Implementation in Real Life" (lecture), World Health Organization, accessed December 18, 2023, https://www.paho.org/en/documents/core-components-infection-prevention-and-control-programs-guidelines-implementation.

39. World Health Organization, *Guidelines on Core Components of Infection Prevention and Control Programmes at the National and Acute Health Care Facility Level* (Geneva: World Health Organization, 2016), https://iris.who.int/bitstream/handle/10665/251730/9789241549929-eng.pdf.

40. "Strategic Priority Infection Prevention and Control Activities for Non-US Healthcare Settings," Centers for Disease Control and Prevention, April 6, 2020. https://public4.pagefreezer.com/browse/CDC%20Covid%20Pages/11-05-2022T12:30/https://www.cdc.gov/coronavirus/2019-ncov/hcp/non-us-settings/ipc-healthcare-facilities-non-us.html.

41. Tolbert Nyenswah, Moses Massaquoi, Miatta Zenabu Gbanya, Mosoka Fallah, Fred Amegashie, Adolphus Kenta, Kumblytee L. Johnson, et al., "Initiation of a Ring Approach to Infection Prevention and Control at Non-Ebola Health Care Facilities—Liberia, January–February 2015," *Morbidity and Mortality Weekly Report* 64, no. 18 (May 2015): 505, https://www.ncbi.nlm.nih.gov/pmc/articles/PMC4584827.

42. FAO, "Part 3: Decontamination Procedures," in *Manual on Procedures for Disease Eradication by Stamping Out* (Rome: FAP, 2001), https://www.fao.org/publications/card/en/c/f264f2ec-c11c-55be-993d-523a9224700c.

43. United States Department of Agriculture, *Foreign Animal Disease Preparedness and Response Plan Standard Operating Procedures: 15. Cleaning and Disinfection* (Washington, DC: United States Department of Agriculture, 2018), https://www.aphis.usda.gov/animal_health/emergency_management/downloads/sop/sop_cd.pdf.

44. "Norovirus (Vomiting Bug)," Health A to Z, British National Health Service, last modified June 17, 2021, https://www.nhs.uk/conditions/norovirus.

45. "Preventing Norovirus," Centers for Disease Control and Prevention, last modified November 9, 2023, https://www.cdc.gov/norovirus/about/prevention.html.

46. Ariella P. Dale, "Outbreak of Acute Gastroenteritis among Rafters and Backpackers in the Backcountry of Grand Canyon National Park, April–June 2022," *Morbidity and Mortality Weekly Report* 71 (September 2022): 1207–11, http://dx.doi.org/10.15585/mmwr.mm7138a2.

47. Luke Runyon, "The CDC Is Looking into a Stomach Bug Outbreak at the Grand Canyon," *Weekend Edition*, National Public Radio, September 24, 2022. Podcast, audio. https://www.npr.org/2022/09/24/1124915552/the-cdc-is-looking-into-a-stomach-bug-outbreak-at-the-grand-canyon.

48. "Health-Care Waste," World Health Organization, last modified February 8, 2018, https://www.who.int/news-room/fact-sheets/detail/health-care-waste.

49. Ministry of Health, Republic of Ghana, *Ghana - Second Health Sector Program Support Center: Environmental Assessment (English)*, Report # E646 (Washington, DC: World Bank Group, 2002), http://documents.worldbank.org/curated/en/316921468749066031/Ghana-Second-Health-Sector-Program-Support-Center-environmental-assessment.

50. Colin S. Brown, Mohamed Elsherbiny, Oliver Johnson, Amardeep Kamboz, Marta Lado, Andrew Leather, Natalie Mounter, et al., "Ebola and Health Partnerships, Action in a Time of Crisis," in *Ebola*, edited by Crtomir Podlipnik (London: Intech, 2016), doi:10.5772/63440.

51. "Terrestrial Animal Health Code, Chapter 4.13: Disposal of Dead Animals," World Organisation for Animal Health, last modified 2010, https://www.woah.org/en/what-we-do/standards/codes-and-manuals/terrestrial-code-online-access/?id=169&L=1&htmfile=chapitre_disposal.htm.

52. International Federation of Red Cross and Red Crescent Societies, *Safe and Dignified Burial: An Implementation Guide for Field Managers* (Geneva: International Federation of Red Cross and Red Crescent Societies, 2019). https://oldmedia.ifrc.org/ifrc/wp-content/uploads/2020/06/IFRC_BurialGuide_web.pdf.

53. "New WHO Safe and Dignified Burial Protocol - Key to Reducing Ebola Transmission." World Health Organization, November 7, 2014, https://www.who.int/news/item/07-11-2014-new-who-safe-and-dignified-burial-protocol---key-to-reducing-ebola-transmission.

54. Pan American Health Organization, *Management of Dead Bodies after Disasters: A Field Manual for First Responders* (Washington DC: Pan American Health Organization, World Health Organization, ICRC, International Federation of Red Cross and Red Crescent Societies, 2009). https://www1.paho.org/english/dd/ped/DeadBodiesFieldManual.pdf.

55. Pandemic Influenza Experts Advisory Committee *Guideline for Burial and Cremation* (United States Pandemic Influenza Experts Advisory Committee, 2007), https://www.mhlw.go.jp/bunya/kenkou/kekkaku-kansenshou04/pdf/09-e14.pdf.

56. International Federation of Red Cross and Red Crescent Societies. *Safe and Dignified Burial.*

57. International Federation of Red Cross and Red Crescent Societies. *Safe and Dignified Burial.*

58. "How to Conduct Safe and Dignified Burial of a Patient Who Has Died from Suspected or Confirmed Ebola or Marburg Virus Disease." World Health Organization, last modified October 30, 2014, https://www.who.int/publications-detail-redirect/WHO-EVD-Guidance-Burials-14.2.

59. Carrie F. Nielsen, Sarah Kidd, Ansumana R. M. Sillah, Edward Davis, Jonathan Mermin, and Peter H. Kilmarx, "Improving Burial Practices and Cemetery Management During an Ebola Virus Disease Epidemic — Sierra Leone, 2014," *Morbidity and Mortality Weekly Report* 64, no. 1 (January 2015): 20. https://www.ncbi.nlm.nih.gov/pmc/articles/PMC4584795.

60. International Federation of Red Cross and Red Crescent Societies. *Safe and Dignified Burial*; World Health Organization. "How to Conduct Safe and Dignified Burial"; Nielsen et al., "Improving Burial Practices."

61. International Federation of Red Cross and Red Crescent Societies. *Safe and Dignified Burial.*

62. "Food Safety," World Organisation for Animal Health, accessed December 17, 2023, https://www.woah.org/en/what-we-do/global-initiatives/food-safety.

63. Food and Agriculture Organization of the United Nations and World Health Organization, *FAO/WHO Framework for Developing National Food Safety Emergency Response Plans* (Rome: Food and Agriculture Organization 2010), https://www.fao.org/3/i1686e/i1686e00.pdf.

64. Kara Rogers, "German E. Coli Outbreak of 2011," Britannica, accessed December 17, 2023, https://www.britannica.com/event/German-E-coli-outbreak-of-2011.

65. Robert Koch-Institute (RKI), *Final Presentation and Evaluation of Epidemiological Findings in the EHEC O104:H4 Outbreak* (Berlin: RKI 2011), https://edoc.rki.de/bitstream/handle/176904/163/23NXL3JomOyAA.pdf.

66. Rogers, "German E. Coli Outbreak of 2011"

67. David Crossland, "Backlash Hits German Government over Handling of Deadly E Coli Outbreak," *National News*, June 7, 2011, https://www.thenationalnews.com/world/europe/backlash-hits-german-government-over-handling-of-deadly-e-coli-outbreak-1.442880.

68. Kai Kupferschmidt, "Cucumbers May Be Culprit in Massive E. Coli Outbreak in Germany," *Science*, May 26, 2011, https://www.science.org/content/article/cucumbers-may-be-culprit-massive-e-coli-outbreak-germany.

69. Eric Kelsey, "Germany E. Coli Cucumber Death Toll Rises to 14," Reuters, May 30, 2011, https://www.reuters.com/article/us-germany-ecoli/germany-e-coli-cucumber-death-toll-rises-to-14-idUSTRE74S12V20110530.

70. "Deadly E. Coli Found on Bean Sprouts," The Local, June 10, 2011, https://www.thelocal.de/20110610/35583.

71. Federal Institute for Risk Assessment, "Samen Von Bockshornklee Mit Hoher Wahrscheinlichkeit Für EHEC O104:H4 Ausbruch Verantwortlich in English: Fenugreek Seeds with High Probability for EHEC O104: H4 Responsible Outbreak' (PDF) (in German)," *Bundesinstitut für Risikobewertung (BfR)*, June 30, 2011, https://mobil.bfr.bund.de/cm/343/samen_von_bockshornklee_mit_hoher_wahrscheinlichkeit_fuer_ehec_0104_h4_ausbruch_verantwortlich.pdf.

72. Elena Köckerling, Laura Karrasch, Aparna Schweitzer, Oliver Razum, and Gérard Krause, "Public Health Research Resulting from One of the World's Largest Outbreaks Caused by Entero-Hemorrhagic Escherichia Coli in Germany 2011: A Review," *Frontiers in Public Health* 5 (December 2017): 332 .https://doi.org/10.3389/fpubh.2017.00332.

73. Judy Dempsey and William Neuman, "Deadly E. Coli Outbreak Linked to German Sprouts," *New York Times*, June 5, 2011, https://www.nytimes.com/2011/06/06/world/europe/06germany.html.

74. Rogers, "German E. Coli Outbreak of 2011".

75. Commission of the European Communities, *Commission Staff Working Document: Lessons Learned from the 2011 Outbreak of Shiga Toxin-Producing* Escherichia coli *(STEC) O104:H4 in sprouted seeds* (Brussels: Commission of the European Communities, 2012), https://food.ec.europa.eu/system/files/2016-10/biosafety_food-borne-disease_cswd_lessons-learned.pdf.

76. Dempsey and Neuman, "Deadly E. Coli Outbreak."

77. "Shiga Toxin-Producing E. Coli (STEC): Update on Outbreak in the EU," European Centre for Disease Prevention and Control, July 27, 2011, https://web.archive.org/web/20111004233651/http:/ecdc.europa.eu/en/activities/sciadvice/Lists/ECDC%20Reviews/ECDC_DispForm.aspx?List=512ff74f-77d4-4ad8-b6d6-bf0f23083f30&ID=1166&RootFolder=%2Fen%2Factivities%2Fsciadvice%2FLists%2FECDC%20Reviews.

78. "*E. Coli*: Rapid Response in a Crisis," European Food Safety Authority, July 11, 2012, https://web.archive.org/web/20181120064044/http:/www.efsa.europa.eu/en/press/news/120711.

79. Rogers, "German E. Coli Outbreak of 2011."

80. "Steps in a Multistate Foodborne Outbreak Investigation," Centers for Disease Control and Prevention, December 13, 2022, https://www.cdc.gov/foodsafety/outbreaks/steps/index.html; Council to Improve Foodborne Outbreak Response (CIFOR), "Chapter 6: Control Measures," in *Guidelines for Foodborne Disease Outbreak Response*, 2nd ed. (Washington, DC: Council to Improve Foodborne Outbreak Response, 2014), http://cifor.us/products/guidelines.

81. CIFOR, "Chapter 6: Control Measures," In *Guidelines*.

82. Public Health Ontario, *Reportable Disease Trends in Ontario* (Ontario: Public Health Ontario, 2018), https://www.publichealthontario.ca/-/media/documents/R/2019/rdto-summaries-2016.pdf?la=en.

83. Heather Hanson, Yvonne Whitfield, Christina Lee, Tina Badiani, Carolyn Minielly, Jillian Fenik, Tony Makrostergios, et al., "Listeria Monocytogenes Associated with Pasteurized Chocolate Milk, Ontario, Canada," *Emerging Infectious Diseases* 25, no. 3 (March 2019): 581, https://doi.org/10.3201/eid2503.180742.

84. "Bovine Spongiform Encephalopathy," World Organisation for Animal Health, accessed December 17, 2023, https://www.woah.org/en/disease/bovine-spongiform-encephalopathy.

85. Douglas J. Lanska, "The Mad Cow Problem in the UK: Risk Perceptions, Risk Management, and Health Policy Development." *Journal of Public Health Policy* 19, no. 2 (1998): 160–83, https://doi.org/10.2307/3343296.

86. "Timeline of Mad Cow Disease Outbreaks," Center for Food Safety, accessed December 17, 2023, https://www.centerforfoodsafety.org/issues/1040/mad-cow-disease/timeline-mad-cow-disease-outbreaks.

87. "BSE Inquiry - The Final Stage Chronology of Events," *BBC News*, June 1999, http://news.bbc.co.uk/hi/english/static/special_report/1999/06/99/bse_inquiry/default.stm.

88. "BSE Inquiry."

89. Gary Finnegan, "The Mad Cow Disease Crisis - How Europe's Health Research Came of Age," Horizon, European Commission, January 29, 2015, https://ec.europa.eu/research-and-innovation/en/horizon-magazine/mad-cow-disease-crisis-how-europes-health-research-came-age.

90. "End to 10-Year British Beef Ban," BBC News, May 3, 2006, http://news.bbc.co.uk/2/hi/4967480.stm.

91. UN Food and Agriculture Organization and World Health Organization, *Codex Alimentarius*, 3rd ed. (Rome: Joint FAO/WHO Food Standards Programme, 2003). https://www.fao.org/3/y5307e/y5307e00.htm#Contents.

92. CIFOR, "Chapter 6: Control Measures," In *Guidelines*.

93. Food and Agriculture Organization of the United Nations/WHO, *FAO/WHO Guide for Developing and Improving National Food Recall Systems* (Rome: Food and Agriculture Organization of the United Nation/ World Health Organization, 2012), 12, https://www.fao.org/3/i3006e/i3006e.pdf.

94. "Monophasic Salmonella Typhimurium Outbreak Linked to Chocolate Products," European Centre for Disease Prevention and Control, April 6, 2022. https://www.ecdc.europa.eu/en/news-events/efsa-and-ecdc-investigate-multi-country-salmonella-outbreak-linked-chocolate-products.

95. Bruce Y. Lee, "Kinder Easter Chocolate Recall after Salmonella Outbreak Leaves 150 Ill, Mostly Young Children," *Forbes*, April 16, 2022, https://www.forbes.com/sites/brucelee/2022/04/16/kinder-easter-chocolate-recall-after-salmonella-outbreak-leaves-150-ill-mostly-young-children/?sh=e5939a323a00.

96. CIFOR, "Chapter 6: Control Measures," In *Guidelines*.

97. Organisation for the Prohibition of Chemical Weapons International Cooperation and Assistance Division Assistance and Protection Branch, *Practical Guide for Medical Management of Chemical Warfare Casualties* (The Hague: Organisation for the Prohibition of Chemical Weapons, 2019), https://www.opcw.org/sites/default/files/documents/2019/05/Full%20version%202019_Medical%20Guide_WEB.pdf.

98. International Atomic Energy Agency, *Preparedness and Response for a Nuclear or Radiological Emergency* (Vienna: International Atomic Energy Agency, 2015), https://www-pub.iaea.org/MTCD/Publications/PDF/P_1708_web.pdf.

CHAPTER 10

1. Centers for Disease Control and Prevention, "Lesson 6: Investigating an Outbreak, Section 2: Steps of an Outbreak Investigation," in *Principles of Epidemiology in Public Health Practice, Third Edition: An Introduction to Applied Epidemiology of Biostatistics* (Washington, DC: Centers for Disease Control and Prevention, 2012), https://www.cdc.gov/csels/dsepd/ss1978/lesson6/section2.html.

2. Michael M. Wagner, Louise S. Gresham, and Virginia Dato, "Case Detection, Outbreak Detection, and Outbreak Characterization," in *Handbook of Biosurveillance* (Amsterdam: Academic Press, 2006), 27–50, doi:10.1016/B978-012369378-5/50005-3.

3. Li Cohen, "Dengue Fever Case in Arizona May Have Been Locally Acquired, Officials Say," *CBS News*, November 16, 2022, https://www.cbsnews.com/news/dengue-fever-case-arizona-maricopa-county.

4. Marilyn J. Field and Kathleen N. Lohr, eds., "Chapter 2, Definitions of Key Terms," in *Clinical Practice Guidelines: Directions for a New Program* (Washington DC: National Academies Press, 1990), https://nap.nationalacademies.org/catalog/1626/clinical-practice-guidelines-directions-for-a-new-program.

5. "Health Emergency Preparedness," World Health Organization, accessed December 18, 2023, https://www.who.int/our-work/health-emergencies.

6. "Isolation of Patients," HSC Public Health Agency, Northern Ireland Regional Infection Prevention and Control Manual, accessed December 19, 2023, https://www.niinfectioncontrolmanual.net/isolation-patients.

7. World Health Organization, *Operational Planning Guidance to Support Country Preparedness and Response* (Geneva: World Health Organization, 2020), https://www.who.int/publications/i/item/draft-operational-planning-guidance-for-un-country-teams.

8. Centers for Disease Control and Prevention, *Public Health Emergency Preparedness and Response Capabilities: National Standards for State, Local, Tribal, and Territorial Public Health* (Atlanta: US Department of Health and Human Services, 2019), https://www.cdc.gov/cpr/readiness/00_docs/CDC_PreparednesResponseCapabilities_October2018_Final_508.pdf.

9. CDC, *Public Health Emergency Preparedness*.

10. "Severe Covid-19 Symptoms: How Ventilators Can Help," COVID-19 Resources, UC Health, June 8, 2020, https://www.uchealth.com/en/media-room/covid-19/ventilators-and-covid-19.

11. Erin Mansfield, "As the Coronavirus Curve Flattened, Even Hard-Hit New York Had Enough Ventilators," *USA Today*, April 28, 2020, https://www.usatoday.com/story/news/2020/04/28/coronavirus-hospitals-avoid-ventilator-shortage-curve-new-york-flattens/3036008001.

12. Leigh Martinez, "Gov. Newsom, Mayor Liccardo Tour Sunnyvale Company Refurbishing Ventilators," FOX KTVU, March 28, 2020, https://www.ktvu.com/news/gov-newsom-mayor-liccardo-tour-sunnyvale-company-refurbishing-ventilators.

13. Lance Williams, Will Evans, and Will Carless, "California Once Had Mobile Hospitals and a Ventilator Stockpile. But It Dismantled Them," *Los Angeles Times*, March 27, 2020, https://www.latimes.com/california/story/2020-03-27/coronavirus-california-mobile-hospitals-ventilators.

14. Nigel Duara and Ana B. Ibarra, "California Ramps Up Output of Ventilators as COVID-19 Cases Grow," *Cal Matters*, March 29, 2020, https://calmatters.org/health/coronavirus/2020/03/newsom-california-can-produce-enough-ventilators-to-meet-covid-19-need.

15. Samantha Masunaga, "California Companies Jump in to Supply Ventilators Needed in Coronavirus Fight," *Los Angeles Times*, March 23, 2020, https://www.latimes.com/business/story/2020-03-23/coronavirus-california-companies-medical-supplies.

16. David Molloy, "Coronavirus: Tech Firm Bloom Energy Fixes Broken US Ventilators," *BBC News*, March 30, 2020, https://www.bbc.com/news/technology-52094193.

17. Cris Barrish, "Bloom Energy Refurbishing Mothballed Ventilators in Delaware and California," WHYY, April 7, 2020, https://whyy.org/articles/bloom-energy-refurbishing-mothballed-ventilators-in-delaware-and-california.

18. "Maintaining Essential Health Services for Tuberculosis, Malaria and HIV During the COVID-19 Pandemic in Low Resource, Non-U.S. Settings," Centers for Disease Control and Prevention, last modified April 29, 2022, https://stacks.cdc.gov/view/cdc/106931.

19. World Health Organization, *Maintaining Essential Health Services: Operational Guidance for the COVID-19 Context: Interim Guidance* (Geneva: World Health Organization, 2020), https://iris.who.int/bitstream/handle/10665/332240/WHO-2019-nCoV-essential_health_services-2020.2-eng.pdf.

20. Kim J. Brolin Ribacke, Dell D. Saulnier, Anneli Eriksson, and Johan Von Schreeb, "Effects of the West Africa Ebola Virus Disease on Health-Care Utilization: A Systematic Review," *Frontiers in Public Health* 4 (October 2016): 222, https://doi.org/10.3389/fpubh.2016.00222.

21. Drew Hinshaw, "Ebola Virus: For Want of Gloves, Doctors Die," *Wall Street Journal*, August 16, 2014, https://www.wsj.com/articles/ebola-doctors-with-no-rubber-gloves-1408142137.

22. CDC, "Maintaining Essential Health Services."

23. World Health Organization, *Coronavirus Disease (COVID-19) Outbreak: Rights, Roles, and Responsibilities of Health Workers, Including Key Considerations for Occupational Safety and Health* (Geneva: World Health Organization, 2020), https://www.who.int/docs/default-source/coronaviruse/who-rights-roles-respon-hw-covid-19.pdf.

24. World Health Organization, "Managing Epidemics."

25. "Response Worker Health and Safety," National Disasters and Severe Weather, Centers for Disease Control and Prevention, September 8, 2017, https://www.cdc.gov/disasters/workers.html.

26. World Health Organization, *WHO Report on Global Surveillance of Epidemic-Prone Infectious Diseases*, no. WHO/CDS/CSR/ISR/2000.1 (Geneva: World Health Organization, 2000). https://iris.who.int/bitstream/handle/10665/66485/WHO_CDS_CSR_ISR_2000.1.pdf.

CHAPTER 11

1. Julian Laufs and Zoha Waseem, "Policing in Pandemics: A Systematic Review and Best Practices for Police Response to COVID-19," *International Journal of Disaster Risk Reduction* 51 (December 2020), https://doi.org/10.1016/j.ijdrr.2020.101812.

2. Wesley G. Jennings and Nicholas M. Perez, "The Immediate Impact of COVID-19 on Law Enforcement in the United States," *American Journal of Criminal Justice* 45, no. 4 (June 2020): 690–701, https://doi.org/10.1007/s12103-020-09536-2.

3. Public Health and Law Enforcement Emergency Preparedness Workgroup, *A Framework for Improving Cross-Sector Coordination for Emergency Preparedness and Response: Action Steps for Public Health, Law Enforcement, the Judiciary and Corrections* (Fairfax, VA: McKing Consulting Corporation, 2008). https://www.cdc.gov/phlp/docs/cdc_bja_framework.pdf.

4. Edward P. Richards, Katerhin C. Rathbun, Corina Sole Brito, and Andrea Luna, *The Role of Law Enforcement in Public Health Emergencies: Special Considerations for an All-Hazards Approach* (Washington, DC: US Department of Justice, Office of Justice Programs, Bureau of Justice Assistance, 2006), https://www.ojp.gov/pdffiles1/bja/214333.pdf.

5. Andrea M. Luna, Corina Solé Brito, and Elizabeth A. Sanberg, *Police Planning for an Influenza Pandemic: Case Studies and Recommendations from the Field* (Washington DC: Police Executive Research Forum, 2007), https://www.publicsafety.gc.ca/lbrr/archives/cnmcs-plcng/cn89173109-eng.pdf; Interpol, *COVID-19 Pandemic: Guidelines for Law Enforcement* (Lyon France: Interpol, 2020), https://www.theiacp.org/sites/default/files/COVID19/COVID19_Pandemic_Guidelines_For_Law_Enforcement.pdf.

6. Jennings and Perez, "Immediate Impact of COVID-19."

7. Katherine Oberholtzer, Laura Sivitz, Alison Mack, Stanley Lemon, Adel Mahmoud, and Stacey Knobler, eds., *Learning from SARS: Preparing for the Next Disease Outbreak: Workshop Summary* (Washington DC: Institute of Medicine, 2004), https://www.ncbi.nlm.nih.gov/books/NBK92462.

8. Julian Fantino, "SARS Outbreak 2003: The Response of the Toronto Police Service," *Police Chief* 72, no. 4 (April 2005): 22–28, https://www.ojp.gov/ncjrs/virtual-library/abstracts/sars-outbreak-2003-response-toronto-police-service.

9. Norimitsu Onishi, "Clashes Erupt as Liberia Sets an Ebola Quarantine," *New York Times*, August 20, 2014, https://www.nytimes.com/2014/08/21/world/africa/ebola-outbreak-liberia-quarantine.html.

10. Marc Silver, "In Riots Sparked by an Ebola Quarantine, a Teen is Shot and Dies," National Public Radio, August 22, 2014, https://www.npr.org/sections/goatsandsoda/2014/08/22/342404795/in-riots-sparked-by-an-ebola-quarantine-a-teen-is-shot-and-dies.

11. Gelila Abraham, Beshea Gelana, Kiddus Yitbarek, and Sudhakar Morankar, "Prevalence of Domestic Violence in a Time of Catastrophic Disease Outbreaks including COVID-19 Pandemic: A Systematic Review Protocol," *Systematic Reviews* 11, no. 1 (March 2022): 1–7, https://doi.org/10.1186/s13643-022-01920-9.

12. Javier Labad, Alexandre Gonzalez-Rodriguez, Jesus Cobo, Joaquim Punti, and Josep Maria Farre, "A Systematic Review and Realist Synthesis on Toilet Paper Hoarding: COVID or Not COVID, That Is the Question," *PeerJ* 9 (January 2021): e10771, https://doi.org/10.7717/peerj.10771.

13. Brad Boserup, Mark McKenney, and Adel Elkbuli, "Alarming Trends in US Domestic Violence during the COVID-19 Pandemic," *American Journal of Emergency Medicine* 38, no. 12 (December 2020): 2753–55, https://doi.org/10.1016/j.ajem.2020.04.077.

14. Council on Criminal Justice, Press Release, "New Analysis Shows 8% Increase in U.S. Domestic Violence Incidents Following Pandemic Stay-at-Home Orders." Council on Criminal Justice, February 12, 2023, https://counciloncj.org/new-analysis-shows-8-increase-in-u-s-domestic-violence-incidents-following-pandemic-stay-at-home-orders.

15. Megan L. Evans, Margo Lindauer, and Maureen E. Farrell, "A Pandemic within a Pandemic—Intimate Partner Violence during COVID-19," *New England Journal of Medicine* 383, no. 24 (December 2020): 2302–4, doi: 10.1056/NEJMp2024046.

16. "The Shadow Pandemic: Violence against Women during COVID-19," UN Women, accessed December 20, 2023, https://www.unwomen.org/en/news/in-focus/in-focus-gender-equality-in-covid-19-response/violence-against-women-during-covid-19.

17. Jonathan M. Berman, "When Antivaccine Sentiment Turned Violent: The Montréal Vaccine Riot of 1885," *Canadian Medical Association Journal* 193, no. 14 (April 2021): E490–E492, https://doi.org/10.1503/cmaj.202820.

18. International Committee of the Red Cross, *Promoting Peer-to-Peer Exchanges on Data Collection Systems to Analyse Violence against Health Care* (Geneva: International Committee of the Red Cross, 2020), https://www.icrc.org/en/publication/4508-promoting-peer-peer-exchanges-data-collection-systems-analyse-violence-against.

19. International Committee of the Red Cross and Health Care in Danger, *Health Care in Danger. ICRC Institutional Health Care in Danger Strategy 2020–2022: Protecting Health Care from Violence and Attacks in Situations of Armed Conflict and Other Emergencies* (Geneva: International Committee of the Red Cross, 2022), https://healthcareindanger.org/wp-content/uploads/2020/10/ICRC-HCiD-strategy-2020-2022.pdf.

20. International Committee of the Red Cross and Health Care in Danger, *Promoting Military Operational Practice that Ensures Safe Access to and Delivery of Healthcare* (Geneva:

International Committee of the Red Cross, 2014). https://healthcareindanger.org/wp-content/uploads/2015/09/icrc-002-4208-promoting-military-op-practice-en-sures-safe-access-health-care.pdf.

21. "Keep Health Workers Safe to Keep Patients Safe: WHO," News Release, World Health Organization, September 17, 2020, https://www.who.int/news/item/17-09-2020-keep-health-workers-safe-to-keep-patients-safe-who; International Committee of the Red Cross, *Protecting Health Care from Violence Legislative Checklist* (Geneva: International Committee of the Red Cross, 2021), https://health-careindanger.org/wp-content/uploads/2021/05/legislative_checklis_on_protect-ing-health-care-from_-violence_web-1.pdf.

22. Vinh-Kim Nguyen, "An Epidemic of Suspicion—Ebola and Violence in the DRC," *New England Journal of Medicine* 380, no. 14 (April 2019): 1298–99, doi: 10.1056/NEJMp1902682.

23. Susan McLellan, Mark G. Kortepeter, Nahid Bhadelia, Erica S. Shenoy, Lauren M. Sauer, Maria G. Frank, and Theodore J. Cieslak, "Ebola in the DRC One Year Later–Boiling the Frog?" *International Journal of Infectious Diseases* 85 (August 2019): 212–13, https://doi.org/10.1016/j.ijid.2019.07.014.

24. "Ending an Ebola Outbreak in a Conflict Zone," World Health Organi-zation, last modified November 29, 2020. https://storymaps.arcgis.com/stories/813561c780d44af38c57730418cd96cd.

25. J. Stephen Morrison and Judd Devermont, "North Kivu's Ebola Outbreak at Day 90: What is to Be Done?," Center for Strategic and International Studies, 2018, https://www.csis.org/analysis/north-kivus-ebola-outbreak-day-90-what-be-done.

26. Nurith Aizenman, "U.S. Government Beefs Up Presence Near Congo's Ebola Epicenter," National Public Radio, March 15, 2019, https://www.npr.org/sections/goatsandsoda/2019/03/15/703758193/u-s-government-beefs-up-presence-near-congos-ebola-epicenter.

27. Owen Dyer, "Escalating Congo Ebola Epidemic Passes 2000 Cases amid Violence and Suspicion," *BMJ* 365 (June 2019), doi:10.1136/bmj.l4062.

28. "WHO Ebola Responder Killed in Attack on the Butembo Hospital," World Health Organization, April 19, 2019, https://www.who.int/news/item/19-04-2019-who-ebola-responder-killed-in-attack-on-the-butembo-hospital.

29. Nurith Aizenman, "Why Health Workers in the Ebola Hot Zone Are Threatening to Strike," *Goats and Soda* (podcast), National Public Radio, April 25, 2019, https://www.npr.org/sections/goatsandsoda/2019/04/25/717079729/why-health-workers-in-the-ebola-hot-zone-are-threatening-to-strike.

30. Michael R. Snyder, "Ebola Response in DRC Undergoes 'Important Shifts' as Violence Intensifies," *Global Observatory*, May 22, 2019, https://theglobalobservatory.org/2019/05/ebola-response-drc-important-shifts-violence-intensifies.

31. Helen Branswell, "Doctors Without Borders Fiercely Criticizes Ebola Outbreak Control Effort," *STAT*, March 7, 2019, https://www.statnews.com/2019/03/07/doctors-without-borders-criticizes-ebola-control-effort.

32. Carley Petesch, "Alarm as Red Cross Workers Attacked in Congo Ebola Efforts," Associated Press News, October 4, 2018, https://apnews.com/article/63fca100669e4bf99447cb1ec5c5c092.

33. Clare Stroud, Kristin Viswanathan, Tia Powell, Robert R. Bass, and Committee on Prepositioned Medical Countermeasures for the Public, "Current Dispensing Strategies for Medical Countermeasures for Anthrax," in *Prepositioning Antibiotics for Anthrax* (Washington, DC: National Academies Press, 2011), https://www.ncbi.nlm.nih.gov/books/NBK190045; "Postal Model for Medical Countermeasures Delivery and Distribution," US Department of Health and Human Services, last modified September 29, 2011, https://www.phe.gov/preparedness/planning/postal/Pages/default.aspx.

34. Centers for Disease Control and Prevention, *Point of Dispensing (POD) Standards* (Atlanta, GA: Centers for Disease Control and Prevention, 2008), https://www.cdc.gov/cpr/documents/coopagreement-archive/fy2008/dispensingstandards.pdf.

35. Christopher Nelson, Edward W. Chan, Anita Chandra, Paul Sorensen, Henry H. Willis, Katherine Comanor, Hayoung Park, Karen A. Ricci, Leah B. Caldarone, Molly Shea, John A. Zambrano, and Lydia Hansell, *Recommended Infrastructure Standards for Mass Antibiotic Dispensing* (Santa Monica, CA: RAND Corporation, 2008), https://www.rand.org/content/dam/rand/pubs/technical_reports/2008/RAND_TR553.pdf.

36. "Hospital Closed Point-of-Dispensing (POD) Plan Template for Medical Countermeasures," Kansas Department of Health and Environment, last modified November 2013, https://www.kdhe.ks.gov/DocumentCenter/View/7161; "Attachment H: Point of Dispensing (POD) Template Plan," Capitol Region Council of Governments, accessed December 20, 2023, https://crcog.org/wp-content/uploads/2017/12/POD-Template-Plan.pdf.

37. "Ciprofloxacin for Post-Exposure Prophylaxis of Anthrax," Centers for Disease Control and Prevention, last modified November 20, 2020, https://www.cdc.gov/anthrax/public-health/cipro-eui-hcp.html.

38. Institute of Medicine, "The Postal Model," in *Medical Countermeasures Dispensing: Emergency Use Authorization and the Postal Model: Workshop Summary* (Washington, DC: National Academies Press, 2010), https://www.ncbi.nlm.nih.gov/books/NBK53124.

39. Oliver Morgan, Morris Tidball-Binz, and Dana Van Alphen, *Management of Dead Bodies after Disasters: A Field Manual for First Responders* (Washington DC: Pan American Health Organization, 2006), https://www.preventionweb.net/files/627_9324.pdf .

40. International Federation of Red Cross and Red Crescent Societies, *Safe and Dignified Burial*; World Health Organization, *How to Conduct Safe*.

41. "Death Is in the Air," episode 13 of *Psych*, season 4.

42. Wouter Graumans, William J. R. Stone, and Teun Bousema, "No Time to Die: An in-Depth Analysis of James Bond's Exposure to Infectious Agents," *Travel Medicine and Infectious Disease* 44 (November–December 2021): 102175, https://doi.org/10.1016/j.tmaid.2021.102175.

43. "Some States Are Imposing Covid-19 Curfews - But Is There Any Science behind Them?" (video), Health, MeredithVideos, December 1, 2020, https://www.yahoo.com/now/states-imposing-covid-19-curfews-160641819.html.

44. Alison Mack, Eileen R. Choffnes, P. Frederick Sparling, Margaret A. Hamburg, and Stanley M. Lemon, eds., *Ethical and Legal Considerations in Mitigating Pandemic Disease: Workshop Summary* (Washington DC: Institute of Medicine Forum on Microbial Threats and National Academies Press, 2007), https://www.ncbi.nlm.nih.gov/books/NBK54167.

45. "Sierra Leone Readies for Controversial Three-Day Nationwide Ebola Curfew," *Straits Times*, September 18, 2014, https://www.straitstimes.com/world/africa/sierra-leone-readies-for-controversial-three-day-nationwide-ebola-curfew.

46. Umaru Fofana, "UPDATE 3—Sierra Leone Wraps Up Three-Day Ebola Lockdown," Reuters, September 21, 2014, https://www.reuters.com/article/health-ebola-leone-idAFL6N0RM0XF20140921.

47. "Sierra Leone Readies."

48. Agence Presse-France, "Sierra Leone Ebola Lockdown Found at Least 200 Infected, Dead: Government," NDTV. September 22, 2014, https://www.ndtv.com/world-news/sierra-leone-ebola-lockdown-found-at-least-200-infected-dead-government-669234.

49. "Sierra Leone Records 130 New Ebola Cases during Three-Day Lockdown," Reuters, September 22, 2014, https://www.reuters.com/article/us-health-ebola-leone/sierra-leone-records-130-new-ebola-cases-during-three-day-lockdown-idUSKBN0HG0NW20140922.

50. "Ebola Outbreak: Sierra Leone Lockdown Declared 'Success,'" BBC News, September 22, 2014, https://www.bbc.com/news/world-africa-29305591.

51. "Sierra Leone Imposes Curfew after Spike in Ebola Cases," Aljazeera, June 13, 2015, https://www.aljazeera.com/news/2015/6/13/sierra-leone-imposes-curfew-after-spike-in-ebola-cases.

52. "Sierra Leone Declares Curfew for Ebola," *Deutsche Welle*, June 13, 2015, https://www.dw.com/en/sierra-leone-enforces-curfew-as-ebola-virus-resurfaces-in-north-west/a-18514943.

CHAPTER 12

1. Rebecca Katz, Aurelia Attal-Juncqua, and Julie E. Fischer, "Funding Public Health Emergency Preparedness in the United States," *American Journal of Public Health* 107, no. S2 (September 2017): S148–S152. https://doi.org/10.2105/AJPH.2017.303956.

2. "WHO Interim Protocol: Rapid Operations to Contain the Initial Emergence of Pandemic Influenza," World Health Organization, October 15, 2009, https://www3.paho.org/hq/dmdocuments/2009/RapidContProtOct15.pdf.

3. S. Saxena and M. Stone. *Preparing Public Financial Management Systems for Emergency Response Challenges*, Special Series on Fiscal Policies to Respond to COVID-19 (Washington, DC: IMF March, 2020), https://www.imf.org/-/media/Files/Publications/covid19-special-notes/special-series-on-covid19-preparing-public-financial-management-systems-for-emergency-response.ashx.

4. Nancy Lee and Rakan Aboneaaj, *MDB COVID-19 Crisis Response: Where Did the Money Go?* (Washington DC: Center for Global Development, 2021), https://www.cgdev.org/publication/mdb-covid-19-crisis-response-where-did-money-go.

5. "FAQs: The Pandemic Fund," World Bank, last modified March 3, 2023, https://www.worldbank.org/en/topic/pandemics/brief/factsheet-financial-intermediary-fund-for-pandemic-prevention-preparedness-and-response.

6. World Health Organization, "Coronavirus Disease (COVID-19) Donors & Partners: WHO Says Thank You!," accessed December 20, 2023, https://www.who.int/emergencies/diseases/novel-coronavirus-2019/donors-and-partners/funding.

7. "The PAHO Covid-19 Response Fund," Pan American Health Organization, accessed December 20, 2023, https://www.paho.org/en/paho-covid-19-response-fund.

8. Ugo Gentilini, "A Game Changer for Social Protection? Six Reflections on COVID-19 and the Future of Cash Transfers," *World Bank Blogs*, January 11, 2021, https://blogs.worldbank.org/developmenttalk/game-changer-social-protection-six-reflections-covid-19-and-future-cash-transfers.

9. Molly Kinder, "Essential but Undervalued: Millions of Health Care Workers Aren't Getting the Pay or Respect They Deserve in the COVID-19 Pandemic," Brookings, May 28, 2020, https://www.brookings.edu/research/essential-but-undervalued-millions-of-health-care-workers-arent-getting-the-pay-or-respect-they-deserve-in-the-covid-19-pandemic.

10. World Health Organization, *Ethical Considerations in Developing a Public Health Response to Pandemic Influenza*, no. WHO/CDS/EPR/GIP/2007.2 (Geneva: World Health Organization, 2007), https://apps.who.int/iris/handle/10665/70006.

11. United Nations Development Program, *Payments Programme for Ebola Response Workers: Cash at the Front Lines of a Health Care Crisis* (New York: United Nations Development Program, 2015), https://www.undp.org/publications/payments-programme-ebola-response-workers.

12. Peter H. Kilmarx, Kevin R. Clarke, Patricia M. Dietz, Mary J. Hamel, Farah Husain, Jevon D. McFadden, Benjamin J. Park, et al., "Ebola Virus Disease in Health Care Workers-Sierra Leone, 2014," *Morbidity and Mortality Weekly Report* 63, no. 49

(December 2014): 1168, https://www.cdc.gov/mmwr/preview/mmwrhtml/mm6349a6.htm.

13. "Payments Programme for Ebola Response Workers," United Nations Development Program, July 27, 2017, https://www.undp.org/publications/payments-programme-ebola-response-workers.

14. T. Dumas, A. Frisetti, and H. W. Radice, *Harnessing Digital Technology for Cash Transfer Programming in the Ebola Response: Lessons Learned from USAID/Office of Food for Peace Partners' West Africa Ebola Responses (2015–2016)* (Oxford: Cash Learning Partnership, 2019), https://www.calpnetwork.org/wp-content/uploads/2020/03/calp-ebola-case-study-web-1.pdf.

15. Joe Abass Bangura, *Saving Money, Saving Lives: A Case Study on the Benefits of Digitizing Payments to Ebola Response Workers in Sierra Leone* (New York: Better Than Cash Alliance, 2016), https://btca-production-site.s3.amazonaws.com/documents/186/english_attachments/BTCA-Ebola-Case-Study.pdf.

16. William Marty Martin, Yvette Lopez, Thomas P. Flannery, and Bill Dixon, "Infectious Disease: Protecting Workers and Organizations—The Role of Compensation & Benefits," *Compensation and Benefits Review* 53, no. 1 (January 2021): 43–55, https://doi.org/10.1177/0886368720947332.

17. Søren Holm, "A General Approach to Compensation for Losses Incurred Due to Public Health Interventions in the Infectious Disease Context," *Monash Bioethics Review* 38, no. 1 (March 2020): 32–46, https://doi.org/10.1007/s40592-020-00104-2.

18. Jeremy Shapiro, "The Impact of Recipient Choice on Aid Effectiveness," *World Development* 116 (April 2019): 137–49, https://doi.org/10.1016/j.worlddev.2018.10.010.

19. UNHCR, UN Refugee Agency, *An Introduction to Cash-Based Interventions in UNHCR Operations* (Geneva: UNHCR, 2012), https://www.unhcr.org/uk/515a959e9.pdf.

20. Justin Sandefur, "Cash Transfers Cure Poverty. Side-Effects Vary. Symptoms May Return When Treatment Stops." *Center for Global Development Blog*, April 19, 2018, https://www.cgdev.org/blog/cash-transfers-cure-poverty-side-effects-vary-symptoms-may-return-when-treatment-stops.

21. Heather Long, "U.S. Now Has 22 Million Unemployed, Wiping Out a Decade of Job Gains," *Washington Post*, April 16, 2020, https://www.washingtonpost.com/business/2020/04/16/unemployment-claims-coronavirus.

22. Paul Morello, "COVID-19 Means a 'New Normal,'" *Feeding America*, May 4, 2020, https://www.feedingamerica.org/hunger-blog/covid-19-means-new-normal.

23. Investopedia Team, "What Is the CARES Act?," Investopedia, last modified October 18, 2023, https://www.investopedia.com/coronavirus-aid-relief-and-economic-security-cares-act-4800707.

24. Tom Simonite, "A Clever Strategy to Distribute COVID Aid—with Satellite Data," *Wired*, December 17, 2020, https://www.wired.com/story/clever-strategy-distribute-covid-aid-satellite-data.

25. United Nations Development Programme, *Assessing the Socio-Economic Impacts of Ebola Virus Disease in Guinea, Liberia and Sierra Leone: The Road to Recovery* (Geneva: United Nations Development Program, 2014), https://www.undp.org/africa/publications/assessing-socio-economic-impact-ebola-west-africa.

26. "Gross Domestic Product," Bureau of Economic Analysis, last modified December 18, 2023, https://www.bea.gov/resources/learning-center/what-to-know-gdp.

27. World Bank, "Chapter 1: The Economic Impacts of the Pandemic and Emerging Risks to the Recovery," in *World Development Report 2022: Finance for an Equitable Recovery* (Washington, DC: World Bank, 2022), https://www.worldbank.org/en/publication/wdr2022.

28. Mario Coccia, "The Relation between Length of Lockdown, Numbers of Infected People and Deaths of Covid-19, and Economic Growth of Countries: Lessons

Learned to Cope with Future Pandemics Similar to Covid-19 and to Constrain the Deterioration of Economic System," *Science of the Total Environment* 775 (June 2021): 145801, https://doi.org/10.1016/j.scitotenv.2021.145801.

29. Caribbean Public Health Agency, *ZIKA: Impacts* (Port of Spain: Caribbean Public Health Agency, 2017), http://missionmosquito.carpha.org/images/CPHD/2017/Zika_impacts.pdf.

30. World Health Organization, *A Checklist for Pandemic Influenza Risk and Impact Management: Building Capacity for Pandemic Response* (Geneva: World Health Organization, 2018), https://apps.who.int/iris/handle/10665/259884.

31. World Bank. *The Economic Impact of the 2014 Ebola Epidemic: Short- and Medium-Term Estimates for West Africa* (Washington DC: World Bank, 2014), https://openknowledge.worldbank.org/bitstream/handle/10986/20592/9781464804380.pdf.

32. Usman Khalid, Luke Emeka Okafor, and Katarzyna Burzynska, "Does the Size of the Tourism Sector Influence the Economic Policy Response to the COVID-19 Pandemic?," *Current Issues in Tourism* 24, no. 19 (January 2021): 2801–20, https://doi.org/10.1080/13683500.2021.1874311.

33. Arlene Alpha and Muriel Figuie, *Impact of the Ebola Virus Disease Outbreak on Market Chains and Trade of Agricultural Products in West Africa: Report for FAO REOWA (Resilience, Emergencies and Rehabilitation in West Africa)* (Dakar: Food and Agriculture Organization, 2016), https://agritrop.cirad.fr/580668/1/FAO-CIRAD-Rapport%20Ebola%20Fili%C3%A8re-final.pdf.

34. Anton Pak, Oyelola A. Adegboye, Adeshina I. Adekunle, Kazi M. Rahman, Emma S. McBryde, and Damon P. Eisen, "Economic Consequences of the COVID-19 Outbreak: The Need for Epidemic Preparedness," *Frontiers in Public Health* 8 (May 2020): 241, https://doi.org/10.3389/fpubh.2020.00241.

35. World Bank. *The Economic Impact of the 2014 Ebola Epidemic.*

36. Khalid et al., "Does the Size of the Tourism Sector."

37. Xiaoyun Wei, and Liyan Han, "The Impact of COVID-19 Pandemic on Transmission of Monetary Policy to Financial Market," *International Review of Financial Analysis* 74 (March 2021): 101705, https://doi.org/10.1016/j.irfa.2021.101705.

38. Ali Zafar, Jan Muench, and Aloysius Uche Ordu, *SDRs for COVID-19 Relief: The Good, the Challenging, and the Uncertain* (Washington, DC: Brookings Institute, 2021), https://www.brookings.edu/articles sdrs-for-covid-19-relief-the-good-the-challenging-and-the-uncertain.

39. D. B. Smorfitt, Steve R. Harrison, and John L. Herbohn, "Potential Economic Implications for Regional Tourism of a Foot and Mouth Disease Outbreak in North Queensland," *Tourism Economics* 11, no. 3 (September 2005): 411–30, https://doi.org/10.5367/000000005774352953.

CHAPTER 13

1. "WHO Issues Best Practices for Naming New Human Infectious Diseases," World Health Organization, May 8, 2015, https://www.who.int/news/item/08-05-2015-who-issues-best-practices-for-naming-new-human-infectious-diseases.

2. "Biological Weapons Convention," United Nations, accessed December 20, 2023, https://www.un.org/disarmament/biological-weapons.

3. Aurelia Attal-Juncqua, Matthew Boyce, and Rebecca Katz, *Assistance Following a Deliberate Biological Event: Operationalizing Article VII of the Biological and Toxins Weapons Convention* (Washington, DC: Georgetown Center for Global Health Science & Security, 2018); "Assistance, Response and Preparedness under the Biological Weapons Convention," United Nations Office for Disarmament

Affairs (UNODA), accessed December 20, 2023, https://www.un.org/disarmament/biological-weapons/assistance-response-preparedness.

4. "Secretary-General's Mechanism for Investigation of Alleged Use of Chemical and Biological Weapons (UNSGM)," UNODA, accessed December 20, 2023, https://www.un.org/disarmament/wmd/secretary-general-mechanism.

5. "Resolution Adopted by the General Assembly on Cooperation between the United Nations and the Organization for the Prohibition of Chemical Weapons, a/RES/55/283" (2020), United Nations General Assembly, accessed December 20, 2023, https://www.opcw.org/sites/default/files/documents/LAO/a55r283.pdf.

6. "Memorandum of Understanding between the World Health Organization and the United Nations Concerning WHO's Support to the Secretary-General's Mechanisms for Investigation of the Alleged Use of Chemical Biological or Toxin Weapons," UNODA, January 31, 2011, https://front.un-arm.org/wp-content/uploads/assets/WMD/Secretary-General_Mechanism/UN_WHO_MOU_2011.pdf.

7. Sanaz Taghizade, Vijay Kumar Chattu, Ebrahim Jaafaripooyan, and Sebastian Kevany, "COVID-19 Pandemic as an Excellent Opportunity for Global Health Diplomacy," *Frontiers in Public Health*, July 2021: 755, https://doi.org/10.3389/fpubh.2021.655021; Sara E. Davies and Clare Wenham, "Why the COVID-19 Response Needs International Relations," *International Affairs* 96, no. 5 (September 2020): 1227–51, https://doi.org/10.1093/ia/iiaa135.

8. Vijay Kumar Chattu, "Politics of Ebola and the Critical Role of Global Health Diplomacy for the CARICOM," *Journal of Family Medicine and Primary Care* 6, no. 3 (September 2017): 463, https://doi.org/10.4103/jfmpc.jfmpc_75_17.

9. Chattu, "Politics of Ebola."

10. "Global Health Security Is Integral to Foreign Policy," World Health Organization Regional Office for the Eastern Mediterranean, accessed December 20, 2023, https://www.emro.who.int/health-topics/health-diplomacy/foreign-policy.html.

11. "Global Level 4 Health Advisory - Do Not Travel (March 19, 2020)," US Embassy in Panama, March 19, 2020, https://pa.usembassy.gov/global-level-4-health-advisory-do-not-travel-march-19-2020.

12. Gavin Bade, Nahal Toosi, and Sam Mintz, "Peru Spars with U.S. over Letting Stranded Americans Fly Home during Coronavirus Outbreak," *Politico*, March 21, 2020, https://www.politico.com/news/2020/03/21/peru-american-citizens-coronavirus-140803.

13. "Health Alert - U.S. Embassy Lima, Peru (Mar. 23, 2020)," US Embassy in Peru, March 23, 2020, https://pe.usembassy.gov/alert-u-s-embassy-lima-peru-mar-21-2020.

14. Eric G. Falls, "Bringing Americans Home - Embassy Lima Responds to the COVID-19 Crisis," *State Magazine*, June 2020, https://statemag.state.gov/2020/06/0620feat02.

15. World Health Organization, *Joint External Evaluation Tool: International Health Regulations (2005)*, 2nd ed. (Geneva: World Health Organization, 2018), https://apps.who.int/iris/rest/bitstreams/1094054/retrieve.

16. World Health Organization, *Joint External Evaluation Tool*.

17. World Health Organization, *Policy Statement on Data Sharing by the World Health Organization in the Context of Public Health Emergencies* (Geneva: World Health Organization, 2016), https://www.who.int/docs/default-source/publishing-policies/who-policy-statement-on-data-sharing.pdf.

18. Sam F. Halabi and Rebecca Katz, eds., *Viral Sovereignty and Technology Transfer: The Changing Global System for Sharing Pathogens for Public Health Research* (Cambridge: Cambridge University Press, 2020).

19. "Global Health Security Partner Engagement. Migration Health Division - Information Sheet," United Nations International Organization for Migration, January 2019,

https://www.iom.int/sites/g/files/tmzbdl486/files/our_work/DMM/Migration-Health/mhd_infosheet_cdc_ghs_13.02.2019.pdf.

20. C. James Hospedales and Lisa Tarantino, "Fighting Health Security Threats Requires a Cross-Border Approach," *Health Systems and Reform* 4, no. 2 (March 2018): 72–76, https://doi.org/10.1080/23288604.2018.1446698.

21. Mary A. Shiraef, Paul Friesen, Lukas Feddern, and Mark A. Weiss, "Did Border Closures Slow SARS-CoV-2?," *Scientific Reports* 12, no. 1 (February 2022): 1–13, https://doi.org/10.1038/s41598-022-05482-7.

22. World Health Organization, *International Health Regulations (2005)* (Geneva: World Health Organization, 2008), https://www.who.int/publications/i/item/9789241580410.

23. Carmen Dolea, "Travel and Trade Restrictions during Outbreaks," World Health Organization, accessed December 20, 2023, https://www.icao.int/EURNAT/Other%20Meetings%20Seminars%20and%20Workshops/CAPSCA%20EUR/CAPSCA-EUR07/CAPSCA%20EUR07%20S3.4.pdf.

24. World Health Organization, *Non-pharmaceutical Public Health Measures for Mitigating the Risk and Impact of Epidemic and Pandemic Influenza: Annex: Report of Systematic Literature Reviews*, no. WHO/WHE/IHM/GIP/2019.1 (Geneva: World Health Organization, 2019), https://apps.who.int/iris/bitstream/handle/10665/329439/WHO-WHE-IHM-GIP-2019.1-eng.pdf.

25. Sharmila Devi, "Travel Restrictions Hampering COVID-19 Response," *Lancet* 395, no. 10233 (April 2020): 1331–32, https://doi.org/10.1016/S0140-6736(20)30967-3.

26. Chiara Poletto, M. F. Gomes, A. Pastore y Piontti, Luca Rossi, Livio Bioglio, Dennis L. Chao, I. M. Longini Jr., M. Elizabeth Halloran, Vittoria Colizza, and Alessandro Vespignani, "Assessing the Impact of Travel Restrictions on International Spread of the 2014 West African Ebola Epidemic," *Eurosurveillance* 19, no. 42 (October 2014): 20936, https://doi.org/10.2807/1560-7917.ES2014.19.42.20936.

27. Shiraef et. al., "Did Border Closures Slow SARS-CoV-2?"

28. Jordan Schermerhorn, Alaina Case, Ellie Graeden, Justin Kerr, Mackenzie Moore, Siobhan Robinson-Marshall, Trae Wallace, Emily Woodrow, and Rebecca Katz. "Fifteen Days in December: Capture and Analysis of Omicron-Related Travel Restrictions," *BMJ Global Health* 7, no. 3 (March 2022): e008642, http://dx.doi.org/10.1136/bmjgh-2022-008642.

29. "COVID-19 and International Trade: Issues and Actions," Organisation for Economic Co-operation and Development (OECD), June 12, 2020, https://www.oecd.org/coronavirus/policy-responses/covid-19-and-international-trade-issues-and-actions-494da2fa.

30. William Alan Reinsch, Sanvid Tuljapurka, and Jakc Caporal, "Trade Symptoms of the Pandemic," *Center for Strategic and International Studies*, April 3, 2020, https://www.csis.org/analysis/trade-symptoms-pandemic.

31. "Updated WHO Recommendations for International Traffic in Relation to COVID-19 Outbreak," World Health Organization, February 29, 2020, https://www.who.int/news-room/articles-detail/updated-who-recommendations-for-international-traffic-in-relation-to-covid-19-outbreak.

32. Christopher A. Casey and Cathleen D. Cimino-Isaacs, "Export Restrictions in Response to the COVID-19 Pandemic," Congressional Research Service, April 23, 2021, https://crsreports.congress.gov/product/pdf/IF/IF11551; "COVID-19 and World Trade," World Trade Organization, accessed December 20, 2023, https://www.wto.org/english/tratop_e/covid19_e/covid19_e.htm.

33. "Risk from Exposure to Hides/Drums Contaminated with Anthrax," Centers for Disease Control and Prevention, last modified November 20, 2020, https://www.cdc.gov/anthrax/animal-products/hides-drums.html.

34. Centers for Disease Control and Prevention. "Cutaneous Anthrax Associated with Drum Making Using Goat Hides from West Africa—Connecticut, 2007," *Morbidity and Mortality Weekly Report* 57, no. 23 (June 2008): 628–31, https://pubmed.ncbi.nlm.nih.gov/18551098.

35. "Past U.S. Cases & Outbreaks," Centers for Disease Control and Prevention, last modified August 29, 2023, https://www.cdc.gov/poxvirus/monkeypox/outbreak/us-outbreaks.html.

36. IASC Reference Group on Mental Health and Psychosocial Support in Emergency Settings, *Mental Health and Psychosocial Support in Ebola Virus Disease Outbreaks: A Guide for Public Health Programme Planners* (Geneva: IASC, 2015), https://reliefweb.int/report/sierra-leone/mental-health-and-psychosocial-support-ebola-virus-disease-outbreaks-guide.

37. United Nations Office for Disaster Risk Reduction, *Sendai Framework for Disaster Risk Reduction 2015–2030* (Geneva: UNISDR, 2015), https://www.undrr.org/publication/sendai-framework-disaster-risk-reduction-2015-2030.

38. Sabine Kuhlmann and Jochen Franzke, "Multi-Level Responses to COVID-19: Crisis Coordination in Germany from an Intergovernmental Perspective," *Local Government Studies*, March 2021, 1–23, https://doi.org/10.1080/03003930.2021.1904398.

39. "The Territorial Impact of COVID-19: Managing the Crisis across Levels of Government," OECD, last modified November 10, 2020, https://www.oecd.org/coronavirus/policy-responses/the-territorial-impact-of-covid-19-managing-the-crisis-across-levels-of-government-d3e314e1.

40. Kuhlmann and Franzke, "Multi-Level Responses to COVID-19."

41. "Conditional Marketing Authorisation," European Medicines Agency, accessed December 20, 2023, https://www.ema.europa.eu/en/human-regulatory/marketing-authorisation/conditional-marketing-authorisation.

42. "Emergency Use Authorization," US Food and Drug Administration, December 20, 2023, https://www.fda.gov/emergency-preparedness-and-response/mcm-legal-regulatory-and-policy-framework/emergency-use-authorization.

43. "Emergency Use Listing Procedure for Vaccines," World Health Organization, accessed December 20, 2023, https://www.who.int/teams/regulation-prequalification/eul/eul-vaccines.

44. "Country Readiness and Delivery Frequently Asked Questions," World Health Organization, accessed December 20, 2023, https://www.who.int/initiatives/act-accelerator/covax/covid-19-vaccine-country-readiness-and-delivery/country-readiness-and-delivery-faqs.

45. "What Is the ACT-Accelerator?," World Health Organization, accessed December 20, 2023, https://www.who.int/initiatives/act-accelerator/about.

46. World Health Organization, *Guidance on Developing a National Deployment and Vaccination Plan for COVID-19 Vaccines: Interim Guidance*, no. WHO/2019-nCoV/Vaccine_deployment/2021.1 (Geneva: World Health Organization, 2021), https://www.who.int/publications/i/item/WHO-2019-nCoV-Vaccine-deployment-2021.1-eng.

47. "Data Sharing in Public Health Emergencies," Georgetown University Center for Global Health Science and Security, accessed December 20, 2023, https://ghss.georgetown.edu/datasharing.

48. Sharon Abramowitz, Tamara Giles-Vernick, Jim Webb, Jennifer Tappan, Elanah Uretsky, Jorge Varanda-Ferreira, Katherine Mason, Molly Beyer, Claire Collin, and Amadou Sall, *Data Sharing in Public Health Emergencies: Anthropological and Historical Perspectives on Data Sharing during the 2014-2016 Ebola Epidemic and the 2016 Yellow Fever Epidemic*, Final report to the Wellcome-DfID joint initiative on epidemic preparedness, November 2018, https://www.glopid-r.org/wp-content/uploads/2019/07/data-sharing-in-public-health-emergencies-yellow-fever-and-ebola.pdf.

49. Ben Goldacre, Sian Harrison, Kamal R. Mahtani, and Carl Heneghan, *WHO Consultation on Data and Results Sharing during Public Health Emergencies* (Oxford: Centre for Evidence Based Medicine, 2015).

50. Allison Black, Duncan R. MacCannell, Thomas R. Sibley, and Trevor Bedford, "Ten Recommendations for Supporting Open Pathogen Genomic Analysis in Public Health." *Nature Medicine* 26, no. 6 (June 2020): 832–41, https://doi.org/10.1038/s41591-020-0935-z.

51. Michelle Rourke, Mark Eccleston-Turner, Alexandra Phelan, and Lawrence Gostin, "Policy Opportunities to Enhance Sharing for Pandemic Research," *Science* 368, no. 6492 (May 2020): 716–18, DOI: 10.1126/science.abb9342.

52. World Health Organization, "WHO's Code of Conduct for Open and Timely Sharing of Pathogen Genetic Sequence Data during Outbreaks of Infectious Disease" (2019), WHO, accessed December 20, 2023, https://moodle2.units.it/pluginfile.php/393844/mod_resource/content/1/WHO_pathogen_sequencing_data_release.pdf.

53. Guy Cochrane, Katharina Lauer, Niklas Blomberg, Rolf Apweiler, and Ewan Birney, "Pathogen Genomics Data Sharing: Public Health Meets Research," *Zenodo*, March 17, 2022, https://doi.org/10.5281/zenodo.6368840.

54. Gian Luca Burci and Frederic Perron-Welch, "International Sharing of Human Pathogens to Promote Global Health Security—Still a Work in Progress," *American Society of International Law* 25, no. 13 (July 2021), https://www.asil.org/insights/volume/25/issue/13#_edn2.

55. Jay Stanley, "Temperature Screening and Civil Liberties during an Epidemic," ACLU, May 19, 2020, https://www.aclu.org/documents/aclu-white-paper-temperature-screening-and-civil-liberties-during-epidemic.

56. World Health Organization, *Guidance for Managing Ethical Issues in Infectious Disease Outbreaks* (Geneva: World Health Organization, 2016), https://apps.who.int/iris/bitstream/handle/10665/250580/9789241549837-eng.pdf.

57. "How Do I Screen for HIV?," Centers for Disease Control and Prevention, accessed December 20, 2023, https://www.cdc.gov/hiv/clinicians/screening/how.html.

58. Jane H. Williams and Angus Dawson, "Prioritising Access to Pandemic Influenza Vaccine: A Review of the Ethics Literature," *BMC Medical Ethics* 21, no. 1 (May 2020): 1–8, https://doi.org/10.1186/s12910-020-00477-3.

59. "Anthrax Vaccine Information Statement | CDC," Centers for Disease Control and Prevention, last modified January 8, 2020, https://www.cdc.gov/vaccines/hcp/vis/vis-statements/anthrax.html.

60. "2009 H1N1 Vaccination Recommendations," Centers for Disease Control and Prevention, October 15, 2009, https://www.cdc.gov/h1n1flu/vaccination/acip.htm.

61. "Pandemic Vaccine Program Distribution, Tracking, and Monitoring," Centers for Disease Control and Prevention, accessed December 20, 2023, https://www.cdc.gov/flu/pdf/pandemic-resources/pandemic-influenza-vaccine-distribution-9p-508.pdf.

62. John Lloyd and James Cheyne, "The Origins of the Vaccine Cold Chain and a Glimpse of the Future," *Vaccine* 35, no. 17 (March 2017): 2115–20, https://doi.org/10.1016/j.vaccine.2016.11.097.

63. Rebecca L. Weintraub, Laura Subramanian, Ami Karlage, Iman Ahmad, and Julie Rosenberg, "COVID-19 Vaccine to Vaccination: Why Leaders Must Invest in Delivery Strategies Now: Analysis Describe Lessons Learned from Past Pandemics and Vaccine Campaigns about the Path to Successful Vaccine Delivery for COVID-19," *Health Affairs* 40, no. 1 (November 2020): 33–41, https://doi.org/10.1377/hlthaff.2020.01523.

64. Weintraub et al., "COVID-19 Vaccine to Vaccination."

65. "Yellow Fever International Travel and Health," World Health Organization, July 1, 2020, https://cdn.who.int/media/docs/default-source/documents/emergencies/

travel-advice/yellow-fever-vaccination-requirements-country-list-2020-en264bd6ca-d536-4835-93be-ef83c10f4b00.pdf.

66. Lawrence O. Gostin, and Lindsay F. Wiley, "Governmental Public Health Powers During the COVID-19 Pandemic: Stay-at-Home Orders, Business Closures, and Travel Restrictions," *JAMA* 323, no. 21 (April 2020): 2137–38, doi:10.1001/jama.2020.5460.

CHAPTER 14

1. "Strengthening Global Health Security at the Human-Animal Interface," World Health Organization, accessed December 20, 2023, https://www.who.int/activities/strengthening-global-health-security-at-the-human-animal-interface.

2. "West Nile Virus - Symptoms, Diagnosis, & Treatment," Centers for Disease Control and Prevention, last modified August 18, 2023, https://www.cdc.gov/westnile/symptoms/index.html.

3. Tracey McNamara, "Lessons Learned from the West Nile Virus Outbreak of 1999: A Pathologist's Perspective," Annual International Association of Aquatic Animal Medicine Conference, New Orleans, LA, 2000, https://www.vin.com/apputil/content/defaultadv1.aspx?pId=11125&meta=generic&catId=29140&id=3981998&ind=113&objTypeID=17.

4. M. J. Studdert, "West Nile Virus Finds a New Ecological Niche in Queens, New York," *Australian Veterinary Journal* 78, no. 6 (October 2008): 400–401, https://doi.org/10.1111/j.1751-0813.2000.tb11826.x.

5. "Top 5 Takeaways from Our Interview with Dr. Tracey Mcnamara," Public Health Landscape, November 2016, https://publichealthlandscape.com/volume-27-november-2016/top-5-takeaways-from-our-interview-with-dr-tracey-mcnamara.

6. Denis Nash, Farzad Mostashari, Annie Fine, James Miller, Daniel O'Leary, Kristy Murray, Ada Huang, et al., "The Outbreak of West Nile Virus Infection in the New York City Area in 1999," *New England Journal of Medicine* 344, no. 24 (June 2001): 1807–14, DOI: 10.1056/NEJM200106143442401.

7. Ronan O'Connell, "The Deadly Irish Epidemic that Helped Bring Dracula to Life," *Atlas Obscura*, June 3, 2020, https://www.atlasobscura.com/articles/irish-epidemic-inspired-dracula.

8. Juan Gómez-Alonso, "Rabies: A Possible Explanation for the Vampire Legend," *Neurology* 51, no. 3 (September 1998): 856–59, DOI: https://doi.org/10.1212/WNL.51.3.856.

9. "Terrestrial Animal Health Code, Glossary," World Organisation for Animal Health, accessed December 20, 2023, https://www.woah.org/en/what-we-do/standards/codes-and-manuals/terrestrial-code-online-access/?id=169&L=1&htmfile=glossaire.htm#terme_surveillance.

10. "Terrestrial Animal Health Code," World Organisation for Animal Health, accessed December 20, 2023, https://www.woah.org/en/what-we-do/standards/codes-and-manuals/terrestrial-code-online-access/?id=169&L=1&htmfile=sommaire.htm.

11. Kate Varela, Jennifer A. Brown, Beth Lipton, John Dunn, Danielle Stanek, NASPHV Committee Consultants, Casey Barton Behravesh, et al., "A Review of Zoonotic Disease Threats to Pet Owners: A Compendium of Measures to Prevent Zoonotic Diseases Associated with Non-Traditional Pets Such as Rodents and Other Small Mammals, Reptiles, Amphibians, Backyard Poultry, and Other Selected Animals," *Vector-Borne and Zoonotic Diseases* 22, no. 6 (June 2022): 303–60, https://doi.org/10.1089/vbz.2022.0022.

12. "The Global Burden of Animal Diseases," World Organisation for Animal Health, accessed December 20, 2023, https://gbads.woah.org; "Moving towards Sustainability: The Livestock Sector and the World Bank," World

Bank, October 18, 2021, https://www.worldbank.org/en/topic/agriculture/brief/moving-towards-sustainability-the-livestock-sector-and-the-world-bank.

13. Stephen Higgs, "Zoonotic Diseases and Nontraditional Pets: Keeping People and Pets Healthy," *Vector-Borne and Zoonotic Diseases* 22, no. 6 (June 2022): 301–2, https://doi.org/10.1089/vbz.2022.29004.hig.

14. "Terrestrial Animal Health Code: Chapter 4.18. Vaccination," World Organisation for Animal Health, accessed December 20, 2023, https://www.woah.org/en/what-we-do/standards/codes-and-manuals/terrestrial-code-online-access/?id=169&L=1&htmfile=chapitre_vaccination.htm.

15. "Oral Rabies Vaccine and Bait Information," Animal and Plant Health Inspection Service, last modified July 22, 2020, https://www.aphis.usda.gov/aphis/ourfocus/wildlifedamage/programs/nrmp/ct_rabies_vaccine_info.

16. Joanne Maki, Anne-Laure Guiot, Michel Aubert, Bernard Brochier, Florence Cliquet, Cathleen A. Hanlon, Roni King, et al., "Oral Vaccination of Wildlife Using a Vaccinia–Rabies-Glycoprotein Recombinant Virus Vaccine (RABORAL V-RG®): A Global Review," *Veterinary Research* 48, no. 1 (September 2017): 1–26, https://doi.org/10.1186/s13567-017-0459-9.

17. Emily G. Pieracci, Christine M. Pearson, Ryan M. Wallace, Jesse D. Blanton, Erin R. Whitehouse, Xiaoyue Ma, Kendra Stauffer, Richard B. Chipman, and Victoria Olson, "Vital Signs: Trends in Human Rabies Deaths and Exposures—United States, 1938–2018," *Morbidity and Mortality Weekly Report* 68, no. 23 (June 2019): 524, http://dx.doi.org/10.15585/mmwr.mm6823e1.

18. "Plague Vaccine Helps Reduce Outbreaks in Prairie Dog Colonies," United States Geological Survey, June 22, 2017, https://www.usgs.gov/news/national-news-release/plague-vaccine-helps-reduce-outbreaks-prairie-dog-colonies.

19. Nate Hegyi, "Biologists with Drones and Peanut Butter Pellets Are on a Mission to Help Ferrets," National Public Radio, December 10, 2017, https://www.npr.org/2017/12/10/569468428/biologists-with-drones-and-peanut-butter-pellets-are-on-a-mission-to-help-ferret.

20. Rindra Randremanana, Voahangy Andrianaivoarimanana, Birgit Nikolay, Beza Ramasindrazana, Juliette Paireau, Quirine Astrid Ten Bosch, Jean Marius Rakotondramanga, et al., "Epidemiological Characteristics of an Urban Plague Epidemic in Madagascar, August–November, 2017: An Outbreak Report," *Lancet Infectious Diseases* 19, no. 5 (May 2019): 537–45, https://doi.org/10.1016/S1473-3099(18)30730-8.

21. K. Heitzinger, B. Impouma, B. L. Farham, E. L. Hamblion, C. Lukoya, C. MacHingaidze, L. A. Rakotonjanabelo, et al., "Using Evidence to Inform Response to the 2017 Plague Outbreak in Madagascar: A View from the WHO African Regional Office," *Epidemiology and Infection* 147 (July 2019), doi:10.1017/S0950268818001875.

22. "2017 – Madagascar," Disease Outbreak News, World Health Organization, November 15, 2017, https://www.who.int/emergencies/disease-outbreak-news/item/15-november-2017-plague-madagascar-en.

23. Heitzinger et al., "Using Evidence to Inform Response."

24. "Plague," World Health Organization, last modified October 23, 2017, https://www.who.int/news-room/questions-and-answers/item/plague.

25. "WHO Provides 1.2 Million Antibiotics to Fight Plague in Madagascar," World Health Organization, October 6, 2017, https://www.who.int/news-room/detail/06-10-2017-who-provides-1-2-million-antibiotics-to-fight-plague-in-madagascar.

26. Margaret Osborne, "Rabid Fox and Her Kits Euthanized after Nine People Were Bitten on Capitol Hill," *Smithsonian Magazine*, April 8, 2022, https://www.smithsonianmag.com/smart-news/rabid-fox-and-her-kits-euthanized-after-nine-people-were-bitten-on-capitol-hill-180979890.

27. "Vector-Borne Diseases," World Health Organization, last modified March 2, 2020, https://www.who.int/news-room/fact-sheets/detail/vector-borne-diseases.

28. "Mosquitoes and Disease," Illinois Department of Public Health, last modified March 29, 2017, http://www.idph.state.il.us/envhealth/pcmosquitoes.htm.

29. Michaeleen Doucleff and Jane Greenhalgh, "Forbidding Forecast for Lyme Disease in the Northeast," *Goats and Soda* (podcast), National Public Radio, March 6, 2017, https://www.npr.org/sections/goatsandsoda/2017/03/06/518219485/forbidding-forecast-for-lyme-disease-in-the-northeast.

30. "Data and Surveillance," Centers for Disease Control and Prevention, last modified August 29, 2022, https://www.cdc.gov/lyme/datasurveillance/index.html?CDC_AA_refVal=https%3A%2F%2Fwww.cdc.gov%2Flyme%2Fstats%2Findex.html.

31. "Results," The Tick Project, accessed December 20, 2023, https://www.tickproject.org/results.html.

32. "Overview," The Tick Project, accessed December 20, 2023, https://www.tickproject.org/the-study.html.

33. Felicia Keesing, Stacy Mowry, William Bremer, Shannon Duerr, Andrew S. Evans Jr, Ilya R. Fischhoff, Alison F. Hinckley, et al., "Effects of Tick-Control Interventions on Tick Abundance, Human Encounters with Ticks, and Incidence of Tickborne Diseases in Residential Neighborhoods, New York, USA," *Emerging Infectious Diseases* 28, no. 5 (May 2022): 957, https://wwwnc.cdc.gov/eid/article/28/5/21-1146_article.

34. Colin Basler, Thai-An Nguyen, Tara C. Anderson, Thane Hancock, and Casey Barton Behravesh, "Outbreaks of Human Salmonella Infections Associated with Live Poultry, United States, 1990–2014," *Emerging Infectious Diseases* 22, no. 10 (October 2016): 1705, doi: 10.3201/eid2210.150765.

35. "Salmonella Outbreaks Linked to Backyard Poultry," Centers for Disease Control and Prevention, last modified November 18, 2021, https://www.cdc.gov/salmonella/backyardpoultry-05-21/index.html.

36. "Outbreak of Salmonella Infections Linked to Pet Hedgehogs," Centers for Disease Control and Prevention, last modified January 13, 2021, https://www.cdc.gov/salmonella/typhimurium-09-20/index.html

37. Marcel A. Müller, Victor Max Corman, Joerg Jores, Benjamin Meyer, Mario Younan, Anne Liljander, Berend-Jan Bosch, et al., "MERS Coronavirus Neutralizing Antibodies in Camels, Eastern Africa, 1983–1997," *Emerging Infectious Diseases* 20, no. 12 (December 2014): 2093, https://doi.org/10.3201/eid2012.141026.

38. "Middle East Respiratory Syndrome Coronavirus (MERS-CoV)," World Health Organization, last modified August 5, 2022, https://www.who.int/en/news-room/fact-sheets/detail/middle-east-respiratory-syndrome-coronavirus-(mers-cov).

39. C. B. Reusken, E. A. Farag, Marcel Jonges, Gert-Jan Godeke, Ahmed M. El-Sayed, S. D. Pas, V. S. Raj, et al., "Middle East Respiratory Syndrome Coronavirus (MERS-CoV) RNA and Neutralising Antibodies in Milk Collected According to Local Customs from Dromedary Camels, Qatar, April 2014," *Eurosurveillance* 19, no. 23 (June 2014): 20829, https://doi.org/10.2807/1560-7917.ES2014.19.23.20829.

40. Fatma Ben Abid, Nada El-Maki, Hussam Alsoub, Muna Al Masalmani, Abdullatif Al-Khal, Peter Valentine Coyle, Mohamed Ali Ben Hadj Kacem, et al., "Middle East Respiratory Syndrome Coronavirus Infection Profile in Qatar: An 8-Year Experience," *IDCases*, no. 24 (May 2021): e01161, https://doi.org/10.1016/j.idcr.2021.e01161; "Update on MERS-CoV Transmission from Animals to Humans, and Interim Recommendations for at-Risk Groups," World Health Organization, last modified January 26, 2018, https://www.who.int/news/item/26-01-2018-update-on-mers-cov-transmission-from-animals-to-humans-and-interim-recommendations-for-at-risk-groups.

41. Jordyn Beazley, "Foot-and-Mouth Disease: Airports to Step Up Precautions as FMD Fragments Found in Meat Products in Australia," *Guardian*, July 20, 2022, https://

www.theguardian.com/australia-news/2022/jul/20/foot-and-mouth-disease-austra-lian-airports-to-step-up-precautions-as-farmers-grow-anxious.

42. "Airport Foot Mats Latest Measure in Australia's FMD Toolkit," Minister for Agriculture, Fisheries and Forestry, last modified July 20, 2022, https://minister.agriculture.gov.au/watt/media-releases/fmd-foot-mats.

43. "Hantavirus Signs & Symptoms," Centers for Disease Control and Prevention, last modified April 5, 2016, https://www.cdc.gov/hantavirus/hps/symptoms.html.

44. Jonathan J. Núñez, Curtis L. Fritz, Barbara Knust, Danielle Buttke, Barryett Enge, Mark G. Novak, Vicki Kramer, et al., "Hantavirus Infections among Overnight Visitors to Yosemite National Park, California, USA, 2012," *Emerging Infectious Diseases* 20, no. 3 (March 2014): 386, https://doi.org/10.3201/eid2003.131581.

45. Mayo Clinic Staff, "Hantavirus Pulmonary Syndrome," Mayo Clinic, last modified January 7, 2022, https://www.mayoclinic.org/diseases-conditions/hantavirus-pulmonary-syndrome/symptoms-causes/syc-20351838.

46. "Yosemite National Park Hantavirus Infection Epi Curves," Centers for Disease Control and Prevention, last modified November 1, 2012, https://www.cdc.gov/hantavirus/outbreaks/yosemite/epi.html.

47. Bruce Barcott, "The Story Behind the Hantavirus Outbreak at Yosemite," *Outside*, December 18, 2012, https://www.outsideonline.com/adventure-travel/national-parks/death-yosemite-story-behind-last-summers-hantavirus-outbreak.

48. Núñez et al., "Hantavirus Infections."

49. Núñez et al., "Hantavirus Infections."

50. Barcott, "The Story behind the Hantavirus."

51. Claire Long and Bill Willis, "Man's New Best Friend: The Opossum," *Kids Environment Kids Health*, June 2015, https://kids.niehs.nih.gov/topics/natural-world/wildlife/animals/opossum.

52. "Opossums: Taking a Bite Out of Lyme Disease," Foundation for Biomedical Research, last modified March 23, 2015, https://fbresearch.org/opossums-taking-a-bite-out-of-lyme-disease-1.

53. FAO, foreword to *Manual on Procedures for Disease Eradication by Stamping Out* (Rome: FAO, 2001), https://www.fao.org/publications/card/en/c/f264f2ec-c11c-55be-993d-523a9224700c; United States Department of Agriculture, *NAHEMS Guidelines: Quarantine and Movement Control FAD Prep: Foreign Animal Disease Preparedness and Response Plan* (Ames, IA: CFSPH, 2016), https://www.aphis.usda.gov/animal_health/emergency_management/downloads/nahems_guidelines/nahems_qmc.pdf; FAO, "Chapter 5: Early Reaction Contingency Planning—Principles and Strategies," in *Manual on the Preparation of National Animal Disease Emergency Preparedness Plans* (Rome: FAO, 1999), https://www.fao.org/publications/card/en/c/830eab8f-0beb-5172-9ec5-7d5ab0e0ebb5.

54. FAO, "Part 1: Destruction of Animals. Chapter 1: Introduction, in *Manual on Procedures*.

55. "Terrestrial Animal Health Code: Chapter 7.6: Killing of Animals for Disease Control Purposes," World Organisation for Animal Health, October 2022, https://www.oie.int/fileadmin/Home/eng/Health_standards/tahc/current/chapitre_aw_killing.pdf.

56. Zohar Lederman, Manuel Magalhães-Sant'Ana, and Teck Chuan Voo, "Stamping Out Animal Culling: From Anthropocentrism to One Health Ethics," *Journal of Agricultural and Environmental Ethics* 34, no. 5 (August 2021): 1–14, https://doi.org/10.1007/s10806-021-09868-x.

57. Malcolm Prior, "Record Avian Flu Outbreak Sees 48m Birds Culled in UK and EU," BBC News, October 3, 2022, https://www.bbc.com/news/science-environment-63097119.

58. "Avian Influenza: Prevention Zone Declared across Great Britain," press release, Department for Environment, Food and Rural Affairs, and Animal and Plant Health Agency, October 17, 2022, https://www.gov.uk/government/news/avian-influenza-prevention-zone-declared-across-great-britain.

59. "Influenza a (H5) - United Kingdom of Great Britain and Northern Ireland," World Health Organization, Disease Outbreak News, January 14, 2022, https://www.who.int/emergencies/disease-outbreak-news/item/influenza-a-(h5)---united-kingdom-of-great-britain-and-northern-ireland.

60. "Investigation into the Risk to Human Health of Avian Influenza (Influenza A H5N1) in England: Technical Briefing 1," UK Health Security Agency, July 14, 2023, https://www.gov.uk/government/publications/avian-influenza-influenza-a-h5n1-technical-briefings/investigation-into-the-risk-to-human-health-of-avian-influenza-influenza-a-h5n1-in-england-technical-briefing-1.

61. "Influenza a (H1N1) Pandemic 2009–2010: Overview," World Health Organization, accessed December 20, 2023, https://www.who.int/emergencies/situations/influenza-a-(h1n1)-outbreak.

62. "No Need to Cull Pigs, Stop Movement: U.N. Food Body," Reuters, April 30, 2009, https://www.reuters.com/article/us-flu-un-pigs/no-need-to-cull-pigs-stop-movement-u-n-food-body-idUSTRE53T6OG20090430.

63. Sameh Seef and Anders Jeppsson, "Is It a Policy Crisis or Is It a Health Crisis?: The Egyptian Context—Analysis of the Egyptian Health Policy for the H1N1 Flu Pandemic Control," *Pan African Medical Journal* 14, no. 1 (February 2013), doi: 10.11604/pamj.2013.14.59.1631.

CHAPTER 15

1. E. N. Hulland, K. E. Wiens, S. Shirude, J. D. Morgan, A. Bertozzi-Villa, T. H. Farag, N. Fullman, et al., "Travel Time to Health Facilities in Areas of Outbreak Potential: Maps for Guiding Local Preparedness and Response," *BMC Medicine* 17, no. 1 (December 2019): 1–16, https://doi.org/10.1186/s12916-019-1459-6.

2. MEASURE Evaluation, *Mapping Community-Based Global Health Programs: A Reference Guide for Community-Based Practice* (Chapel Hill, NC: Caroline Population Center, 2014), https://www.measureevaluation.org/resources/publications/ms-13-76/at_download/document.

3. World Health Organization *Mass Casualty Management Systems: Strategies and Guidelines for Building Health Sector Capacity* (Geneva: World Health Organization, 2007), https://apps.who.int/iris/handle/10665/43804.

4. Spectrum News Staff and Zack Fink, "NYC Subways to Close from 1 AM to 5 AM Daily for Full Cleanings," *Spectrum News NY 1*, May 1, 2020, https://www.ny1.com/nyc/all-boroughs/news/2020/04/30/cuomo-announces-mta-to-close-nyc-subway-system-overnight-for-daily-full-cleanings-.

5. "Curbing COVID-19 in Kenyan Public Transport," WHO Regional Office for Africa, last modified July 15, 2021, https://www.afro.who.int/photo-story/curbing-covid-19-kenyan-public-transport.

6. Al Sanders, "King County Executive Recognizes Metro Program for Safely Transporting COVID Patients," *King County Metro* (blog), September 3, 2021, https://kingcountymetro.blog/2021/09/03/king-county-executive-recognizes-metro-program-for-safely-transporting-covid-patients.

7. "Guidance on Air Medical Transport (AMT) for Patients with Ebola Virus Disease (EVD)," Centers for Disease Control and Prevention, last modified September 19, 2023, https://www.cdc.gov/vhf/ebola/clinicians/emergency-services/air-medical-transport.html.

8. "Guidance on Air Medical Transport."

9. APIC, *Guide to Infection Prevention in Emergency Medical Services: Association for Professionals in Infection Control and Epidemiology* (United States: APIC 2013), https://nasemso.org/wp-content/uploads/Guide-to-Infection-Prevention-in-EMS-APIC.pdf.

10. Olive C. Kobusingye, Adnan A. Hyder, David Bishai, Eduardo Romero Hicks, Charles Mock, and Manjul Joshipura, "Emergency Medical Systems in Low- and Middle-Income Countries: Recommendations for Action," *Bulletin of the World Health Organization* 83, no. 8 (August 2005): 626–31, https://www.scielosp.org/pdf/bwho/v83n8/v83n8a17.pdf.

11. Vipul Mishra, Richa Ahuja, N. Nezamuddin, Geetam Tiwari, and Kavi Bhalla, "Strengthening the Capacity of Emergency Medical Services in Low and Middle Income Countries Using Dispatcher-Coordinated Taxis," *Transportation Research Record* 2674, no. 9 (July 2020): 338–45, https://doi.org/10.1177/0361198120929024; Aditya C. Shekhar, "Ambulance Allocation: What's the Right Balance?" *EMS World*, February 7, 2020, https://www.hmpgloballearningnetwork.com/site/emsworld/article/1223842/ambulance-allocation-whats-right-balance.

12. "Transportation for Pandemic Response (TPR) COVID-19 Mobility Services," King County Metro, April 7, 2020, https://www.apta.com/wp-content/uploads/Transport-for-Pandemic-Response-Briefing-Paper.-4.7.2020.pdf.

13. World Food Programme, *United Nations Humanitarian Air Service* (*UNHAS*) *2020 Overview* (Rome, Italy: World Food Programme, 2021), https://docs.wfp.org/api/documents/WFP-0000129673/download/?_ga=2.238847360.142005940.1634011689-605403308.1634011689.

14. "Humanitarian Air Services Factsheet," European Civil Protection and Humanitarian Aid Operations, accessed December 20, 2023, https://civil-protection-humanitarian-aid.ec.europa.eu/what/humanitarian-aid/humanitarian-air-services_en.

15. "Humanitarian Air Services Factsheet."

16. "Airbus Military Aircraft Perform Life-Saving Medevac Missions during the COVID-19 Pandemic," Aerospace Security and Defence Industries Association of Europe, May 21, 2020, https://www.asd-europe.org/airbus-military-aircraft-perform-life-saving-medevac-missions-during-the-covid-19-pandemic.

17. Jeremy Hsu, "SARS Outbreak Isolators Helped 'Ebola Air' Fly Infected Patients," *Scientific American*, September 18, 2014, https://www.scientificamerican.com/article/sars-outbreak-isolators-helped-ebola-air-fly-infected-patients.

18. Cameron McWhirtere, "Special Planes Are Lifeline for Ebola Patients," *Wall Street Journal*, March 13, 2015, https://www.wsj.com/articles/special-planes-are-lifeline-for-ebola-patients-1426276096.

19. Robert Roos, "Very Few Aircraft Equipped to Evacuate Ebola Patients," Center for Infectious Disease Research and Policy, September 16, 2014, https://www.cidrap.umn.edu/ebola/very-few-aircraft-equipped-evacuate-ebola-patients.

20. Josh Hicks, "The Whole World Relies on This One U.S. Company to Fly Ebola Patients," *Washington Post*, October 28, 2014, https://www.washingtonpost.com/news/federal-eye/wp/2014/10/28/the-world-relies-on-this-one-company-to-fly-ebola-patients.

21. Roos, "Very Few Aircraft Equipped."

22. Roos, "Very Few Aircraft Equipped."

23. Hicks, "The Whole World Relies."

24. McWhirtere, "Special Planes Are Lifeline."

25. "Contagious Disease Transport," Phoenix Air, accessed December 20, 2023, https://phoenixair.com/air-ambulance/contagious-disease-transport.

26. "The Latest Technology in Biocontainment Systems," MRIGlobal, accessed December 20, 2023, https://www.mriglobal.org/the-latest-technology-in-biocontainment-systems.

27. "Contagious Disease Transport."

28. World Food Programme, *United Nations Humanitarian Air Service*.

29. "Vital Air Service Delivers Life-Saving Assistance during COVID-19 Pandemic," World Food Programme, August 19, 2021, https://reliefweb.int/report/world/vital-air-service-delivers-life-saving-assistance-during-covid-19-pandemic.

30. "EU Humanitarian Air Bridge: Helping Aid Reach the People in Need During the Coronavirus Pandemic," European Civil Protection and Humanitarian Aid Operations, accessed December 20, 2023, https://civil-protection-humanitarian-aid.ec.europa.eu/eu-humanitarian-air-bridge-helping-aid-reach-people-need-during-coronavirus-pandemic_en.

31. Rebecca F. Denlinger, Martha H. Marsh, and Bruce A. Rohde, *The Prioritization of Critical Infrastructure for a Pandemic Outbreak in the United States Working Group: Final Report and Recommendations by the Council* (Washington DC: National Infrastructure Advisory Council, 2007), https://www.dhs.gov/xlibrary/assets/niac/niac-pandemic-wg_v8-011707.pdf.

32. "Emergency Support Function #1 – Transportation Annex," FEMA, June 2016, https://www.fema.gov/sites/default/files/2020-07/fema_ESF_1_Transportation.pdf.

33. World Health Organization, *COVID-19 Supply Chain System: Requesting and Receiving Supplies* (Geneva: World Health Organization, 2020), https://www.who.int/publications/m/item/covid-19-supply-chain-system-requesting-and-receiving-supplies.

34. Neelam Sekhri, *Forecasting for Global Health: New Money, New Products and New Markets* (Washington, DC: Center for Global Development, 2006): 1–51, https://cgdev.org/sites/default/files/archive/doc/ghprn/Forecasting_Background.pdf.

35. Stroud et al., "Current Dispensing Strategies."

36. "Project Last Mile," Coca Cola Company, accessed December 20, 2023, https://www.coca-colacompany.com/social/project-last-mile.

37. "Delivery Innovation: Coca-Cola Company," The Global Fund, accessed December 20, 2023, https://www.theglobalfund.org/en/private-ngo-partners/delivery-innovation/coca-cola.

38. World Health Organization, "Content Sheet 4-1," in *Laboratory Quality Management System: Handbook* (Geneva: World Health Organization, 2011), https://www.who.int/publications/i/item/9789241548274.

39. National Academies of Sciences, Engineering, and Medicine, *Impact of the Global Medical Supply Chain on SNS Operations and Communications: Proceedings of a Workshop* (Washington, DC: National Academies Press, 2018), https://www.ncbi.nlm.nih.gov/books/NBK525648; Fiona A. Miller, Steven B. Young, Mark Dobrow, and Kaveh G. Shojania, "Vulnerability of the Medical Product Supply Chain: The Wake-Up Call of COVID-19," *BMJ Quality and Safety* 30, no. 4 (March 2021): 331–35, http://dx.doi.org/10.1136/bmjqs-2020-012133.

40. "COVID-19 and the Global Supply Chains for Medical Supplies," Global Financing Facility, and World Bank Group, accessed December 20, 2023, https://www.globalfinancingfacility.org/sites/gff_new/files/documents/COVID-19-Supply-Chain-ENGLISH.pdf.

41. Miller et al., "Vulnerability of the Medical Product Supply Chain."

42. Jane Feinmann, "PPE: What Now for the Global Supply Chain?," *BMJ* 369 (May 2020), https://doi.org/10.1136/bmj.m1910.

43. "COVID-19: Agencies Are Taking Steps to Improve Future Use of Defense Production Act Authorities," US Government Accountability Office, December 16, 2021, https://www.gao.gov/products/gao-22-105380.

44. "Global Vaccine Action Plan," World Health Organization, accessed December 20, 2023, https://www.who.int/teams/immunization-vaccines-and-biologicals/strategies/global-vaccine-action-plan.

45. "Best Practices in Supply Chain Preparedness for Public Health Emergencies," technical report, USAID, March 1, 2019, https://www.ghsupplychain.org/best-practices-supply-chain-preparedness-public-health-emergencies.

46. Zeina Najjar, Emma Quinn, Teresa Anderson, Vicky Sheppeard, and Leena Gupta, "Surveillance Methods to Detect the Impact of a Significant Cold Chain Breach," *Vaccine* 37, no. 30 (July 2019): 3950–52, https://doi.org/10.1016/j.vaccine.2019.05.091.

47. Australian Government Department of Health, *National Vaccine Storage Guidelines "Strive for 5,"* 3rd ed. (Canberra: Commonwealth of Australia, 2019), https://www.health.gov.au/resources/publications/national-vaccine-storage-guidelines-strive-for-5.

48. "The Challenging Journey to Reach Nepal's Hillside Communities with Vaccines," UNICEF, accessed December 20, 2023, https://www.unicef.org/stories/delivering-vaccines-and-building-trust-in-nepal; Solomon Yimer, "No Mountain High Enough: Ethiopian Vaccinators Climb to Reach Missed-Out Children," Gavi, the Vaccine Alliance, February 7, 2023, https://www.gavi.org/vaccineswork/no-mountain-high-enough-ethiopian-vaccinators-climb-reach-missed-out-children; "Trekking through the Snow to Deliver Vaccines: Vaccinators Tackle Winter Conditions and Challenging Contexts during Afghanistan's Last Polio Campaign of the Year," GPEI, December 23, 2020, https://polioeradication.org/news-post/trekking-through-the-snow-to-deliver-vaccines.

49. Jennifer Houdek, "The Serum Run of 1925," LitSite Alaska Digital Archives Partnership, University of Alaska Anchorage, November 27, 2010, http://www.litsitealaska.org/index.cfm?section=Digital%20Archives&page=Land%20Sea%20Air&cat=Dog%20Mushing&contentid=2559&viewpost=2.

50. Lucy Breakwell, Edna Moturi, Louisa Helgenberger, Sameer V. Gopalani, Craig Hales, Eugene Lam, Umid Sharapov, et al., "Measles Outbreak Associated with Vaccine Failure in Adults—Federated States of Micronesia, February–August 2014," *Morbidity and Mortality Weekly Report* 64, no. 38 (October 2015): 1088–92, doi: 10.15585/mmwr.mm6438a7.

51. Breakwell et al., "Measles Outbreak."

52. Craig M. Hales, Eliaser Johnson, Louisa Helgenberger, Mark J. Papania, Maribeth Larzelere, Sameer V. Gopalani, Emmaculate Lebo, et al., "Measles Outbreak Associated with Low Vaccine Effectiveness among Adults in Pohnpei State, Federated States of Micronesia, 2014," *Open Forum Infectious Diseases* 3, no. 2 (March 2016), https://doi.org/10.1093/ofid/ofw064.

53. Jamison Pike, Ashley Tippins, Mawuli Nyaku, Maribeth Eckert, Louisa Helgenberger, and J. Michael Underwood, "Cost of a Measles Outbreak in a Remote Island Economy: 2014 Federated States of Micronesia Measles Outbreak," *Vaccine* 35, no. 43 (September 2017): 5905–11, https://doi.org/10.1016/j.vaccine.2017.08.075.

54. "Company History," Dippin Dots, accessed December 20, 2023, https://www.dippin-dots.com/about/company-history.

55. Valerie McNamara, "The Unexpected Companies Involved in COVID-19 Vaccine Distribution," Global Edge, January 14, 2021, https://globaledge.msu.edu/blog/post/56953/the-unexpected-companies-involved-in-cov.

56. Maddie Bender, "What the Dippin' Dots 'Cold Chain' Can Teach Us about COVID-19 Vaccines," *Popular Science*, December 15, 2020, https://www.popsci.com/story/health/covid-vaccine-cold-chain-dippin-dots-ice-cream.

57. Terri Rebmann, Kyle McPhee, Leslie Osborne, Daniel P. Gillen, and Gabriel A. Haas, "Best Practices for Healthcare Facility and Regional Stockpile Maintenance and Sustainment: A Literature Review," *Health Security* 15, no. 4 (August 2017): 409–17, https://doi.org/10.1089/hs.2016.0123.

58. "The 2009 H1N1 Pandemic: Summary Highlights, April 2009–April 2010," Centers for Disease Control and Prevention, June 16, 2010, https://www.cdc.gov/h1n1flu/cdcresponse.htm.

59. National Academies of Sciences, Engineering, and Medicine, "The Strategic National Stockpile: Origin, Policy Foundations, and Federal Context," in *The Nation's Medical Countermeasure Stockpile: Opportunities to Improve the Efficiency, Effectiveness, and Sustainability of the CDC Strategic National Stockpile: Workshop Summary* (Washington, DC: National Academies Press, 2016), https://www.ncbi.nlm.nih.gov/books/NBK396378.

60. "Influenza Pandemic: Lessons from the H1N1 Pandemic Should Be Incorporated into Future Planning," US Government Accountability Office, June 27, 2011, https://www.gao.gov/products/gao-11-632.

61. "An HHS Retrospective on the 2009 H1N1 Influenza Pandemic to Advance All Hazards Preparedness," US Department of Health and Human Services, last updated June 15, 2012, https://www.phe.gov/Preparedness/mcm/h1n1-retrospective/Documents/h1n1-retrospective.pdf.

62. Catherine Yen, Terri B. Hyde, Alejandro J. Costa, Katya Fernandez, John S. Tam, Stéphane Hugonnet, Anne M. Huvos, Philippe Duclos, Vance J. Dietz, and Brenton T. Burkholder, "The Development of Global Vaccine Stockpiles," *Lancet Infectious Diseases* 15, no. 3 (February 2015): 340–47, https://doi.org/10.1016/S1473-3099(14)70999-5.

63. "Protecting You from Monkeypox: Information on the Smallpox Vaccination," UK Health Security Agency, last modified September 6, 2022, https://www.gov.uk/government/publications/monkeypox-vaccination-resources/protecting-you-from-monkeypox-information-on-the-smallpox-vaccination#ref; "Japan OKs Smallpox Vaccine to Prevent Monkeypox," *Arab News*, July 29, 2022, https://www.arabnews.jp/en/japan/article_77241; "Acam2000 (Smallpox Vaccine) Questions and Answers," US Food and Drug Administration, last modified August 19, 2022, https://www.fda.gov/vaccines-blood-biologics/vaccines/acam2000-smallpox-vaccine-questions-and-answers; "Fact Sheet: Biden- Harris Administration's Monkeypox Outbreak Response," The White House, June 28, 2022, https://www.whitehouse.gov/briefing-room/statements-releases/2022/06/28/fact-sheet-biden-harris-administrations-monkeypox-outbreak-response.

64. "Mpox (Monkeypox)," World Health Organization, last modified April 18, 2023, https://www.who.int/news-room/fact-sheets/detail/monkeypox.

65. World Health Organization, *A Systematic Review of Public Health Emergency Operations Centres (EOC)* (Geneva: World Health Organization, 2013), https://iris.who.int/bitstream/handle/10665/99043/WHO_HSE_GCR_2014.1_eng.pdf.

66. S. Arunmozhi Balajee, Omer G. Pasi, Alain Georges M. Etoundi, Peter Rzeszotarski, Trang T. Do, Ian Hennessee, Sharifa Merali, Karen A. Alroy, Tran Dac Phu, and Anthony W. Mounts, "Sustainable Model for Public Health Emergency Operations Centers for Global Settings," *Emerging Infectious Diseases* 23, suppl. 1 (December 2017): S190, https://doi.org/10.3201/eid2313.170435.

67. Daniel J. Brencic, Meredith Pinto, Adrienne Gill, Michael H. Kinzer, Luis Hernandez, and Omer G. Pasi, "CDC Support for Global Public Health Emergency Management," *Emerging Infectious Diseases* 23, suppl. 1 (December 2017): S183, https://doi.org/10.3201/eid2313.170542.

68. World Health Organization, *Systematic Review.*

69. Jeffrey L. Bryant, Daniel M. Sosin, Tim W. Wiedrich, and Stephen C. Redd, "Emergency Operations Centers and Incident Management Structure," in *The CDC Field Epidemiology Manual* (Atlanta, GA: CDC, 2018), https://www.cdc.gov/eis/field-epi-manual/chapters/EOC-Incident-Management.html.

70. World Health Organization, *Systematic Review.*

71. "CDC Emergency Operations Center (EOC)," Centers for Disease Control and Prevention, last modified September 26, 2023, https://www.cdc.gov/cpr/eoc/eoc.htm

72. "Deactivating the EOC," Federal Emergency Management Institute, accessed December 20, 2023, https://emilms.fema.gov/is_2200/groups/142. html; Federal Emergency Management Agency, *Emergency Operations Center Skillsets User Guide* (Washington, DC: FEMA, 2018), https://www.fema.gov/sites/default/files/2020-05/fema_nqs_eoc-skillset-guide_0.pdf.

73. Centers for Disease Control and Prevention, "Progress toward Poliomyelitis Eradication-Nigeria, January 201–September 2012," *Morbidity and Mortality Weekly Report* 61, no. 44 (November 2012): 899–904, https://pubmed.ncbi.nlm.nih.gov/23134973.

74. Joseph Okeibunor, Peter Nsubuga, Mbaye Salla, Richard Mihigo, and Pascal Mkanda, "Coordination as a Best Practice from the Polio Eradication Initiative: Experiences from Five Member States in the African Region of the World Health Organization," *Vaccine* 34, no. 43 (October 2016): 5203–7, https://doi.org/10.1016/j.vaccine.2016.05.066.

75. Scott Desmarais, "Eradicating Polio in Nigeria," McKinsey, February 1, 2016, https://www.mckinsey.com/industries/healthcare-systems-and-services/our-insights/eradicating-polio-in-nigeria.

76. Jefcoate O'Donnell, "Nigeria Just Won a Complex Victory over Polio," *Foreign Policy*, August 21, 2019, https://foreignpolicy.com/2019/08/21/nigeria-just-won-a-complex-victory-over-polio.

77. Okeibunor et al., "Coordination as a Best Practice."

78. "Global Polio Eradication Initiative Applauds WHO African Region for Wild Polio-Free Certification," news release, World Health Organization, August 25, 2020, https://www.who.int/news/item/25-08-2020-global-polio-eradication-initiative-applauds-who-african-region-for-wild-polio-free-certification.

79. "Contingency Fund for Emergencies (CFE)," World Health Organization, accessed December 20, 2023, https://www.who.int/emergencies/funding/contingency-fund-for-emergencies.

80. "Global Humanitarian Response Plan COVID-19 (April–December 2020) GHRP July Update," United Nations Office for the Coordination of Humanitarian Affairs, accessed December 20, 2023, https://www.unocha.org/sites/unocha/files/Global-Humanitarian-Response-Plan-COVID-19.pdf.

81. "How We Work," United Nations Sustainable Development Group, accessed December 20, 2023, https://unsdg.un.org/about/how-we-work.

82. United Nations High Commissioner for Refugees, *IASC Protocol for the Control of Infectious Disease Events* (New York: IASC, 2019), https://data.unhcr.org/en/documents/details/74754.

83. "Global Outbreak Alert and Response Network," GOARN, accessed December 20, 2023, https://goarn.who.int.

84. Republic of Sierra Leone, *National Communication Strategy for Ebola Response in Sierra Leone* (Freetown: Republic of Sierra Leone, 2014), http://ebolacommunicationnetwork.org/wp-content/uploads/2014/10/National-Ebola-Communication-Strategy_FINAL.pdf.

85. Landry Ndriko Mayigane, Cindy Chiu de Vázquez, Candice Vente, Denis Charles, Frederik A. Copper, Allan Bell, Hilary Kagume Njenge, et al., "The Necessity for Intra-Action Reviews During the COVID-19 Pandemic," *Lancet Global Health* 8, no. 12 (October 2020): e1451–e1452, https://doi.org/10.1016/S2214-109X(20)30414-9.

86. Federal Emergency Management Agency, *Effective Coordination of Recovery Resources for State, Tribal, Territorial and Local Incidents* (Washington, DC: FEMA, 2015), https://www.fema.gov/sites/default/files/2020-07/fema_effective-coordination-recovery-resources-guide_020515.pdf.

87. Federal Emergency Management Agency, *Pre-Disaster Recovery Planning Guide for Local Governments* (Washington, DC: FEMA, 2017), https://www.fema.gov/sites/default/files/2020-07/pre-disaster-recovery-planning-guide-local-governments.pdf.

88. Federal Emergency Management Agency, *Pre-Disaster Recovery Planning Guide.*

89. Federal Emergency Management Agency, *Effective Coordination of Recovery Resources.*

90. Federal Emergency Management Agency, *Long-Term Community Recovery Planning Process* (Washington, DC: FEMA, 2005), https://www.fema.gov/pdf/rebuild/ltrc/selfhelp.pdf.

91. World Health Organization, *Pandemic Influenza Preparedness and Response: A WHO Guidance Document* (Geneva: World Health Organization, 2009), https://apps.who.int/iris/bitstream/handle/10665/44123/9789241547680_eng.pdf.

92. Sam Tozay, William Fischer, David Wohl, Kayla Kilpatrick, Fei Zou, Edwina reeves, Korto Pewu, et al., "Long-Term Complications of Ebola Virus Disease: Prevalence and Predictors of Major Symptoms and the Role of Inflammation," *Clinical Infectious Diseases* 71, no. 7 (Nov. 2019): 1749–55, https://doi.org/10.1093/cid/ciz1062.

93. Bridge M. Kuehn, "Registry Tracks ZIKA-Related Birth Defects in US," *JAMA* 327, no. 10 (March 2022): 910, https://doi:10.1001/jama.2022/2206.

94. "HHS Announced the Formation of the Office of Long COVID Research and Practice and Launch of Long COVID Clinical Trials through the RECOVER Initiative," press release, US Health and Human Services, July 31, 2023, https://www.hhs.gov/about/news/2023/07/31/hhs-announces-formation-office-long-covid-research-practice-launch-long-covid-clinical-trials-through-recover-initiative.html.

95. G. W. Parker, "Best Practices for After-Action Review: Turning Lessons Observed into Lessons Learned for Preparedness Policy," *Revue scientifique et technique* 39, no. 2 (August 2020): 579–90, https://doi.org/10.20506/rst.39.2.3108.

96. World Health Organization, *The Global Practice of After Action Review: A Systematic Review of Literature*, no. WHO/WHE/CPI/2019.9 (Geneva: World Health Organization, 2019), https://www.who.int/publications/i/item/WHO-WHE-CPI-2019.9.

97. "Lessons Learned and After Action Assessments," Centers for Disease Control and Prevention, accessed December 20, 2023, https://www.cdc.gov/niosh/erhms/pdf/LessonsLearned.pdf.

98. Parker, "Best Practices for After-Action Review."

99. World Health Organization, *Guidance for After Action Review (AAR)*, no. WHO/WHE/CPI/2019.4 (Geneva: World Health Organization, 2019), https://www.who.int/publications/i/item/WHO-WHE-CPI-2019.4.

WRAPPING UP

1. Jaason M. Geerts, Donna Kinnair, Paul Taheri, Ajit Abraham, Joonmo Ahn, Rifat Atun, Lorena Barberia, et al., "Guidance for Health Care Leaders during the Recovery Stage of the COVID-19 Pandemic: A Consensus Statement," *JAMA Network Open* 4, no. 7 (July 2021): e2120295–e2120295, doi:10.1001/jamanetworkopen.2021.20295.

ACKNOWLEDGMENTS

Global expert advisors from a variety of fields involved in outbreak response and numerous researchers have contributed over the years to the development of the Georgetown Outbreak Activity Library (GOAL). The initial online tool had an advisory group that included a medical epidemiologist from European Centers for Disease Control, the World Health Organization team lead for MERS, who eventually became the technical lead for the global COVID-19 response for WHO, a virologist who coordinated response efforts for Ebola in both West Africa and in the DRC, a program manager for surveillance projects around the world, and an infectious disease physician who had provided direct response for multiple outbreaks and supported the emergency program at the WHO.

We would like to recognize the valuable work performed by current and former staff and students at the Center for Global Health Science and Security and their contributions to the Georgetown Outbreak Activity Library, our online tool. Their research and writing inspired many of the activities in this book. Aurelia Attal-Juncqua, Matthew Boyce, Ellen Carlin, Claire Standley, Jessica Lin, Jordan Schermerhorn, Juliana St. Goar, Hannah Todd, Kate Toole, Aika Wojt, and Emily Woodrow—we are grateful for your belief in the GOAL project and your commitment to capturing the rationales behind public health action to share with the world. Thanks also go to the Data Lab team at the Center for Global Health Science and Security (formerly Talus Analytics) led by Ellie Graeden, supported by Hailey Robertson, Tess Stevens, Ryan Zimmerman, Justin Kerr, Kelsey Smith, Nicole Stephan, and Micahael Van Maele, who designed and built the online tool.

Many thanks also to the students who worked on GOAL case studies, including Madison Alvarez, Madison Berry, Emily Sherman, Hannah Todd, and Mark Wilcox. Several of their case studies were adapted and used in the book.

ABOUT THE AUTHORS

Rebecca Katz, PhD, MPH, is a professor and the director of the Center for Global Health Science and Security at Georgetown University; she holds joint appointments in Georgetown University Medical Center and the School of Foreign Service. She has spent more than two decades working on pandemic preparedness and response and on the domestic and global implementation of the International Health Regulations, as well as global governance of public health emergencies. She has taught courses on emerging infectious diseases and global health security and diplomacy, and advised on the response to multiple outbreaks. She was asked to support President Biden's response to the COVID-19 pandemic.

Years ago, while sitting in meetings related to outbreak response in Geneva, Switzerland, with diplomats from around the world, Dr. Katz realized that many of the diplomats did not have a complete understanding of the range of activities critical to preventing, detecting, and responding to outbreaks and other public health emergencies. In other international meetings, she witnessed public health and response professionals struggle to find resources to help guide the entire range of outbreak response activities, as well as to see the dynamics of all of the stakeholders involved. This drove Dr. Katz and her colleagues to create a suite of tools, including an online outbreak activity library and tools to help map stakeholders to different parts of an outbreak response, from the local to the global scale.

Throughout the COVID-19 pandemic, Dr. Katz was asked to advise a range of organizations and governments around the world, on issues from developing plans to keep employees and clients safe at a casino in Las Vegas, to advising mayors on their response activities, to working on international agreements. These experiences, coupled with two decades teaching about health security, led her to develop a commitment to improving public literacy in public health, and outbreak response in particular, across the learning continuum.

Dr. Katz has authored more than one hundred peer-reviewed manuscripts and six books (this is the seventh), in addition to numerous op-eds, blogs, white papers, and book chapters. From 2004 to 2019, Dr. Katz was a consultant to the Department of State, working on issues related to the Biological Weapons Convention, pandemic influenza, and disease surveillance. She returned to the Department of State in January 2021 as a senior advisor to the Secretary on the global COVID-19 response and global health security and in 2023 moved to become a senior advisor in the newly established Bureau of Global Health Security and Diplomacy. In 2019, Dr. Katz co-convened the first international scientific conference on global health security, bringing together more than nine hundred participants from around the world to form a community of practice. Dr. Katz received her undergraduate degree from Swarthmore College, an MPH from Yale University, and a PhD from Princeton University. She is a member of the Council on Foreign Relations and the Cosmos Club.

Mackenzie S. Moore, MSc, is an epidemiologist and scientist driven by questions about how humans' interactions with their communities, environment, and animals influence the dynamics of infectious disease and the emergence of old and new pathogens. Inspired by her great-grandmother's work as a nurse in California tuberculosis sanatoriums, she explores topics in epidemic intelligence, pandemic preparedness and response, and outbreak policy and develops evidence-based training courses and knowledge hubs.

Ms. Moore has worked as a global health and biosecurity consultant at a number of organizations, including USAID, the International Organization for Migration Central America Office, the World Bank, and the Global Fund to Fight AIDS, Tuberculosis and Malaria. Ms. Moore worked with Dr. Katz as a senior research associate at the Center for Global Health Science and Security at Georgetown University. She started working with the Center as a Global Health Initiative Fellow while completing her graduate degree, writing for GOAL, the interactive online tool that identifies all activities and actors involved in outbreak response, a heavy inspiration for this book. She worked as a writer, coder, and data manager, and served as GOAL project manager. While at the Center, she also worked on global health security governance projects; designed and piloted Field Epidemiology Training Program exercises; served as technical lead conducting field work in the Pacific mapping and evaluating health systems and health security; and coded and analyzed a range of pandemic policies. She has published her work in peer-reviewed journals and presented it as posters and on speaker panels at international conferences. She is deeply committed to enhancing public health literacy among the general public and inspiring curiosity by making scientific concepts and research accessible and understandable. Writing *Outbreak Atlas* is an integral part of that mission.

Ms. Moore is pursuing her PhD at the University of Edinburgh in Scotland as a Wellcome Trust scholar. She received an MSc in global health, specializing in disease control and prevention, from Georgetown University, and a BA in anthropology from the University of California, Berkeley, where she was a Regents' and Chancellor's Scholar, graduated with highest honors, and was awarded the Frankenberg Prize for Outstanding Honors Thesis in Critical Medical Anthropology.

ABOUT THE ILLUSTRATOR

Madelyne Adams is an illustrator and hand lettering artist based in Washington, DC, who contributed illustrations to this book.

INDEX

Guinea, 11, 105, 111, 161. *See also* West Africa Ebola
    outbreak (2014–2016)
Guinness Brewery, 19

H1N1 influenza
    emergency declaration and, 83
    emergency funding and, 154
    emergency operations and logistics and,
        219–20
    as emerging zoonotic disease, 186
    governance and, 167, 182
    outbreak response and, 199–200
    surveillance and, 32
Haiti, 61
hand hygiene materials, 122
hand washing, 96, 125. *See also* hygiene
handwashing, 193
hantavirus pulmonary syndrome (HPS), 197–98
Health Canada, 20–21
health care services and facilities
    humanitarian response and, 67
    outbreak operations and, 134–38
    security and, 144–46
health care workers
    emergency funding and, 157–58
    emergency operations and logistics and, 205–6
    governance and, 181, 182
    role and importance of, 138–39
    security and, 144–46
health care–associated infections (HAI), 117
Health Surge Capacity Initiative, 136
Health Workforce Estimator (HWFE), 104
Henipavirus diseases, 86
hepatitis, 4–5
Herwaldt, Barbara L., 21
highly pathogenic avian influenza (HPAI), 186,
    199
Hornbrook, R. W., 66
hotlines, 91
housing, 70–71
human remains, 120–23
humanitarian data, 64, 66, 75. *See also* data collec-
    tion and management
humanitarian response, 59, 63–71
hygiene
    burials and, 122
    communication and, 96
    community engagement and, 68–70
    food safety and, 123–27

importance of, 19, 110–11
    lab analysis and, 44–45
    zoonotic diseases and, 193–94
hypoxemia, 136–37

identification of human remains, 120
imports, 160, 175
incident command systems (ICSs), 222
indicator-based surveillance (IBS), 29–31, 61
indirect transmission, 15. *See also* mosquitoes
infection prevention and control (IPC), 111, 117–20,
    132, 134–35
influenza, 47. *See also* H1N1 influenza
information. *See* communication; data collection
        and management
information sharing, 172, 179–80
informed consent, 181
interagency committees, 176–77
Inter-Agency Standing Committee (IASC), 225
Inter-American Development Bank, 155
International Atomic Energy Agency (IAEA), 129
International Centre for Diarrhoeal Disease
        Research, 31
International Committee of the Red Cross (ICRC),
        69–70
International Federation of Red Cross and Red
        Crescent Societies (IFRC), 225–26
international financial system, 162
International Health Regulations (IHR)
    emergency operations and logistics and, 225
    governance and, 166–68, 173, 175
    notification of outbreak and, 85–86
    surveillance and, 32–33, 35
International Monetary Fund (IMF), 155
International Organization for Migration (IOM),
        33, 225
international organizations
    emergency funding and, 156
    notification of outbreak to, 85–86
    See also specific organizations
international public health treaties, 166–70
International Reagent Resource (IRR), 53
International Rescue Committee (IRC), 69–70
International Sanitary Conferences, 166
interviews, 7, 9
Ireland, 19
isolation, 70–71, 114. *See also* physical distancing;
        quarantine
isoniazid (INH), 115

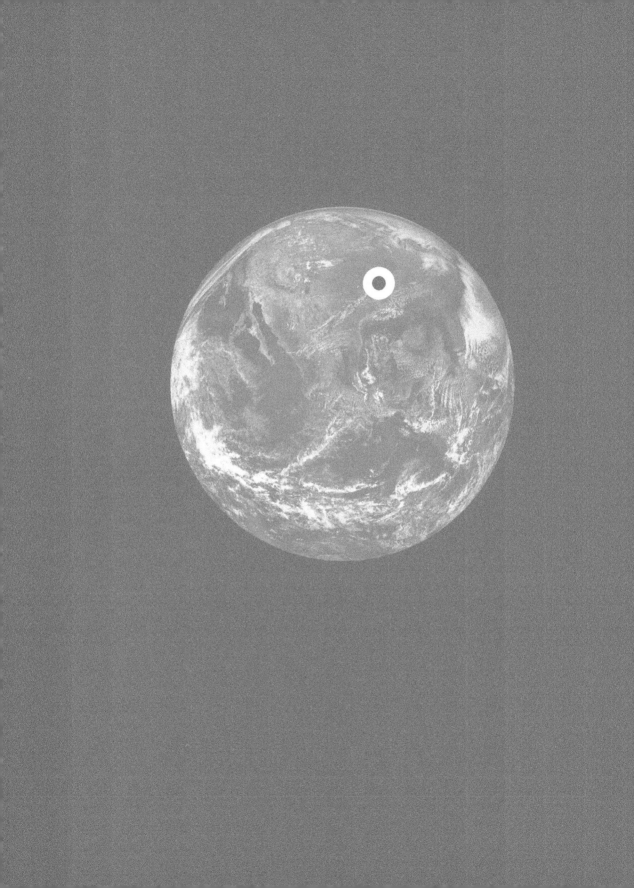

USER'S GUIDE

Think of this book as a guide to the who, what, when, where, why, and how of outbreaks. Outbreaks occur in different places, present in different ways, and require different responses around the world. As a result, there is no exact list followed by governments and responders regarding what goes on before, during, and after an outbreak. We have attempted here to condense our experience in outbreak preparedness and response, along with the guidance and feedback from our colleagues across the globe and from the wide variety of fields involved in epidemics, into a comprehensible guide.

As an armchair epidemiologist's guide to outbreaks, we have designed this book to welcome you into the world of outbreaks. You are meant to jump around. Some sections of this book are more interesting than others—and that is okay. Start with what seems interesting to you, whether it is one field of outbreak response or a specific outbreak case study. You will find that each section connects to another, as it happens in real life during a response. These links, indicated with the icon shown in the margin here, serve to show how the activities involved in detecting, responding, and recovering from outbreaks are interconnected and may occur at different times or in different ways depending on the context of the infectious disease, such as the geographic location, mode of transmission, and availability of medicines, responders, and other resources.

When you see this icon, know that the activity you are reading about may also occur during another phase of outbreak response, or is connected to another activity or topic.

Public health professionals are urgently calling on citizen scientists to engage as outbreaks occur more frequently and in increasingly complex environments, thereby expanding the number of stakeholders and types of activities required to control the spread of disease, and requiring active participation by the impacted populations. Successful outbreak response relies heavily on public support and community engagement.

Public engagement comes from an educated public. Access to this information can bolster the participatory process of public health by creating a more informed, engaged population. This book lifts the curtain on the rationale and interconnectedness of actions across different fields and at various levels to respond to disease outbreaks by presenting outbreak activities in a way that ensures a shared understanding of the essential activities to control an outbreak.

We hope this book will be of interest to every armchair epidemiologist, public health student, and self-selecting scientist that emerged during the pandemic. Maybe it will even answer some of our families' questions!

INTRODUCTION

At the start of the COVID-19 pandemic, our friends and family started asking questions. Lots of questions. We work in pandemic preparedness and response—a field that was considered so niche that most of our family members didn't quite understand what we did for a living. But as the SARS-CoV-2 virus started to spread, people were looking for help understanding what was happening, figuring out how to protect themselves and their loved ones, and making sense of policy decisions.

Our friends and family, along with the rest of the population, watched the COVID-19 response with a new level of interest in public health, learning epidemiologic terms and developing diverse levels of expertise and facilities with the tools used in outbreak response. Terms we taught in graduate level epidemiology courses were now overheard in banter at the grocery store (under masks and behind plexiglass). Yet the success of the response efforts was uneven. The public was seized by coverage of the pandemic and the decisions made by governments, public health officials, businesses, and communities—but not necessarily provided with a guide to understand the rationale behind the requested or required public health actions.

Over previous years we had curated an interactive online tool for professionals that identifies the activities and actors involved across all phases of an outbreak, capturing what needs to get done, when, and by whom.[1] We created this book to translate the content behind that tool for a broader audience by comprehensively mapping the enormous complexity of outbreak response and detailing the necessary actions required for disease prevention and mitigation.

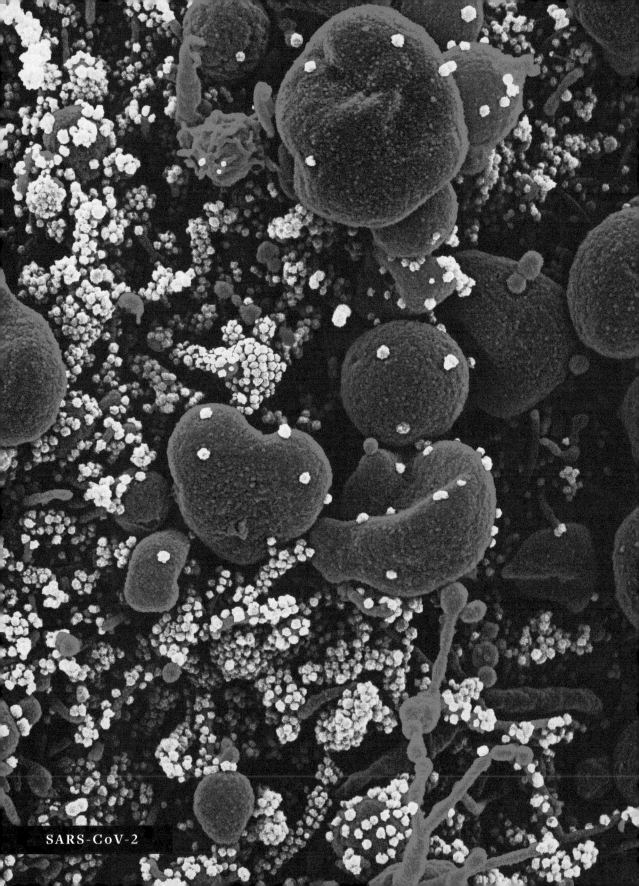
SARS-CoV-2

MSF: Médecins Sans Frontières / Doctors Without Borders

NFP: national focal point

NGO: nongovernmental organization

NIH: National Institutes of Health

NPI: nonpharmaceutical intervention

OCHA: UN Office for the Coordination of Humanitarian Affairs

OPCW: Organization for the Prohibition of Chemical Weapons

OR: odds ratio

PCR: polymerase chain reaction

PEP: post-exposure prophylaxis

PHEIC: Public Health Emergency of International Concern

PHEOC: public health emergency operations center

PFGE: pulsed-field gel electrophoresis

POC: point of care

POD: point of dispense

POE: points of entry

PPE: personal protective equipment

PPR: pandemic prevention, preparedness, and response

RMSF: Rocky Mountain spotted fever

RR: risk ratio

RRT: rapid response team

RSV: respiratory syncytial virus

RT-PCR: reverse transcriptase-polymerase chain reaction

RVF: Rift Valley fever

SARS: severe acute respiratory syndrome

SNS: strategic national stockpile

SOP: standard operating procedures

STD: sexually transmitted disease

STI: sexually transmitted infection

TB: tuberculosis

TSE: transmissible spongiform encephalopathy / prion disease

UN: United Nations

UNDP: United Nations Development Programme

UNHCR: United Nations High Commissioner for Refugees

UNICEF: United Nations Children's Fund

UNSG: United Nations Secretary General

UNSGM: United Nations Secretary General's Mechanism for Investigating Allegations of Chemical or Biological Weapons Use

US CDC: United States Centers for Disease Control and Prevention

US FDA: United States Food and Drug Administration

VCJD: variant Creutzfeldt-Jakob disease

WASH: water, sanitation, and hygiene

WFP: World Food Programme

WGS: whole genome sequencing

WHO: World Health Organization

WOAH: World Organisation for Animal Health (previously went by the acronym OIE)

WPV: wild poliovirus

WTO: World Trade Organization

XDR: extensively drug resistant

ZIKAV: Zika virus

ACRONYMS

AAR: after-action report

AMR: antimicrobial resistance

AMT: air medical transport

BSE: bovine spongiform encephalopathy / mad cow disease

BSL: biosafety level

BWC: Biological and Toxin Weapons Convention

CASPER: Community Assessment for Public Health Emergency Response

CBD: Convention on Biological Diversity

CBS: community-based surveillance

CFR: case fatality rate; case fatality ratio

CHW: community health worker

CJD: Creutzfeldt-Jakob disease

COV: coronavirus

CSW: community surveillance worker

CWD: chronic wasting disease

DR: drug resistant

EBS: event-based surveillance

ECDC: European Centre for Disease Control

EOC: emergency operations center

ERP: emergency response plan

EVD: Ebola virus disease

FAO: Food and Agriculture Organization

FDI: foreign direct investment

FETP: Field Epidemiology Training Program

FMD: foot and mouth disease

GDP: gross domestic product

GISAID: Global Initiative on Sharing All Influenza Data

GOARN: Global Outbreak Alert and Response Network

GPEI: Global Polio Eradication Initiative

GSD: genetic/genomic sequence data

HAI: healthcare-associated infection

HIV/AIDS: human immunodeficiency virus, acquired immunodeficiency syndrome

HPAI: highly pathogenic avian influenza

IBS: indicator-based surveillance

ICS: incident command system

ICRC: International Committee of the Red Cross

ICU: intensive care unit

IFRC: International Federation of Red Cross and Red Crescent Societies

IHR: International Health Regulations

INGO: international nongovernmental organization

IOM: International Organization for Migration

IPC: infection prevention and control

IDP: internally displaced people

IRC: International Rescue Committee

IRR: International Reagent Resource

JEE: Joint External Evaluation

LAI: laboratory-acquired infection

LMIC: low- and middle-income country

LPAI: low pathogenicity avian influenza

MCM: medical countermeasure

MDB: multilateral development bank

MDR: multi-drug resistant

MERS: Middle Eastern Respiratory Syndrome (also MERS-CoV)

MOH: Ministry of Health

In the last few decades,
the number of
infectious disease outbreaks
has more than tripled.

CONTENTS

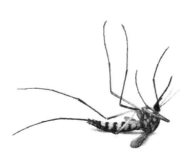

This book is dedicated to every person who wished
they understood more during an outbreak.

And to our families and friends, whose questions
inspired us, and for their support and encouragement
while we brought this information together.